A
Genetic Counseling
Casebook

A
Genetic Counseling
Casebook

Eleanor Gordon Applebaum
and
Stephen K. Firestein

THE FREE PRESS
A Division of Macmillan, Inc.
New York

Collier Macmillan Publishers
London

The Free Press
A Division of Macmillan, Inc.
866 Third Avenue, New York, N. Y. 10022

Collier Macmillan Canada, Inc.

Printed in the United States of America

printing number
1   2   3   4   5   6   7   8   9   10

Library of Congress Cataloging in Publication Data
Main entry under title:

A genetic counseling casebook.

   Bibliography: p.
   Includes index.
   1. Genetic counseling—Case Studies.   I. Applebaum,
Eleanor Gordon.   II. Firestein, Stephen K.
RB155.G364   1983   362.1′96042   82–48605
ISBN 0–02–900860–3

To Cecily, Conrad, and Lesley.

To Herb, Jan, Rob, Walter, Eben, Ruth, and Victor.

To the families of all who labored to assemble this book.

Contents

Acknowledgments   ix

Introduction   1

1. Counseling in Cystic Fibrosis: Easing the Burden
   of Self-Incrimination   13

2. Second-Guessing Counselees' Motives: Osteogenesis
   Imperfecta Congenita   22

3. Refusing to Accept the Diagnosis of Down Syndrome:
   A Family in Hiding   30

4. Complete Acceptance of a Recurring Disorder in a Large
   Extended Family: Mandibulofacial Dysostosis   36

5. First Things First: Denial in Someone at Risk
   for Charcot-Marie-Tooth Disease   44

6. Neonatal Death and Counseling Error: Potter Syndrome   53

7. Multiple Miscarriage and Translocation   66

8. Resisting Counselee Pressure for Decision by Others:
   Duchenne Muscular Dystrophy   73

9. Hazardous Pathways in Nondirective Counseling   83

10. A Child with 47,XYY and Fetal Alcohol Syndrome:
    Not Being Allowed to Help   101

11. Helping the Counselee to Focus Her Feelings:
    Chondroectodermal Dysplasia   113

12. Dealing with the Specifics of Amniocentesis
    and Elective Abortion   119

13. Counseling After Multiple Infant Deaths   135

14. Genetic Counseling Within the Framework of Individual
    Cultural Needs: Orofaciodigital Syndrome Type I   145

15. A Young Married Woman Discovers That She Has XO
    and XY Cell Lines: 45,XO/46,XY Mosaicism   157

16. Counseling with Unexpected Disclosure   167

17. A Face of Her Own: Down Syndrome Mosaicism   173

18. Uninterrupted Pregnancy with Prenatal Diagnosis of Open
    Neural Tube Defect: Cultural Influences on Access to Self-Help   180

19. The Prenatal Diagnosis 47,XXX: Two Cases, Two Decisions   194

20. The Need for Time to Work Through an Agonizing Decision:
    Werdnig-Hoffmann Disease   204

21. A Divided Family: Counseling for Huntington's Disease   222

22. Waiting for the Axe to Fall: A Rare Late-Onset Neurological
    Disorder   235

23. The Undiagnosable Child: Special Counsel for the Parents   246

24. A Counselee Looks Back at Twelve Years of Counseling:
    G_{M1}-Gangliosidosis, Type II   268

    Glossary   279

    Index   285

Acknowledgments

The editors wish to express their gratitude to the following group of genetic counselors who contributed narratives drawn from their clinical practice for this casebook. An additional contributor, not a professional counselor, has favored us with a report of great value to this collection. Without the cooperation of all, this book could not have been assembled.

The contributors' names have not been attached to their specific reports, as an additional measure to safeguard the privacy of the counselees, all of whose identities have already been appropriately disguised.

Naomi Fisher Bartnoff, M.S.	Cyril P. Legum, M.D.
Carolyn Bay, M.S.	Ellen S. Marcus, M.S.
Myrna Ben-Yishay, M.S.	Elsa Reich, M.S.
Caroline L. Clow	Margaret Riggs, M.S.
Virginia L. Corson, M.S.	Beverly R. Rollnick, M.S., Ph.D.
Mary Danca, M.S.	Sylvia P. Rubin, M.S.
Judith Rand Dichter, M.S.	Susan Schmerler, M.S.
Cynthia Dolan, M.S.	Niecee Singer, M.S.
Gary S. Frohlich, M.S.	Ann C. M. Smith, M.A.
Muriel M. Gluckson, M.A., M.S.	Lorraine Suslak, M.S.
Rosalie B. Goldberg, M.S.	Phyllis Taterka, M.S.
Audrey Heimler, M.S.	Sherry E. Wallace, M.S.
Felicia M. Jock	Joan O. Weiss, M.S.W.,
Patricia M. LaGrua, M.S.N.	A.C.S.W., L.C.S.W.

The editors are additionally indebted to Jessica Davis, M.D., for assistance concerning descriptions of specific genetic maladies, and to Joan Marks, director of the Human Genetics Program at Sarah Lawrence College, for her consistent encouragement from the outset of this project.

Introduction

The Scope of Genetic Problems

Clinical genetics is the branch of medicine concerned with heritable disorders. Its research activities seek to enlarge our knowledge of genetically determined disorders through study of affected groups in the population by clinical encounter and by related laboratory investigation.

A direct clinical encounter involves provision of numerous diagnostic, therapeutic, and counseling services to individuals grappling with genetic disorders. These helping functions are offered by professional teams of clinicians and laboratory scientists whose activities tend to center in major medical facilities. Because of the special problems encountered, the variety of counseling in this area of medicine is conveniently called "genetic counseling."

When referring to heritable disorders as a group, how large a category are we concerned with, and how important is it in relation to the general health of the population? A recent report notes responses to both these questions: "Health statistics from wealthier countries, including the United States, show that congenital disease has now become the major cause of infant mortality, accounting for 25 percent to 35 percent of all infant deaths" (Council on Scientific Affairs, AMA, 1982). In the same summarizing report by the Council, reference is made to the cataloging of inherited defects by Victor McKusick, as follows:

> . . . 736 inherited defects that are definitely transmitted by autosomal dominant inheritance and a similar number that have been suspected of being inherited in this way. He has labeled 521 conditions known to be definitely transmitted as autosomal recessive characteristics and 596 more in which this possibility may exist. There are 107 definite and 98 suspected recessive disorders that are X-linked, so that the abnormality is manifested only in sons of carrier mothers. There are many other disorders that are probably multifactorial in origin, but may yet have a strong hereditary component, e.g., hypertension, schizophrenia, diabetes mellitus, asthma, and peptic ulcer. (Council on Scientific Affairs, 1982)

1

Genetic problems share with many other medical problems the qualities of being tragic and bewildering. For parents, however, genetic problems pose certain additional burdens: They undermine self-esteem by exhibiting to the rest of the world demonstrably flawed reproductive capacity. Frequently parents must make difficult decisions regarding genetic disorders, decisions with major life repercussions. The sequelae of these choices are lived with indefinitely—sometimes contentedly or tolerably, at other times with sorrow and depression. The consequences of deciding *not* to have a child may be as influential upon future marital and family life as the decision to proceed with childbearing in the face of the more than ordinary risks of bearing a defective baby. For individuals already affected with a genetic disorder, or at risk for developing one later in life, uncertainty persists over long periods of time.

Genetic Counseling: What It Is and Where to Get It

Genetic counseling has been defined as follows:

> Genetic counseling is a communication process which deals with the human problems associated with the occurrence, or the risk of occurrence, of a genetic disorder in a family. This process involves an attempt by one or more appropriately trained persons to help the individual or family (1) comprehend the medical facts, including the diagnosis, the probable course of the disorder, and the available management; (2) appreciate the way heredity contributes to the disorder, and the risk of recurrence in specified relatives; (3) understand the options for dealing with the risk of recurrence; (4) choose the course of action which seems appropriate to them in view of their risk and their family goals, and act in accordance with that decision; and (5) make the best possible adjustment to the disorder in an affected family member and/or to the risk of recurrence of that disorder. (Ad Hoc Committee on Genetic Counseling, 1975)

The reader will note that in the first sentence of the quoted definition the term "process" is used, and it is the nature of this process that prompted us to assemble this casebook. The process is initiated in a number of ways. Aside from the more sophisticated counselees, who are self-selected, we see patients referred by family physicians, obstetricians, ante-partum clinics, pediatricians, neurologists, nurses, social workers, clergy, parents of children other than the one directly affected, and members of large families who believe relatives to be at risk for some problem with which they already contend. There are many entrances for counselees into the counseling process, and, as has been noted, there are many problems that serve as tickets of admission.

The process begins with the very first counselee contact. From then on, *everyone* dealing directly with the counselees has an impact on the totality of the process.

As in any discipline that is evolving, there has been a gradual shift in attitude regarding the boundaries of the genetic counseling function. Initially, making available medical information regarding diagnosis, risks, options, and disorder management were the counseling goals. To these considerable tasks has been added a new dimension: consideration of the psychological ramifications of this information for the individuals being counseled. Items 4 and 5 of the genetic counseling definition hint at this additional task. Stronger evidence of this shift in thought is given by the recently incorporated American Board of Medical Genetics (1980) in its listing of skills required of those seeking Board certification. The three subspecialties which are patient-oriented rather than laboratory-oriented (clinical geneticist, Ph.D. medical geneticist, and genetic counselor) are required to have the following "skills in interviewing and counseling techniques" in common:

> (1) to elicit from the patient or family the information necessary to reach an appropriate conclusion; (2) to anticipate areas of difficulty and conflict; (3) to help families and individuals recognize and cope with their emotional and psychological needs; (4) to recognize those situations requiring psychiatric referral; and (5) to transmit pertinent information effectively, i.e., in a way that is meaningful to the individuals or family. (The American Board of Medical Genetics, 1980, pp. 9, 13, 20)

Where is genetic counseling offered? The counselors whose reports follow are practicing in a variety of settings. Medical genetics clinics are usually part of large university medical centers. The need for sophisticated evaluative studies involving laboratory procedures and medical consultation with other specialties makes this a practical arrangement. Sparsely populated areas are, however, usually quite distant from major medical centers. Outreach or satellite programs are attempting to serve outlying regions by arranging to visit specified subclinics periodically. Counselees are directed to such subclinics by local health personnel. This satellite system is also employed within some very large cities where there are numerous medical centers with genetics clinics. In these latter areas satellite clinics are needed because of the large numbers of potential counselees who are seen in hospitals not forming part of university medical centers, and not equipped to provide comprehensive genetic diagnostic and counseling services.

The Professional Status Committee of the National Society of Genetic Counselors has recently surveyed its membership to gather information for identifying trends in practice of this specialty. The survey discovered, among other things, that whereas in times past genetic counseling services were concentrated within major medical centers, increasingly they are being provided by public health facilities, outreach programs, and for-profit organizations.

The rapid multiplication of counseling centers was statistically summarized in the report already cited of the Council on Scientific Affairs of the American Medical Association: "In the United States, there were said to be ten counseling centers in 1951; 25 in 1961; and 400 in 1974" (Council on Scientific Affairs, AMA, 1982).

The development of new counseling facilities is being spurred by advances in knowledge and by increasing demand for services as the public learns that something is known, and something can be done, about many defects and disorders that hitherto have been so often hidden away with shame, embarrassment, and chronic depression.

Those Who Are Counseled

Families or individuals who seek or are referred to genetic counseling services have usually experienced a reproductive misfortune, or for some other reason such as an item in their family history, are believed to be at risk for such a calamity in the future. The specific questions that bring people to counseling include many related to prenatal testing, diagnosis, treatment and management of defective children, and family planning when there is above-average risk of genetic disorder in future children. This book includes examples drawn from all categories.

Those Who Serve as Counselors

Those who are designated as genetic counselors have arrived at this functional characterization via a number of routes. First there were medical geneticists, pediatricians, and certain psychiatrists. As time passed, and the work of the genetic clinic proliferated along with new knowledge, more of the counseling was offered by social workers, psychologists, and some nurses (all of whom learned what they needed to know about genetic diseases informally), and, increasingly, by specially trained professionals who had pursued graduate-level curricula leading to the designation of Genetic Associate.

The Genetic Counselor's Knowledge and Skills

As a special form of crisis intervention, genetic counseling demands a great deal from its practitioners. Naturally, counselors must be fully familiar with the manifestations of genetic disorders and with their inheritance patterns, including penetrance and expressivity characteristics; the changing status of diagnostic, preventive, management, and treatment procedures; the derivation of risk estimates; the availability of helping health and social services and parent help groups; and the ethical and legal issues stemming from the availability of new technology. This is the substantive background particularized for counseling for genetic disorders. But there is much more.

The counselor is continually respectful of the fact that disorders of reproductive life are traumas striking powerfully at marital unity, threatening the individual psychological equilibriums of parents and children in different ways. Counselees can be expected to be wary of having their dreaded fear of being found to be inherently flawed confirmed by the counseling. The counselor is aware that counselees are going to be encountered in states of shock, anxiety, mourning, rage, depression, or some combination of these; and that alternations between these states and replacement of one by another are to be expected. The counselor must, therefore, maintain continuing sensitivity to the counselees' emotional condition at any moment of an interview in order to be able to decide the most useful style, dose, and timing of whatever genetic information is to be conveyed. In addition to the counselees' emotional state the counselor must consider such factors as the seriousness of the particular condition involved, specific family reproductive goals and history, and the counselees' educational, ethnic, religious, and socioeconomic background. The expectable number of contacts with particular counselees also influences the way the counseling is conducted.

When dealing with counselees from an ethnic subculture, counselors must try to learn as much as possible of the attitudes toward family life and toward counseling experience reported as characteristic of that group. Although there are great interindividual variations of attitude and belief within a given subculture, it is still of great value for the counselor to be aware of certain typical attitudes and beliefs. It is quite arresting to learn how differently the members of certain ethnic groups behave in conversational settings with strangers—in terms of verbal/nonverbal behaviors and openness or reserve. Most genetic counselors still tend to be white, middle-class professionals, and through ignorance they may seriously misinterpret responses from members of ethnic or cultural groups other than their own. Social scientists have been according increasing attention to this area of study, and counselors will gain much from such works as Sue (1981).

Effective genetic counselors, like other counseling practitioners, require knowledge of the different forms taken by counselees' spontaneous psychological self-protective mechanisms ("defenses") as revealed by conversation and behavior. The counselor respects the need for the counselee to make use of these self-protections, temporarily or permanently, and must acquire the interviewing skills that incorporate this respectful attitude. Investigation of what anticipated emotional distress these psychological defenses are warding off must be gentle, in the service of helping counselees to grapple with difficult choices and realities.

To have command of the substantive information and interpersonal skills described may strike the reader as a tall order for any one person to fill. It is. Yet properly trained and experienced genetic counselors are able to do the job remarkably well.

Since the clinical situations are very distressing, the strain upon the counselor's emotional composure is considerable. Yet the counselor is obliged to maintain sufficient equilibrium to be able to function effectively during interviews. Hopefully, the nature of the interaction will not press the counselor to mobilize his or her own psychological defenses and withdraw from empathic contact with the counselees before an interview is concluded.

Characteristics of the Genetic Counseling Interaction

We have already indicated the multiple routes of referral by which prospective counselees reach diagnostic and counseling services for problems in human genetics. Once a patient has arrived at the genetic counseling facility, some objective for the counseling interaction must be selected to permit focused work.

Sometimes patients are in ignorance of the reason for referral for genetic counseling, arriving at the clinic in compliance with a directive from another clinic of a medical center. If, for example, a pregnant woman older than 35 years of age comes to the genetic clinic unaware of the reason for referral, the counselor will probably need to explain the use of amniocentesis for mothers of her age. This will be the counseling objective for that very first encounter.

In other instances counselees do have specific worries and questions which may immediately shape the objective of the counseling, and in line with which all communicated substantive information must be arrayed. A young adult may, for example, wish to learn if he or she is at risk for development of a late-onset neurological disorder transmissible to children yet unborn.

As all who work in a counseling format soon learn, it is essential for counselor and counselee to agree on the objective of the counseling, regardless of its source. Only then can they work toward that designated goal with harmony and reciprocal respect. When there is a disparity in objectives for the interaction, the counselees' objective will carry the day. A counselor who tries to work in the face of such a disparity usually discovers that he or she is not understood, is "not getting through"; the information offered is left behind in the office, so to speak, or the counselee breaks off the contact altogether through failing to keep subsequent appointments.

The above comments lead to a consideration of two counseling styles, referred to as "directive" and "nondirective." In the field of genetic counseling debate continues as to the preferable style to employ. It is the editors' conviction that nondirective counseling is far more effective as a source of medical benefit to counselees, and the reports in this casebook all demonstrate variations of nondirective counseling.

To clarify, the directive approach is the style with which most people are more familiar, as it is patterned after our usual experience with medical care. We are accustomed to presenting ourselves to a physician with some complaint; then we are usually questioned for additional historical details, subjected to physical and laboratory examinations, and, hopefully, given a diagnosis. Finally, a list of recommendations is presented and we are sent on our way with the full force of professional authority urging us to follow the recommendations and achieve improved health. It is a quite variable matter whether the physician learns if the recommendations have been followed, or whether we even heard without distortion what he told us. Fortunately for us all, this approach to helping a patient is effective in the vast majority of instances—fortunately, because a physician can rarely allot sufficient time to an individual patient for clarifying and answering all questions. In instances of directive counseling, the shared objective of the interaction is rapidly perceived, and if counselor and counselee "speak the same language," it can be achieved in many instances.

With the nondirective approach in counseling, we do not present a counselee with our private agenda of interview content. Rather, we search for the counselee's agenda, and try to help the counselee achieve his or her objective by making available our knowledge of all facets and ramifications of genetic disorders. We have a special concern to discover whatever difficulties counselees may have in assimilating what is being told to them. Appreciating the emotionally loaded nature of the knowledge being conveyed, we are alert to difficulties in comprehending it, since undigested counseling is utterly useless and makes the entire undertaking a waste of time for all concerned. "Nondirective" does *not* mean that counselees may make any use they please of the interview opportunity. It does mean that the counselor does not seek to superimpose his own objective upon that of the counselees.

By proceeding in this manner, we believe, maximum autonomy in decision making is preserved for the counselees, the ones who live out the consequences of their frequently very difficult decisions.

The opening moves in the counseling experience are fairly standardized, but from then on the unfolding process varies endlessly. With great patience the counselor seeks to help the counselees contend with every obstacle to understanding and making use of the available information, whether the impediments be cognitive or emotional. Owing to the limitless variations in individual reaction to serious reproductive dilemmas, there will probably be some unique features in almost every counseling experience. Counseling with regard to the very same malady is unlikely to follow the same course with different individuals. This casebook presents a number of examples of variations in connection with the same diagnosis. The genetic counseling experience, involving as it does a process of inquiry, explanation, assimilation, and often decision making, requires a span of time. Counseling will, therefore, usually necessitate multiple visits, although sometimes logistics preclude more than a single contact with the counselees. Such stringent limitation of contact opportunities makes the work more difficult, even if the counselor tries to facilitate integration of information conveyed through follow-up letters and telephone contacts.

The counselor cannot presume to know what is the ''best'' decision for the counselees to make. ''Best'' is an ambiguous adjective, and should mean a course of action that the counselees can live with after having been helped to understand the problem and available options. The particular option chosen by a counselee will be governed not only by the natural history of the malady concerned, but by factors such as age, strength of the marital bond, number and health of children, the counselee's personal health, expectations of family size, and various ethnic, religious, and socioeconomic considerations. Sometimes the counselor is pressed by bewildered counselees to state what he or she would do in their circumstances. Counselors must resist the temptation to respond to this pressure, because in all honesty no outsider, professional or other, can do more than *imagine* what he would decide if placed in the counselees' shoes. Such a speculation could well be very different from what the outsider would *actually* decide if he faced the counselees' dilemma. And after all, no outsider can ever duplicate the counselees' experience of life within the circle of their own family.

The Counselor's Burdens and Satisfactions

The application of counselor skills through the counseling process is done in an atmosphere that is often depressing or anxiety-provoking. Not every professional can tolerate such a milieu, nor is it any dishonor to prefer a more lighthearted kind of work. Yet the field is very stimulating. To help a family successfully grapple with difficult choices, knowing that the reverberations of constructive steps continue indefinitely, is a source of great professional and personal satisfaction.

Who Should Read This Casebook?

This annotated casebook is designed to provide a much-needed collection of clinical reports for all who may be interested in the field of genetic counseling. We hope for a readership comprising five groups: (1) professionals and trainees in the field of genetic counseling who are actively struggling with clinical problems similar to those to be described; (2) non-geneticist physicians and other health service personnel who may be brought into contact with prospective or actual counselees (this group of readers will include family physicians, obstetricians, pediatricians, endocrinologists, dentists, nurses, psychotherapists, and social workers); (3) students of professions whose career paths may bring them into contact with prospective counselees, (e.g., medical, dental, nursing, psychology, and social work students); (4) religious leaders called upon for pastoral counseling; (5) interested individuals among the general public whose curiosity concerning genetic counseling has, for whatever reason, led them to seek additional information about it.

This is an audience of greatly varied backgrounds. For those who approach the casebook without the advantage of educational background in biology, a glossary of special terminology appearing in the book has been appended.

What the Reader Will Find

The case reports that follow are stories of the struggles of different families with serious reproductive problems. Our aim has been less to offer a range of genetic maladies—in a number of instances the genetic diagnosis is the same—than to offer a spectrum of counseling interactions. From these the reader may develop by increments a mental model of what the genetic counseling interaction is about.

For those preparing to become professional genetic counselors we hope that these reports will stimulate question and discussion. As every counseling situation is an interaction between two or more specific individuals, we anticipate readers will at times disagree as to the strategies, tactics, and emphases described. From such disagreements we expect sharpened perspectives to emerge.

Each report includes a note on the reason for its selection, and the nature of the particular genetic malady is described. At various points of the narrative the psychoanalyst editor has provided annotations to clarify features of the interaction, and to highlight some application of underlying counseling principles.

These comments will be indicated by vertical lines in the margins and by the use of sans serif type face, illustrated here. The editor's Further Comments, which appear at the end of each chapter, will be indicated by the sans serif type face only.

In each narrative one or another variable of the process interaction may be the focus of the reporting counselor's attention. We have placed few constraints upon the reporting counselors, and so the reports differ from one another in keeping with different levels of experience, varied communicative styles, and the personalities of the counselors themselves.

Since the counselor contributors were asked to report with the fullest realism, the reader will encounter details of referral, appointment setting, medical record search, determination of diagnosis and risk estimates, impact of counselor and counselee upon one another, remembered dialogue, inferences as to unverbalized or unconscious conflicts, and all manner of special problems discovered only as the counseling proceeded. If the counseling required multiple interviews, as is common, some condensation was inescapable, but an effort was always made to preserve the essential features and emotional nuances of the case.

What the Reader Will Not Find

It is uncommon to learn very much of the private reflections of counselees in these usually short-term interactions with the reporting professionals. Ought we to expect more in the way of private reflections about the interactions from the counselors? We believe so, and many of the narratives reflect this expectation.

The professional needs time and considerable experience in order to feel sufficiently secure to display to the general public a detailed account of what he or she said and did. An even longer experience is required for the seasoned practitioner to consider sharing with outsiders his private impressions of and reflections about the counselees, other professionals, or himself in the interaction. Such personal dimensions may be shared with colleagues in private conferences, but infrequently with larger groups. A few detailed accounts concerning parents of defective children have been reported with much greater psychological depth, but these reports appear mostly in the literature of the psychological, rather than genetic, disciplines. Essays by Solnit and Stark (1961) and Lax (1972) are examples.

Nor will readers discover in these pages much in the way of generalized presentation of a syllabus of counseling principles. Such discussions are already available in the literature, as in the recent volumes by Kessler (1979) and Hsia et al. (1979). Rather, we have chosen to lead readers through twenty-four complicated situations anticipating that this exposure will result in a broadened awareness of the realities of the genetic counseling process.

We have not sought to give the impression that the process described in any report is *the way* to help the counselee in question. Rather, we consider that there is no one "correct" way to handle every situation, but a number of suitable strategies. Since a counselor's clinical experience always includes some unique encounters, every counselor approaches a new clinical situation from a slightly different vantage point. Probably no two counselors will handle a situation identically, and even the same counselor will handle certain situations differently at different points of his or her career.

No true names of counselees, counselors, or other professionals will be found in this casebook. All names are pseudonyms. The reporting counselors are distributed throughout the United States, Canada and Israel. For further assurance of counselee privacy, all counselors' names have been detached from their case reports.

A Brief Note on Credentials

Our group of counselor contributors includes professionals who hold M.D., M.A., M.S., Ph.D., M.S.W., and M.S.N. degrees. Some of our contributors refer to themselves as genetic counselors, others as genetic associates, terms to be regarded as interchangeable.

> Eleanor Gordon Applebaum, M.A., M.S.
> Genetic Associate
>
> Stephen K. Firestein, M.D.
> Faculty, The Psychoanalytic Institute
> New York University Medical Center

References

Ad Hoc Committee on Genetic Counseling (1975). Genetic counseling. *Amer. J. Human Genetics* 27: 240–242.

American Board of Medical Genetics (1980). Information for candidates: certification procedure, eligibility and examination information.

Council on Scientific Affairs, American Medical Association (1982). Genetic counseling and prevention of birth defects. *JAMA* 248: 221–224.

HSIA, Y.; HIRSCHHORN, K.; SILVERBERG, R.; and GODMILOW, L., eds. (1979). *Counseling in genetics.* New York: Alan Liss.

KESSLER, S. (1979). *Genetic counseling.* New York: Academic Press.

LAX, R. (1972). Some aspects of the interaction between mother and impaired child: mother's narcissistic trauma. *International J. Psycho-Analysis* 53: 339–344.

National Society of Genetic Counselors (1981). The state of the Society. Perspectives in genetic counseling 3 (no. 4): 4–5.

NOTMAN, M., and NADELSON, C., eds. (1978). *The woman patient, medical and psychological interfaces.* Vol. 1: *Sexual and reproductive aspects of women's health care.* New York: Plenum Press.

SOLNIT, A., and STARK, M. (1961). Mourning and the birth of a defective child. In R. Eissler; A. Freud; H. Hartmann; and M. Kris, eds., *The psychoanalytic study of the child,* Vol. 16, pp. 523–537. New York: International Universities Press.

SUE, D. (1981). *Counseling the culturally different.* New York: Wiley.

1

Counseling in Cystic Fibrosis: Easing the Burden of Self-Incrimination

This report of the experience of the O'Reillys is offered to illustrate the impact of the birth of a child with a genetic disorder, the reverberations of that occurrence on parental self-esteem and marital harmony, and how a genetic counselor goes about providing assistance for dealing with all consequences, such as planning for the care of the affected child, and living through a subsequent, anxiety-laden pregnancy.

Cystic fibrosis (CF) is the most prevalent serious chronic genetic disease of Caucasian children and young adults. Estimates of the incidence range from one in 1,600 to one in 2,500 live births, with a carrier rate of one in 20 to one in 25. The basic molecular defect is unknown. CF is a systemic disorder characterized by a dysfunction of the exocrine glands which results in abnormal amounts of electrolytes in sweat, insufficient secretion of pancreatic digestive enzymes, and progressive obstructive pulmonary disease. CF shows a wide range of symptomatic expression, but there is no method of predicting in advance the severity or outcome. With increased understanding of the pathophysiology, and improved methods of treatment, remarkable progress in patient survival rate has been achieved. The National Data Registry of the Cystic Fibrosis Foundation reported in 1976 that 50 percent of patients with CF had survived until the age of 21, whereas twelve years before 50 percent survived to the age of 3.

Genetic counseling does not have the advantage of accurate carrier identification and prenatal diagnosis. Counseling must focus upon gradually helping parents to understand the pathophysiology of CF, how heredity contributes to their child's disease, and how recurrence risks are calculated from the Mendelian autosomal recessive pattern of inheritance. The family requires considerable assistance to be able to grapple with the complicated program for managing an affected child, and to integrate the reality of CF into their planning for more children.

Most patients are referred to specialized team-treatment centers by pediatricians who suspect CF because of recurrent pulmonary infections, malabsorption and/or diarrhea, and failure to thrive. A quantitative sweat test in conjunction with a clinical evaluation is used to confirm the diagnosis. The family of a newly diagnosed patient requires the support of the entire staff during the difficult period when members are suffering from the initial emotional impact of the diagnosis and at the same time are trying to learn the complex daily regimen of pulmonary therapy and home medical management. The family introduced below did not have any professional assistance during the difficult six weeks following the diagnosis.

Kathleen Bradley, mother of the affected child, had arrived in the United States from Ireland in April 1975 to prepare for her wedding to Tommy O'Reilly. They had been engaged for two years when Tommy emigrated to New York City to seek a job and save sufficiently to be able to send for Kathleen. Tommy had found a steady job delivering bakery products to a local supermarket chain. As planned, Kathleen came to New York to reside until the wedding in the home of her brother, Brian. Brian had never informed anyone in his extended family that his son, Brian, Jr., was afflicted with cystic fibrosis.

Two months after arriving, Kathleen was married to Tommy. Only two months later their nephew, Brian, Jr., died suddenly as a consequence of heat prostration and acute diarrhea. Kathleen was already pregnant with Brigit. During the next seven months Kathleen and Tommy were understandably anxious about the outcome of this pregnancy, but were unwilling to discuss their fears with others. The occurrence of cystic fibrosis in the family was carefully concealed from their small, tightly knit group of friends newly arrived from Ireland.

Brigit O'Reilly was born in a major metropolitan hospital that performs sweat tests, but does not provide care for patients with CF. The parents, on their own initiative, requested a sweat test when Brigit was 7 days old, and the test was positive. At that hospital the procedure following a positive sweat test is for a pediatric pulmonary physiologist to describe briefly to the parents the nature of CF and the fact that it is inherited as a Mendelian autosomal recessive disorder. He then strongly recommends seeking regular medical care at a CF treatment center. Our center was recommended as the nearest. Clear instructions to telephone the center to arrange for a repetition of the sweat test were given to the O'Reillys. Instead of following this advice, the O'Reillys brought Brigit to a local pediatrician who had no specialized knowledge of CF. This delay deprived the family of the full professional support they so urgently needed at that time.

This delay in following the physiologist's advice was regrettable as regards the assistance needed by infant and parents. It was at the same time an entirely human response, possibly to be understood as an effort to deny through action the serious import of the information already received.*

Our first contact with this family occurred six weeks later when Brigit was admitted with pneumonia to our hospital's Pediatric Section. The needs of each family determine the priority of support services offered to parents. The first day the baby was in the hospital a CF staff physician asked me to go up to the floor and arrange a meeting with the parents. Tommy and Kathleen were in Brigit's room. I introduced myself, explaining my role within the CF group, and suggested we go into the conference room to discuss CF, the disease, and the genetics. Kathleen, standing in front of the crib so I could not see the baby, responded loudly and with obvious hostility.

KATHLEEN: We will not be needing to talk to you. The baby's sickness is my fault. Tommy should leave me and find someone who can give him healthy children.

G.C.: Tommy, how do you feel about this? Do you agree with your wife about the sickness, that it's all her fault?

TOMMY: The doctors have been saying two parents have to have something or other, but I'm fine. I feel fine; no one in my family has sick children. The way Katie has been crying and carrying on I'll not argue with her about it. If she thinks it's all her doing, let it be her doing!

G.C.: Kathleen, have you been sick? Is that another reason you believe just you are the cause?

KATHLEEN: No, I'm strong as an ox, but my blood is bad. All my children will have the sickness.

G.C.: Neither of you has given the "sickness" a name. It's cystic fibrosis. Didn't the Bradleys talk to you about it?

TOMMY: No, they were always hiding it from everyone. They put away some kind of pump and tubes when anyone came into the apartment.

G.C.: I'd like to tell you a little about cystic fibrosis; that's the name of the illness. You should start by calling it cystic fibrosis or CF because that will be better for you, and in the future, better for the baby. It's also important for us to talk to each other in words we know. Did either of you ever study biology?

TOMMY: No, we both only finished grade school in Ireland.

*Editors' Comment.

The counselor's work is now cut out for her: to explain all the needed facts to a couple who are altogether unfamiliar with such concepts as "gene," "chromosome," or "reduction division"—no mean feat.

The counselor has made an important additional assessment to guide herself in conducting this initial interview: She appreciates that the dose of new information to be conveyed to the couple must be restricted because of their limited educational background, because they are in emotional turmoil, and because they have only made her acquaintance a few minutes previously.

G.C.: Have you ever thought about why children look something like both of their parents, but not exactly like either one?

KATHLEEN and TOMMY: No.

G.C.: Well, nature has a very accurate system for making this happen. One-half of everything that decides how a baby will be formed comes from the mother, and one-half from the father. Scientists have named these things that do the deciding "genes." Genes work in pairs to direct the formation of every substance that makes the body chemistry work. A person can have one gene of a pair working, the other not. Parents of CF children each carry one nonworking gene and one that is working correctly. Carriers themselves are healthy. Unfortunately there is no way at present to tell if a person is a carrier of this nonworking gene. If both parents contribute their *nonworking* gene to the baby, then the child will have CF. When you are feeling better, I can draw a picture of the kinds of combinations that can result when both parents are carriers. For example, you can have healthy children who are carriers like yourselves—or CF children like Brigit who have received two nonworking genes. We will talk about the risk of CF in future children. This system of two genes is true for all our traits, from eye color to blood types.

Kathleen, you have taken all the guilt and responsibility onto your shoulders, and Tommy seems willing to go along with it, but the inheritance of CF just doesn't work that way. I think time and our staff can help you to overcome the feelings of resentment and despair which are so crushing now. . . . Could I see the baby?

The counselor's interest in examining the baby, and her calm acceptance of the infant as a child with a medical problem, yet not less lovable for it, usually helps counselees along the path to a comparable attitude.

Kathleen moved away from the crib, and for the first time I could see Brigit. She was a beautiful baby, and, happily, had blue eyes, Kathleen's were brown but Tommy's blue. Kathleen picked up the baby to change her diaper. I asked Kathleen if she would try to think about how the baby could have inherited blue eyes. When Brigit was back in her crib, I suggested we sit down comfortably so I could draw some diagrams for them. This time they accepted my offer, and Kathleen took Tommy's arm as they walked out of the room. We talked for an hour, in very simple terms, about heredity. I asked if I could draw a family pedigree, and while I was taking down the information about the offspring of Tommy's twin sister, Anne, he explained that she had had two miscarriages because of an Rh blood problem. When I asked him what type of problem, he explained Rh incompatibility very clearly. I diagrammed what he had said and showed them how the inheritance of blood types could be applied to understanding the inheritance of CF. This was the beginning of a true realization by Tommy that CF was a recessive disease. I gave the O'Reillys the diagrams I had drawn.

Giving the counselees the diagrams employed to explain an inheritance pattern is the counselor's further acknowledgment of a limit to the dose of information that can be assimilated in one interview. The counselees can look at the diagrams as often as they need for the gradual digestion of the counselor's explanation.

I ended the discussion by talking about the emotional crisis they were going through. I asked if they believed they had had a good and happy marriage before Brigit was born. They both said they were "wonderful happy." I tried to reassure them that their feelings of help-lessness and anxiety could be ameliorated gradually through a slow and often difficult process, making it possible for them to work out their future together.

I explained that their adjustment might be made even more difficult because of three factors: Brian, Jr.'s death; the pattern of hiding CF set by the Bradleys; and Brigit's being a first child in a family whose goals included having many children. I suggested that setting up a step-by-step practical daily plan of management would be the beginning of their ability to cope with CF.

I cautioned them to be patient with each other because we had learned from other couples that at least six months to a year is required for parents to start handling the disbelief, depression, and anxiety created by the diagnosis. It often takes just as long for the explanations about genetics to be clearly understood. The O'Reillys were encouraged to write down their questions as they arose so that answers could be pro-vided during this turbulent period of learning. An appointment was ar-ranged for the next day.

Writing down questions is a very useful measure. Interviews with the counselor are, for some time, tense experiences, and important questions are readily forgotten except if there is a written reminder.

The second counseling session proceeded very much the same way as the first: Mrs. O'Reilly's anger and self-blame, tears, then gradually lessened tension. Tommy was hostile until Kathleen's tears stopped, but he no longer agreed that CF was only her fault.

During the remaining twelve days of Brigit's hospitalization the O'Reillys had four more arranged counseling sessions. Each interview began with Kathleen crying for a few minutes. With succeeding sessions she became more rapidly composed.

Brigit was gaining weight and progressing very well. Our staff respiratory physical therapist taught both parents inhalation and pulmonary therapy; they learned the techniques rapidly.

Tommy has by this point been able to digest enough of his own disappointment, sorrow, and rage at fate so that he no longer needs to try to protect his self-esteem by placing on Kathleen the full responsibility for the misfortune.

What this sequence illustrates is the psychological work of mourning, which goes on within the mind of the one who has experienced serious loss. In this situation the loss has many dimensions, but most notably there is loss of the dream of the perfect baby, complicated as soon as the baby is brought home by the burdensome reality of the afflicted infant requiring special care. The clinic appointments and the daily care regimen can readily rekindle painful emotions of sorrow, grief, and anxiety. With the passage of time the reminders become less painful.

In discussions with the O'Reillys we explored their feelings regarding contraception, abortion, and family size. Mrs. O'Reilly said they both wanted many children. "Raising a large and happy lot" was the dream that comforted Kathleen during her separation from Tommy before they married. She said that their religion would prevent any use of contraception or consideration of abortion even if prenatal diagnosis was available.

When the hospital stay was over, weekly clinic appointments were prearranged for the following month. The first two weeks both parents came with Brigit, and in spite of the complex, often tedious registration procedure, everything went smoothly. At our weekly case conference the doctors reported that the parents' pattern of emotional response was the same as what we had observed during Brigit's hospitalization: an angry, tense Tommy, Katie crying for the first few minutes, then both gradually relaxing and paying careful attention to the medical questions and instructions.

The third visit presented a crisis. Mrs. O'Reilly arrived with Brigit, red-eyed and distraught. Tommy had not come with them. She asked to speak with me privately. Her first question was whether there was any new research in prenatal diagnosis for CF. This clearly indicated that she was pregnant, but it took almost an hour of crying and talking around the subject before she told me she was "two months gone." Tommy, she said, was not unhappy about the pregnancy, but he was "furious angry" because she couldn't stop crying. Katie's fear about having another CF child had overwhelmed her completely. She said she could barely get out of bed to care for Brigit. I asked her permission to invite the unit's clinical psychologist to join our conversation. She answered, "Nothing can help me but a healthy baby," but agreed to include him in our talk. We gently and gradually explained that her second pregnancy had brought on acute and overwhelming anxiety. Her depression and tears served to increase Tommy's feelings of helplessness, which he expressed as anger. She told us Tommy wanted their second child and had wanted to come to the clinic with her that morning. He had tried to be comforting. We told Katie that by not allowing him to help she was adding to his frustration and anger.

Kathleen is correct as regards her doubts concerning her reproductive capacity: Only the birth of a healthy infant will eventually reassure her. But this assertion does not nullify another correct assertion: It works out far better for all concerned if the mother of a defective infant takes some time to (1) complete the psychological work of mourning the misfortune and (2) assimilate the demanding tasks of caring for an ill infant *before* adding an inevitably anxiety-laden new pregnancy. For most women an interval of six to twelve months would not be too long for this purpose.

One may question whether feelings of helplessness are being transmuted into expressions of anger. More likely, Tommy's frustration over his inability to successfully comfort his grieving wife leads him to angrily urge that she stop weeping and thereby cease reminding him of his limitation as comforter. The counselor's attention to Tommy—so often the father is left out—is very valuable. A week, after all, includes 168 hours, of which clinic visits constitute only a few. Helping the more available husband/father to be more helpful, and the mother to accept that help, aids the family unit tremendously.

By this time regular clinic hours were over and Brigit needed feeding. We all shared lunch, after which Brigit had her scheduled medical examination. We suggested that Tommy be telephoned. He arrived shortly, and we repeated much of our earlier discussion. Katie made an effort to limit her tears and promised that she would "work towards talking, not bawling."

This was not easily achieved. We met with the O'Reillys each afternoon for the remainder of that week. Then we scheduled a telephone support schedule, every morning for the next two weeks, then three mornings weekly, and finally every Monday morning. As the pregnancy approached term, we planned to increase the level of support.

Even in the very early sessions with the O'Reillys, we sought to encourage them to be more open about their problems. We suggested that they try to discuss them with relatives and friends if appropriate opportunities arose. Apparently we were successful, as the O'Reillys asked for CF literature to give to visiting family members.

At our clinic new families are seen weekly for two months, monthly for the balance of the first year. These frequent meetings permit individualized assessment of the effectiveness of the counseling and attention to factors limiting that effectiveness. During the early period all of the supporting staff—which includes a social worker, a clinical psychologist, and a pulmonary therapist—try to see the family at each visit. Occasionally explanatory letters are written, with permission, to siblings, aunts, and uncles who live out of state.

Further Comment

The account offered here may be characterized as the story of how a couple begins to go about digesting and accommodating to three "hammer blows" in rapid succession. The first smash is the unexpected birth of a little girl afflicted with cystic fibrosis. The second blow, almost simultaneous with the first, is confrontation with the complicated task of providing proper nutritional and medical care for the newborn. And the third, following close behind, is the information about the inheritance pattern for CF and its impact on this couple, for whom birth control is proscribed on religious grounds.

The news of the diagnosis stimulates both parents in the direction of self-reproaches. It can be uncanny for a parent to reflect on the information that he or she can be quite robust and feel entirely well, yet transmit genetic material that produces a dreadful disease. Kathleen proclaims that the entire onus is on her. In so doing she offers Tommy an "out," which, in the stress of the situation, he is understandably willing to take. When Kathleen asserts that she will give the malady to every child, that every child will be affected, she speaks of something that is possible, but not likely, for the chance is the same with each pregnancy, 25 percent.

In dealing with this traumatized couple the counselor decides to defer most of the details of instruction concerning the genetic inheritance pattern until she has acquired a better sense of the couple's background in biological knowledge. To omit this step would be an error, possibly nullifying the usefulness of subsequent conversations.

The O'Reillys' agitation is partly stimulated by the fact of Brian, Jr., the son of Kathleen's brother and sister-in-law. The closeness of Brigit's birth to the terminal illness of Brian, Jr., must generate worries that a similar fate may await Brigit, despite every health-promoting effort.

The concealment of the medical truth regarding Brian, Jr., exemplifies the common belief that genetic illness represents parental defectiveness and is therefore shameful and embarrassing. Naturally, the maintenance of the demanding regimen of dietary and pulmonary treatment required for an infant with CF becomes even more difficult if parents believe it all must be done covertly. Rationalized, self-imposed social isolation may be the outcome of persisting feelings of shame.

To deliver an infant with CF is always upsetting. If, however, a mother has already borne a healthy baby, she *knows* she has the capability. Such knowledge mitigates the anxiety of the question "Am I able to become the mother of a healthy baby?" Kathleen will have to wait for that reassurance.

The reader will note the careful attention to follow-up contacts with this family. This policy is in keeping with the experience that without follow-up visits and/or telephone contacts the counselor cannot know how useful the counseling has been. Not to conduct such follow-up appraisals courts self-deception about effectiveness, and if the process falls short of usefulness, should we bother with it?

References

DENNING, C.; GLUCKSON, M.; and MOHR, I. (1976). Psychological and social aspects of cystic fibrosis. In J. Mangos, and R. Talamo, eds., *Cystic fibrosis: projections into the future,* pp. 127–151. New York: Stratten Intercontinental Medical Books.

WOOD, R.; BOAT, T.; and DOERSHUK, C. (1976). State of the art: cystic fibrosis. *Amer. Rev. Respiratory Dis.* 113:833–878.

2

Second-Guessing Counselees' Motives: Osteogenesis Imperfecta Congenita

This report on the Muller family was selected because it points up the magnitude of the dilemma of an average couple, not manifesting severe neurosis, faced with the disclosure that they are presumably both carriers for a usually lethal disorder. They are eager to have more children, and the prospect of prenatal diagnosis and elective abortion is for a number of reasons quite complicated.

The report also illustrates the benumbed initial state in which the counselor encountered the counselees, and the consequent necessity for multiple contacts with them spread over time. Further, it illustrates how mistaken the professional may sometimes be in drawing inferences to predict counselee behavior; and how for some parents even the possibility of lethal defects in another child will not dissuade them from conceiving.

When Joanne Muller was born with blue sclerae and multiple fractures of all limbs, several ribs, and the skull, the diagnosis of osteogenesis imperfecta congenita (OIC) was assigned. As there was no family history of easily fractured bones, and as Joanne's arms and legs had short, broad bones, the disorder was categorized as an autosomal recessive variety.

In the majority of families where there is OIC a single infant is the only affected individual, and the mode of inheritance cannot be determined. The term "osteogenesis imperfecta" is applied to a heterogeneous group of hereditary disorders characterized by increased bone fragility. Of the group, Joanne's disease would probably be Type II.

Marie and Michael Muller, an unrelated white couple of German and Czechoslovakian background, Roman Catholic, are ages 25 and 26 respectively. Marie has a high school diploma and she worked as a clerk before her first child was born. Michael is a plumber and is attending college part-time, majoring in accounting. Both the Mullers have large, close families living nearby. Their son, Robert, is a normal 2-year-old.

Following a cesarean section, performed because of lack of progress of labor, the Muller's second pregnancy resulted in a daughter, Joanne, with OIC. X-ray findings were compatible with the autosomal recessive form of the disorder.

Soon after the baby's delivery, the Mullers' pediatrician, Dr. S., informed the parents that he suspected osteogenesis imperfecta. He told them that it was a genetic disorder present in the baby from the moment of conception and that genetic counseling would be made available to them. He explained the baby's difficulties but said he was uncertain in regard to her life expectancy. Dr. S. immediately began arranging for Joanne to be placed in a children's convalescent and rehabilitative hospital, explaining to the parents that because of the continuing potentiality for fractures it would be difficult to care for the baby at home. At first Mrs. Muller was reluctant, but when Dr. S. suggested that she regard the placement as a stopgap measure, she agreed.

The situation for the Mullers was quadruply calamitous from the first moments: (1) Nonprogressing labor necessitated a cesarean section. (2) The couple was informed that their daughter had significant genetic defects. (3) They were then told that the baby had to be separated from them for the sake of its welfare, that for a while they would be deprived of her. Such a separation so early cannot help but impede the initial period of mother-child interaction. (4) The Mullers were put on notice that they were at risk for repetition of the catastrophe. Fortunately, they were informed *jointly*, which provided the possibility of reciprocal emotional support as they shared the shocking news.

Mrs. A., the genetic associate at the hospital, was informed about this baby the day after the Mullers received the diagnosis. Mrs. A. introduced herself to the couple in Mrs. Muller's hospital room and explained that the full range of genetic counseling services was available; she did not intend to become involved at that time in a lengthy description of inheritance patterns. However, Mr. Muller's questioning led her to explain that the type of osteogenesis imperfecta Joanne had was probably autosomal recessive in inheritance pattern. Since neither of the parents had experienced any fractures, other than a football injury by Mr. Muller, the likelihood of dominant inheritance was remote. Therefore, the couple was tentatively reassured in regard to their normal son.

During the explanation, Mrs. Muller said very little. This pattern continued during two subsequent visits by Mrs. A. On one occasion, Mrs. Muller excused herself to go to the nursery.

Ordinarily such laconic behavior on the counselee's part will alert the genetic counselor to the possibility of a state of shocked numbness that impedes assimilation of emotionally loaded information. The hasty departure to the nursery also suggests that for Mrs. Muller the interviews were hard to bear.

The genetic consultant, Dr. O., and Mrs. A. met with the parents the day before Mrs. Muller was discharged from the hospital. Dr. O. confirmed the diagnosis of OIC with autosomal recessive inheritance pattern. He reassured the Mullers that their normal son would not be affected inasmuch as he had had no manifestations up to that time, and confirmed that there was no cure for Joanne's condition. He told the parents that in future pregnancies fetal X-rays taken between sixteen and twenty-four weeks of gestation might be used for prenatal diagnosis, but the absence of visible fractures at that time could not completely rule out the condition in a fetus. Dr. O. also said that an affected baby would probably not live very long.

Joanne was moved by ambulance to the specialized children's hospital the same day Mrs. Muller went home. Mr. Muller's oldest sister came with him to bring Mrs. Muller home.

Mrs. Muller visited and cared for Joanne at the other hospital daily. She was almost always accompanied by another adult member of her own or Mr. Muller's family. Joanne died of respiratory complications at the age of four weeks.

Mrs. Muller's involvement in her ill daughter's care was very important for her. It tended to mitigate some of the pain of the obligatory separation from Joanne and reassured her about the quality of care offered by the institution. It gave her some sense that she was not altogether helpless in the situation, but could do something, something important. Being accompanied on trips to the hospital by a relative provided emotional support.

Ten days after Joanne's death, Mr. and Mrs. Muller came to Mrs. A.'s office to discuss options and risks concerning future children. Both appeared to understand well the autosomal recessive pattern of inheritance involved.

After the introductory pleasantries, Mrs. Muller immediately stated that she wanted to adopt a child but her husband did not. When the couple was encouraged to discuss this, Mrs. Muller turned to her husband and said, "You're involved with your career, but I want to raise children."

Both parents agreed that they were unwilling to take the risk of having another child with OIC. They referred to Dr. O.'s suggestion that future pregnancies might be monitored by X-rays from the sixteenth to twenty-fourth weeks. They were a bit skeptical of relying on this technique since Dr. O. had not *guaranteed* the identification of an affected fetus.

Mrs. A asked if they had considered other alternatives besides adoption. When they said they had not, she mentioned artificial insemination by a donor. Both Mr. and Mrs. Muller replied that this had occurred to them, but they had not discussed it. Mr. Muller said that he was definitely not in favor of this alternative since the child would be completely unrelated to him. Mrs. Muller was less definite but did indicate that she did not think she wished to undergo the procedure.

Mrs. A. had been hesitant about bringing up artificial insemination so early and had wanted to see if the subject would be raised by one of the Mullers. Afterward, she wondered whether she should have waited until another session.

Another topic brought up by the Mullers was the safety of abortion in the second trimester, should an affected fetus be discovered by X-ray. Mrs. A. reassured them in this regard. Both the Mullers said that having to decide about abortion would be an emotionally charged issue, and they were not sure they wished to place themselves in that position.

Even in the best of hands, second-trimester abortion carries an increased risk.

They were, in addition, quite fearful that if they had another affected infant it might survive longer than Joanne had, only to keep on suffering with the disorder.

In reviewing autosomal recessive inheritance, Mrs. A. repeated that all of us carry between six and ten very harmful recessive genes. Mr. Muller murmured, "What a hell of a thing to have in common!"

As stated, this comment about harmful recessive genes may have a somewhat misleading impact. The context of the remark is, of course, the consequences to progeny of mother and father both contributing the same gene. That is clear.

To the carrier who bears the gene, however, it is not harmful. Recently it has been considered that certain recessive genes may even be beneficial to the carrier, despite the potential for making trouble for offspring. It is now believed, for example, that the bearer of sickle-cell trait may be somewhat protected against certain forms of malaria.

Mrs. Muller asked if her siblings were in danger of having children with OIC and was reassured that even if they carried the OIC gene, their unrelated spouses would be unlikely to have the same gene. Because the extended family knew Joanne had a genetic disorder, there was concern about the prospective children of Mrs. Muller's brother and sister.

Mrs. A. asked the Mullers how they had reacted to her visits while Mrs. Muller and Joanne were both still hospitalized. Mrs. Muller replied that she had virtually ignored Mrs. A.'s visits. "I heard your voice but I wasn't listening. I was thinking about the baby and wanting to be with her."

> This report confirms the earlier comment about the parents' initial state of shock and numbness. Multiple counseling visits are therefore essential to effective work.

Mrs. Muller said that both her own and her husband's families had been very supportive while Joanne was in the specialized hospital and also at Joanne's funeral. She appreciated the fact that a family member always accompanied her when she visited Joanne.

The Mullers said that one of Mr. Muller's older sisters had been pressing them to take Joanne to other specialists in the hope of a cure. However, all of their inquiries concerning orthopedists and geneticists had been rewarded with the names of the same physicians who had already seen Joanne. Therefore, the Mullers accepted the diagnosis and the prognosis.

Mrs. Muller was very satisfied with the care Joanne had received at the specialized hospital and was happy that she had spent as much time with the infant as possible. The couple felt that everything possible had been done for their daughter.

During the interview neither of the Mullers displayed much emotion, either about their daughter's death or toward each other. Mrs. Muller did most of the talking. Mr. Muller appeared depressed.

Two weeks later the Mullers returned to meet with Mrs. A. and Dr. O. Again Mrs. Muller was more talkative than her husband, and she returned to her anxious question about the survivability of another affected child. Dr. O. confirmed that another affected child would most likely (95 percent probability) be afflicted as severely as Joanne and would probably not survive longer than she had. The doctor reaffirmed that serial X-rays of a pregnancy from the sixteenth to twenty-fourth weeks would probably, but not certainly, identify fractures in the fetus. He warned that adoption of normal children is difficult in this country and said that artificial insemination would require a carefully weighed decision on their part.

> The unvarnished facts presented here make the Mullers' consideration of having another baby in the usual manner a very tough choice. The ques-

tion is not merely "Is one chance in four of having another OIC baby an acceptable risk?" Rather, it is "Could we bear the experience of losing another infant following nine months of pregnancy and a repeat cesarean section?"

As matters stood at the time of Joanne's death, all options provoked conflicts, and the team's hope was that additional follow-up visits would help the Mullers resolve some of those conflicts. Feelings about adoption or artificial insemination were prominent issues for both. It was speculated that Mrs. Muller might consider revising her dream of a large family and try to develop alternative major interests. There was suspicion that after an interval the Mullers would be willing to take the risk of another pregnancy monitored by X-rays during the sixteenth to twenty-fourth weeks.

Although Mrs. A. telephoned Mrs. Muller twice in the next four months, the Mullers failed to make an appointment for a follow-up visit. About seven months after Joanne's death, Mrs. A. was informed by Dr. S., the Mullers' pediatrician, that the couple was expecting another child. Mrs. A. waited to hear about this pregnancy from the Mullers or from their obstetrician, so that prenatal diagnosis by radiology and possibly ultrasonography might be undertaken. She was disappointed that no contact was made and concluded that her genetic counseling had been ineffective.

At approximately thirty-four weeks' gestation, Mrs. Muller phoned to inform Mrs. A. of the pregnancy and to set up an appointment. Mrs. A. was curious about the purpose of the appointment at that late date, but did not ask about this during their conversation. When they met a few days later, Mrs. Muller stated that she wished to find out if it would be possible to determine radiologically whether her unborn baby was affected with OIC. Mrs. A. promised to speak to the radiologist about this and telephone Mrs. Muller with his answer. When Mrs. Muller was asked why she wished this information, she said that the obstetrician was not certain a cesarean section was necessary. If a choice existed, Mrs. Muller's decision would be influenced by the findings as to whether or not the baby already manifested OIC. Mrs. A.'s unspoken reaction to this reply was that the Mullers would probably choose vaginal delivery for an affected child, if given the choice, in order to reduce the chance of its survival. She was therefore surprised to hear Mrs. Muller continue," If the baby has broken bones already, I'll have a cesarean so I won't hurt it unnecessarily."

Mrs. A. believed that the Mullers had indeed misunderstood the genetic counseling received earlier, and that they were under the mistaken impression that an affected child with minimal manifestations had a good chance to survive. She therefore asked Mrs. Muller whether she was aware that with an affected child the family might again undergo the tragic experience they had endured with Joanne, including almost inevitable death in the early weeks or months of life. Mrs. Muller said that she understood this but felt the need to do the best she could for the child, and that included prolonging its survival.

She was also aware of the 25 percent risk of having an affected child, but she and her husband had decided to take that chance. The interview concluded with Mrs. A.'s promising to supply the information the Mullers desired. By the time the information had been obtained—that an affected fetus might or might not be identifiable—Mrs. Muller had already visited her obstetrician. The decision had been made that in any event a cesarean section would be performed. Prior to the actual procedure X-rays were taken which revealed no fractures. A normal boy was delivered. Mrs. Muller subsequently conveyed to Mrs. A. her joy at having decided to risk the pregnancy.

Two weeks later Mrs. A. met Dr. S. and inquired about the Mullers' baby. He said that the baby was fine but he did not expect to have him in his care, since Mrs. Muller's older sister had convinced the couple that Dr. S.'s recommendation for Joanne's placement at the children's specialized hospital had resulted in poor care, possibly leading to her death. This lack of confidence in the pediatrician was borne out when the Mullers brought their 2-month-old infant son to us to be rechecked for OIC. We confirmed the original findings that the child was indeed free of the disorder.

The follow-up information in this instance was very valuable to the counselor. First, she learned that her appraisal of the counseling as ineffective, because the Mullers decided not to have mid-trimester prenatal diagnosis, was erroneous. The Mullers had understood the counseling fairly well, but had made use of it in ways other than anticipated by the counselor. Their own sense of the seriousness of the painful loss of Joanne was not what the counselor had imagined, since it did not preclude the new pregnancy.

Equally erroneous was the counselor's private assumption that the Mullers would opt for vaginal delivery to reduce the child's chances for survival if X-rays revealed a defective fetus. Counselor and counselee attitudes do not always correspond, making alertness to the unique makeup of counselees a professional requirement that is never suspended.

Further Comment

Surprises of every variety are everyday experiences in the field of genetic counseling. With appropriate humility the genetic counselor of the Mullers observes that her expectations of how the Mullers would use the information conveyed to them in the counseling sessions turned out to be wide of the mark.

In view of the traumatic impact of their daughter's early death the counselor had presumed the Mullers desired at whatever cost to avoid any possible repetition of the experience. Alternatives to natural child-bearing were reviewed. Yet it quickly became clear that the alternatives were unappealing. The literature includes positive reports of parental satisfaction with donor artificial insemination, but it is not a technique for everyone. Nor does every genetic counselor feel at ease recommending it.

Nor can every couple elect abortion. Naturally, this must color the utility for a given couple of prenatal diagnostic evaluations. On the other hand, a preliminary statement against abortion may be changed in the face of report of a damaged fetus.

All the options are difficult. The alternatives must be presented so that a couple does not feel hopeless about selecting the pathway emotionally "right" for them. It is very hard to guess what path will be chosen when mourning over the catastrophe has ended. Plainly, the misfortune pro-vides a severe challenge to the strength of the marital bond.

The Mullers understood everything they had been told. The mixture of unavailability or unacceptability of alternative pathways, their under-standing of the risk percentages, and their drive to have their own children led to the new pregnancy. Their preparation for another cesarean section "to help the baby as much as possible" if it were affected, just as though it might survive better than Joanne, may be evidence of the emotional self-protection of denial. Luck was with them this time.

Related to the mechanism of denial just described, the Mullers revised their perspective of past history, blaming their former physician for judg-ment contributory to Joanne's death. To lose confidence in a physician after a fatality is not rare, though, as here, it may be quite irrational. The attribution of the fatality to bad advice, rather than disease, may have been precisely what permitted the Mullers to go ahead with the new preg-nancy, determined to persist no matter what.

References

Lubs, H., and Travers, M. (1981). Genetic counseling in osteogenesis imperfecta. *Clinical Orthopedics* 159: 36–41.

Miller, T. (1978). Intrauterine diagnosis of fetal disease by X-ray. *J. National Med. Assoc.* 70:875–876.

Sillence, D., et al. (1979). Genetic heterogeneity in osteogenesis imperfecta. *J. Med. Genetics* 16:101–116.

3

Refusing to Accept the Diagnosis of Down Syndrome: A Family in Hiding

This is the first of a number of chapters that focus on Down syndrome. The situation of the Toyama family illustrates how the psychological defense of "denial" can operate powerfully even in an individual—in this case, the mother—with the medical sophistication of a trained nurse. Yet the daily perception of the child's problem gradually wore away the strength of that denial, at least for the mother, and permitted her to benefit from counseling.

The story further illustrates how it is even possible to work effectively with one spouse despite evidence that doing so must be generating tension between the husband and wife. This is not always possible, since in some instances there must be peace at home between the spouses at any price, even if that price is discontinuance of counseling.

One of the most common referrals to our Pediatric Genetics Clinic is the case of suspected Down syndrome. Pediatricians in private practice or at well-baby clinics notice the typical facies of a child and suggest to the parents that chromosome studies be done to clarify their suspicions. Under the best of circumstances, conveyance of the diagnosis of Down syndrome—with its implications of mental retardation, possible cardiac and respiratory problems, and long-term expectations of the need for a sheltered adult life—is difficult and results in great family unheaval. Parents' response to this frightening suggestion regarding their child may include any or all of the following: denial, anger, guilt, shame, and grief for the normal child that might have been.

A family seen at our clinic posed some additional problems. They were referred to us by the Neurological Department of a neighboring facility for the handicapped. The child, Lee, had been seen there at age 11 months because of slow development and floppy muscle tone. The resident physician suspected Down syndrome and sent a sample of Lee's blood to our cytogenetics laboratory for chromosome studies. When a diagnosis of trisomy 21 confirmed his suspicions, he arranged to see Mrs. Toyama and told her that the child had a chromosomal disorder. He recommended that the family attend the Genetics Clinic the following day in order for Lee to be seen by the Genetics Unit and for the family to be given more detailed information. Mrs. Toyama agreed to this and an appointment was arranged.

As we met for clinic that day, I noted that Mrs. Toyama and Lee had come without Mr. Toyama. This was not usual for a first counseling session of this type. After Lee had been examined by Dr. D., I came in to greet Mrs. Toyama. Since we had a visiting medical student at our clinic (as is often the case), I asked if the student might sit in while we talked. Mrs. Toyama's response that she would prefer to be alone was the first clue that she was very upset.

We began the counseling session by my obtaining a family history. Mr. Toyama was 33 years old and an assistant professor of mathematics, and Mrs. Toyama, 28, was a nurse. Both parents were of Japanese ancestry and this was their first pregnancy. The remainder of the history was unremarkable.

Next we discussed the concerns that had brought Mrs. Toyama to the Neurological Department. She explained that she believed her son to have unusually floppy muscle tone for his age and to have a somewhat unusual-looking face. In addition to epicanthal folds, other hallmarks of the chromosome abnormality such as simian creases, a flat facial profile, upward-slanting eyes, and small, oddly shaped ears were noted by us.

G.C.: Mrs. Toyama, Lee's blood studies have given us an explanation for his poor muscle tone and slow development.

[Through the use of normal karyotypes I explained that normally a person has 46 chromosomes, or 23 pairs, in all of his body cells with the exception of the sperm or egg, but that in the mechanics of cell division accidents sometimes occur. Babies can be born with an abnormal number of chromosomes in their cells. Medical problems can then be expected, since these chromosomes are strings of transmitted genetic information, and additional or missing information usually has serious consequences.]

G.C.: Lee has an additional chromosome in all the cells of his body. It is a small chromosome and can be identified as a #21. This condition is known as Down syndrome or trisomy 21, "trisomy" meaning three of one particular chromosome rather than the usual pair. Having the extra #21 means that there are a number of consequences for Lee's development. . . . Mrs. Toyama, have you ever heard of Down syndrome?

MRS. TOYAMA: Yes; at M.G. Hospital, where I work, I once met a woman whose child had Down syndrome. She told me about some of the difficulties the family was having.

G.C.: Mrs. Toyama, let's look at Lee's karyotype now. The laboratory looked at Lee's blood sample in a special way, enabling them to see the chromosomes in many cells and count them. Then they took pictures of some cells so that the chromosomes could be removed from the photo, identified, arranged, and glued onto this cardboard. Do you see the #21 chromosomes on Lee's karyotype? There are three of them. Let's look back at a normal karyotype; it has two #21 chromosomes.

MRS. TOYAMA: Is Lee's problem my fault?

This question is the most expectable from any mother of an afflicted baby. More often than not, irrational elements contribute to this doubt in the mother's mind: Even when (1) it may be impossible to decide which parent is the responsible one or (2) both parents may share the responsibility, the mother by virtue of the fact that *she* was the pregnant one tends to arrogate the major—or, indeed, the only—responsibility to herself.

G.C.: This kind of chromosome abnormality is no one's fault, but is an accident or error that occurs in the egg *or* the sperm when the chromosomes do not divide evenly. [Diagrams of such a nondisjunctive event were shown to Mrs. Toyama. These seemed to help her visualize how trisomy could occur when a cell containing 24 chromosomes united with a cell containing 23 chromosomes at conception.]

MRS. TOYAMA: What will the extra chromosomes mean for Lee's future?

G.C.: Lee has done well so far. He does not have the heart or digestive problems that some Down children have. His delayed development will become more apparent as he grows older and you compare his skills with those of other children. He will go to special classes and need much attention. Lee will never be able to live all on his own making independent decisions, but he may work in a sheltered environment and live in a supervised group home.

[The finality of this information brought tears to Mrs. Toyama's eyes, and I shifted the discussion to another important area.]

G.C.: How does your husband feel about your concerns?

MRS. TOYAMA [with difficulty]: He does not believe that Lee has a problem and refuses to talk to me whenever I bring up my worries. He would not come to clinic with me today.

This expectation that the developmental pace of a Down child will diverge increasingly from that of his normal age mates has obvious impact on a family's planning. Before that point—especially if other anomalies are not present—the impact of the retardation is *blunted* by the fact that normal children of the same age have not developed very far either. The family's confrontation with this new social-developmental reality may spur long-range planning in the direction of a sheltered setting.

Mr. Toyama's response indicates a major unavoidable focus in further counseling interaction. His reaction to the dreadful news is a total denial, which he both *states* to his wife and also enacts through his refusal to come to the clinic at all. It is tempting to consider forgetting about him and offering assistance only to Mrs. Toyama, the accessible spouse. As a practical matter such a strategy is likely to be foredoomed. A counselor spends only an *occasional* hour with a mother, while the woman's husband spends *many* hours with her. The husband can readily undermine the clinic's work, because the mother feels, at home, the full pressure of her own need to accommodate to him simply so that the couple can reside together.

G.C.: Have you been able to talk to anyone else in your family about your worries?

Mrs. Toyama [tearfully]: We have no relatives in the United States, and I could never tell my family about Lee. They are so proud of our little son.

G.C.: It must have been very difficult for you to deal with your suspicions and worries by yourself. We must try to help your husband understand Lee's problem.

The availability of prenatal diagnosis was discussed during that first session, as was the possibility of an infant stimulation program for Lee. Mrs. Toyama borrowed our recommended family source material, *The Child with Down's Syndrome* (Smith and Wilson, 1973). When we told Mrs. Toyama that we would like to send a letter to Lee's pediatrician summarizing our findings and discussion, she requested that Lee's diagnosis be kept in the strictest confidence and not be given to any other physicians including her obstetrician. We suggested that she return with her husband in six weeks to discuss questions they might have about Lee's problem and the counseling.

The sense of embarrassment and shame that this request bespeaks is relatively common. In time, of course, the truth of the situation can hardly be denied through concealment of the child.

During the postclinic conference the Toyama family was discussed, and it was suggested that Dr. M., a Japanese doctor in our Genetics Unit, speak with the couple on their return. Although there was no language barrier, we thought that someone of similar cultural background might better understand this family and offer additional support.

At the second counseling session Dr. M. spoke with Mrs. Toyama, who once again had come without her husband. Fuller information regarding Lee's perinatal history was given to Dr. M. The Toyamas had been given the diagnosis of Down syndrome shortly after Lee's birth (almost a year before) by their pediatrician. Mrs. Toyama changed pediatricians at once, and the new physician agreed with her that Lee seemed normal.

This reaction to the bad news is so reminiscent of the accounts of the fate in ancient times of bearers of bad tidings: They were killed! The first pediatrician was "killed" by being discharged summarily.

Subsequently this new pediatrician, investigating Lee's hospital records, recommended that Lee be seen in our Genetics Clinic. Mrs. Toyama did not follow this advice. Months later, when she could no longer ignore Lee's slow development, Mrs. Toyama arranged to take Lee to the Neurology Clinic at the neighboring medical facility, fearing the consequences of going to a Genetics Clinic. From the time of Lee's birth she had been very anxious about him, yet unable to face the possibility that there was something ''not right'' with him. She had been unable to share with anyone the burden she carried. At this session she reiterated her feelings of guilt that had built up over a year of anxiety. Mrs. Toyama expressed her willingness to do everything she could for her son. She would not consider the possibility of foster care or institutionalization. Neither would she consider an infant stimulation program or participation in a parents' group.

As it became increasingly apparent that Mr. Toyama would not come to the Genetics Clinic, phone contact was initiated with him by Dr. M. It would take much time and discussion for the father to come to terms with his son's problems. We felt that we could have been much more helpfull to this family if they had been able to come as a unit. Communication, however, was solidly established with Mrs. Toyama, enabling her to begin to accept the dreaded diagnosis and to deal with her feelings of guilt. We were fortunate to be able to offer her the possibility of prenatal diagnosis by amniocentesis to allay the family's fear of recurrent trouble in future pregnancies.

Three months later Mrs. Toyama sought me out on clinic day with news of a suspected pregnancy and a request for referral to a new obstetrician, someone outside the Japanese community of the city. We recommended a physician who works closely with our Genetics Unit, and he followed Mrs. Toyama through an amniocentesis and a successful conclusion of the pregnancy.

Further Comment

After the initial diagnosis of Down syndrome there was a lengthy period before Mrs. Toyama found her way to suitable genetic counseling — an interval that is impressive and assuredly meaningful. She required quite a bit of time to begin to grapple actively with the verdict on Lee. Shock and denial had to run their course first, and we must remind ourselves that this process had to proceed without emotional support from her husband. Mr. Toyama was even less able to contend with the diagnosis, and still is.

Mrs. Toyama offers a good illustration of the distinction between "understanding" something and "accepting" it. She understands the diagnosis and the stated implications, but has the greatest difficulty in accepting them. Acceptance would mean taking those steps that might enhance Lee's developmental movement. In so doing, she might well have to struggle with her husband's denial of any difficulty.

We are not often presented with counselees in an optimal emotional state for counseling, and have no choice but to work with them as we find them. We may need to offer many suggestions to the spouse who is there, to help her or him deal with the more resistant marriage partner.

We hope that the Toyamas were able to smooth over their situation before adding a new baby to the family. Mrs. Toyama has now demonstrated that she can produce a normal child, an achievement of enormous value to her self-esteem and emotional equilibrium. It is striking that although the clinic staff thought rapport with the Toyamas would be enhanced through inclusion of Dr. M., a Japanese physician, Mrs. Toyama expressed her preference to work with an obstetrician outside the Japanese community. The strong preference for all possible privacy, generated by distress about Lee, in all likelihood required such a choice. However, Mrs. Toyama did agree to have the pregnancy monitored by amniocentesis rather than denying that a mishap had occurred or could happen again.

References

DE LA CRUZ, F., and GERALD, P., eds. (1981). *Trisomy 21*. Baltimore: University Park Press.

SMITH, D., and WILSON, A. (1973). *The child with Down's syndrome*. Philadelphia: W. B. Saunders.

4

Complete Acceptance of a Recurring Disorder in a Large Extended Family: Mandibulofacial Dysostosis

Wendell and his family illustrate how a family can accept to a considerable degree a disfiguring genetic malady that affects different people in different ways. Acceptance is made possible through mutual identification as members of an extended family group that shares the disorder, and through erroneous attribution of the disorder to the family's ethnic origin.

Wendell himself demonstrates the great relief that may accrue to an individual when he is finally supplied with a true medical diagnosis for what until then he has regarded as a private peculiarity, with who knows what private meanings. When one considers the situation of the Toyama family in light of this case, one can appreciate that peculiarity of appearance alone cannot be regarded as a complete explanation for the need of some families to hide.

A 28-year-old man named Wendell, with a severely malformed physical appearance, came to our specialized clinic to see if help was available to correct surgically his serious facial disfigurement. He had defective hearing and unusually poor speech. In a rather rehearsed manner he was able to give a complete history of his multiple physical handicaps and many hospitalizations, and the frequent surgical procedures he had undergone. In addition to a disfiguring cleft lip he had a repaired cleft palate. There was residual scarring from earlier surgical repair of his nose and lip. His hearing loss was severe and uncorrected, and he was wearing his deaf mother's hearing aid. (We later learned that his mother's deafness was unrelated to Wendell's disorder.) His teeth had been in severe malocclusion, necessitating more than a decade of orthodontic care. His palatal repair had not been completely successful, and had to be followed by years of speech therapy.

Wendell's many problems had not been neglected, but his condition had never been given a name or explained as a genetic disorder until he consulted our clinic.

This particular case was chosen to illustrate the enormous positive impact that genetic counseling had on Wendell—benefits which he gleefully tried to extend to his large family. For four generations they had been unaware that their many affected members had indeed inherited their special problems. This naiveté on the family's part is somewhat understandable for two reasons: First, the variable expressivity of this heritable autosomal dominant disorder, mandibulofacial dysostosis, resulted in family members having considerable variation in disfigurement and functional loss, ranging from hardly perceptible manifestations to very serious stigmata such as Wendell's. Second, so many family members were affected that it seemed quite acceptable to them to resemble one another in appearance. This was borne out by a photograph which Wendell brought to the clinic when we had become better acquainted. It is a formally posed photograph of a bride and groom (Wendell's mother and father) and a small wedding party. Two of Wendell's father's relatives are included in the photo. It is obvious that two of these three people have mandibulofacial dysostosis. Neither, however, bears Wendell's severe stigmata. What remains difficult to understand, in view of Wendell's extensive medical history, is that he was undiagnosed for twenty-eight years.

The mental mechanism of denial takes innumerable forms in different contexts. Considering that mandibulofacial defects are difficult or impossible to conceal, the subject cannot deny the *fact* of their existence. Yet it may be possible to deny the emotional import of this fact, pointing as it does to defective inheritance. Notions of being in *any* way "defective" are for all of us among the most powerful stimuli to activate mental mechanisms such as denial to protect or repair wounded self-esteem. Denial does not operate alone, but usually in conjunction with other automatic self-protective mechanisms. In Wendell's family there appears to be auxiliary rationalization: "This is the way we look in our family." Why term this a "rationalization?" Like every rationalization the statement has its nucleus of truth: They do indeed look that way. We call it a rationalization because it is a way of avoiding the truth that this is not just any family trait, like dark hair or swarthiness, but a genetic defect. The various family members bolster one another's defensiveness.

Why need a counselor note this mental defensiveness? Because it *may* be an impediment to counseling that has to be dealt with.

Why no correct diagnosis in twenty-eight years? This is hard to say, and one could offer many untestable hypotheses.

Mandibulofacial dysostosis, also known as Treacher Collins syndrome, in its severe form is a well-recognized craniofacial anomaly. It has been described extensively in the medical and dental literature. The syndrome has most often been described as a single gene autosomal dominant disorder. At least 60 percent of cases occur sporadically, while the other 40 percent present a family history. The salient features of Treacher Collins are: a typical facies characterized by malformed ears; a downward slant of the palpebral fissures; a prominent nose with absence of the fronto-nasal angle; deficient cheek and orbital bones or absent cheekbones; and colobomas of the lower eyelids. The chin typically is receded and the mouth is open at rest, revealing an open bite. Conductive deafness is common. Often the palate is highly arched, and occasionally it is cleft. Mental deficiency has only been reported rarely. The penetrance of the Treacher Collins gene is high, meaning that carriers of the abnormal gene will usually have some detectable manifestation of the syndrome. Any single manifestation may vary in its clinical severity, a phenomenon referred to as "variable expressivity."

Wendell was referred to our clinic by his new family physician for evaluation, counseling, and (hopefully) treatment. The counselor saw him frequently over a period of one and a half years.

At our first meeting Wendell was accompanied by his sister, Janet (age 27), and his cousin Dottie. This first session lasted two and a half hours, during which we were able to inform Wendell of the name for his condition and explain its genetics. His immediate response was gratitude beyond and disproportionate to the actual counseling received. This exuberance lasted throughout the entire counseling session, as we easily defined thirteen additional affected family members and several other likely cases. In this affected group were Wendell's deceased father and his sister, Janet, who was very mildly affected. Although she had significant hearing loss, downward-slanting palpebral fissures, and flattened cheekbones, her appearance was not obviously abnormal. In contrast to Wendell's chatty cheerfulness Janet's demeanor was somber, reflective, and attentive.

Their cousin, Dottie, served as family historian as well as family chauffeur. By avocation she was an ambulance driver for a voluntary rescue service, a job she reportedly enjoyed thoroughly. She, too, was examined during this first visit to the clinic and was found to be free of the "family disease." In her mid-thirties Dottie had married a much older man who had been a victim of cerebral palsy. She said that she had considered it important *not* to marry anyone of her own nationality, for she had always felt that the family problem was a "Danish disease." (Her analysis tells us inheritance *was* suspected as a cause of the family disorder by at least one family member, even though the implication was broadened and softened by erroneously regarding the disorder as ethnic, common to an entire people!).

Wendell and Janet impressed the counselor as giving evidence of similar personality problems that seemed to be importantly linked to their both having Treacher Collins syndrome. Neither seemed assertive or independent. Both relied heavily on Dottie, who did not seem to mind, and even appeared to enjoy their dependence. Wendell worked full-time as a clerk in an office, and lived with his mother and stepfather.

Wendell, Janet, and Dottie expressed a strong determination to spread the news of the diagnosis to other family members. The session concluded with plans to meet again two weeks later. The counselor decided to permit ample time to mull over and start to digest the emotionally charged information provided by all parties during this first meeting.

In a clinical situation of *this* type the two-week interval should be very useful, as it will permit the counselees to react and churn around the new information and some of its implications. Questions often will occur to them in the privacy of their homes that would not occur to them while still at the clinic. On subsequent contact the counselor will be able to assess how the counselees' needs for emotional self-protection have distorted the conveyed information. Correction can then be offered so that counseling effectiveness is enhanced.

Clinical situations more acute than Wendell's require much more frequent contacts with the counselor—because of counselee distress or the need for rapid and momentous decisions.

During the second session Wendell continued to be cheerful and optimistic, Janet again appeared serious; in fact she was more troubled than during our first meeting. At 27 she is married and the mother of a 5-year-old son. For three and a half years she has been actively trying to become pregnant, without success. She is certain that her son is unaffected by the family malady and brought photographs of him to confirm this.

Wendell was extremely verbal and open about his feelings. He remarked, "I feel as if God has given me something very special. He has singled me out! He has given me something unusual that I did not even know about until you told me." (Wendell was referring to the counselor's naming of his problem.) He said he felt a kind of dignity, almost an importance, related to the fact that he had such a rare genetic condition. He inquired if we were planning to publish his case.

It is quite notable with many counselees that supplying a correct name for their difficulty is experienced as a benefaction of a sort. What has hitherto been regarded as a private quirk or a personal peculiarity, the source of which stimulates all manner of fantasy, has now been given a new meaning in a broader context. Wendell's family has learned that the phenomena that plague them are describable and explainable according to certain biological laws. Wendell's question about possible publication of his case suggests he now appreciates that the study of his burdensome condition may even benefit others: a heavy wound to pride transmuted into a particular variety of virtue.

Between regular counseling visits for evaluation or treatment Wendell would sometimes bounce into the office to say "Hi." He proved to be consistently cooperative in getting together a family album with pictures and information of all first-, second-, third-, and even fourth-degree relatives.

At the third counseling session Wendell brought Janet, her husband, Al, his mother, Cousin Dottie, and her sister, Eve. Once again we reviewed the genetics of Treacher Collins syndrome. Wendell registered the impression that he was immensely enjoying his visits to the clinic and all the attention he was receiving. Although nothing had yet changed in terms of his facial appearance, his hearing, or his speech problems, *everything* had seemingly changed subjectively for this severely stigmatized young man. He now had the dignity and comfort of a name for his condition, making it easier for him to accept it. He now understood that he had inherited his disorder from his father, although he never voiced any complaints directed at his father. The burden of responsibility for his condition was lifted from Wendell.

We spoke in detail of the meaning of a family, of a person at risk for inheriting and transmitting a defective gene. We discussed alternatives for childbearing for an affected woman or for the wife of an affected man. Surprisingly, Wendell's reaction to the knowledge he might transmit a defective gene was one of unconcern. He said he would not hesitate to have children. Of course, all this was hypothetical since Wendell was not expecting to marry or have a family in the near future. But he definitely planned to marry *and* have children. His sister was less philosophical and more immediately concerned about her future, as she was now at a decision-making stage of her life. Should she continue to plan a family? Janet said that in the final analysis "It is God's decision." After three counseling sessions she fully understood the possible consequences of a 50 percent risk for any child conceived. She understood, yet at the same time expressed great faith that she and her family would be spared!

The reporting counselor's exclamation point implies that if she were in her counselees' position, she believes she could not adopt such a bland, optimistic outlook. Such counselee responses tell us that the meaning of a particular clinical condition in human terms is experienced very differently by different people. The desire to have one's own children in the usual biological manner is surpassingly strong and colors reaction even to 50 percent probability. Compare this reaction to that of the Mullers, the family at risk for osteogenesis imperfecta congenita.

Some months later a meeting was arranged with Wendell, Dottie, Wendell's paternal great-aunt, Elsie, her 39-year-old daughter, Fran, and her 18-year-old grandson, Bill. The great-aunt and grandson were obviously affected with the disorder, but minimally so. The daughter, Fran, was quite beautiful and seemingly unaffected, although we knew that she was an obligate carrier, since her son, Bill, was affected. Fran had two other children, whom we did not meet.

Initially, this little group showed reluctance in discussing the family disorder. Sensing this, the counselor separated them from Wendell and Dottie by sending Dottie on a contrived mission and having Wendell examined in another room. Once privacy was established, Elsie, Fran, and Bill were more willing to contribute. They were rather reserved about establishing a relationship with the same medical professionals who were treating other family members. They seemed to follow the genetic explanation. They were counseled as to Bill's hearing problem and the precautions that must be taken with anesthesia for surgery because of airway hypoplasia in Treacher Collins syndrome. Bill had already come dangerously close to death as a result of breathing complications when his tonsils were removed. To date we have not heard again from these three. It is this counselor's strong impression that they deliberately elected not to investigate further the ramifications of the family disorder.

At present Wendell has undergone three surgical procedures on his upper and lower face and on his ears. He has grown a mustache and looks considerably better. His ear surgery has improved his hearing. Wendell continues to be cheerful and hopeful. He tells us that Janet has *adopted* a child. Dottie no longer chauffeurs Wendell to the clinic. We do not hear from any other family members.

—Which just goes to show that despite what counselee responses may be during an ongoing interview, the later digestion and assimilation of information may lead a counselee to an altogether unexpected path of action.

In our earlier experience, counseling for mandibulofacial dysostosis has not usually resulted in the beneficial impact on personality functioning exhibited by Wendell. Most often the propositus is a young child who is diagnosed and treated, and the counseling is predominantly addressed to the parents. They tend to exhibit all forms of denial when informed that their offspring has a genetic disorder, and that they have a possible responsibility for having transmitted that disorder to the child. Many times, of course, neither parent is affected, and the case is a sporadic occurrence. In one vividly recalled family with a severely affected child, the father was suspected of being affected but would have had to submit to various studies to confirm or negate this suspicion. The tests were never permitted. Any suggestions to alert other family members were met with horror. Secrecy was paramount, evidently because the parents could not imagine how they would grapple with all the distressing emotions stirred up by the ramifications of the child's diagnosis.

It may seem to the reader quite a straightforward matter for a counselee to undergo indicated diagnostic studies and to notify family members. Yet some counselees are very resistant to such suggestions, and only laborious work in the context of strong rapport with their counselor will induce them to change their minds.

Further Comment

In regard to acceptance of a condition, the story of Wendell and his family contrasts sharply with the situation of the Toyamas struggling to deal with Down syndrome.

Here are individuals of several generations variably afflicted with the same kind of trouble. Having some sense of its familial nature, they attribute it somewhat ambiguously to their ethnic background. Then they are offered a specific technical name for what they have always known. It can be quite striking to outsiders, like the professionals caring in different capacities for this family, to discover how subjective the response to disfigurement may be.

There is an apocryphal story of the visit of a genetic counselor to the bedside of a woman who has just delivered an infant with polydactyly. With some uneasiness the counselor approaches the new mother and as tactfully as possible informs her that the baby has an extra digit on each extremity. Expecting a strong show of distress, the counselor is surprised by the mother's buoyant reply: "Oh, he's just like his old man!"

Certainly, in Wendell's family acceptance of the defect is strongly based upon its being shared. Other factors also militate toward acceptance. The expressivity in different individuals ranges from mild to severe affliction, so one may individually be lucky. Disfigurement, malocclusion of the teeth, and hearing impairment without mental retardation or deteriorative trend do not have the same impact as certain other more devastating forms of autosomal dominant disorder. Even without knowing the technical name for their difficulty, Wendell's family had tried to help him by pursuing corrective surgery, orthodontia, and speech therapy.

Contrast mandibulofacial dysostosis with another autosomal dominant disorder, Huntington's disease. Afflicted members of families with this disease are hard to hide, not because of disfigurement but because of notable neurological signs and disturbed behavior. Deteriorative trends are expected, with suicide, psychosis, and death among the manifestations. With such a problem in the family, compounded by the fact that the disorder is not detected till the middle years, even the unaffected members are burdened with anxiety about themselves, let alone their possible progeny. Familial though it may be, Huntington's disease is hardly "acceptable." (A family's struggle with this disease will be reported later in the casebook.)

References

Gorlin, R.; Pindborg, J.; and Cohen, M. (1976). Mandibulofacial dysostosis. In *Syndromes of the head and neck,* 2nd ed., pp. 453–458. New York: McGraw-Hill.

Smith, D. (1976). *Recognizable patterns of human malformation,* 2nd ed., pp. 134–135. Philadelphia: W. B. Saunders.

5

First Things First: Denial in Someone at Risk for Charcot-Marie-Tooth Disease

Another example demonstrates the operation of denial to maintain relative composure in the face of a frightening reality that just refuses to go away. Charcot-Marie-Tooth disease is the first of the late-onset neurological disorders to be encountered in this collection. The combination of concern about offspring along with concern about whether the parents themselves are free of the disease is presented rather directly.

It is apparent that this counseling experience inescapably generated so much discomfort that it rendered follow-up contacts unattractive to the counselees. Whether such an outcome was altogether avoidable is moot; in any event, the situation of counseling people about the disease in question presents the counselor with a very difficult challenge.

Charcot-Marie-Tooth disease is a neurological disorder which presents special counseling problems because of the variability in age of onset. The symptoms can initially manifest themselves during adult years or during the second or first decade of life. There is some tendency toward later onset in males. This disorder begins insidiously with weakness and eventual atrophy of the peroneal muscles of the leg. The condition advances slowly to involve other distal leg and arm muscles. In some families gastrointestinal symptoms have been observed. The inheritance pattern of Charcot-Marie-Tooth disease is heterogeneous: Autosomal dominant, autosomal recessive, and X-linked patterns of transmission are known to occur.

Mrs. Lois Andros initially came to the hospital's Genetics Department at the urging of her grandmother. Both Mrs. Andros and her grandmother had been visiting the former's grandfather, an inpatient at the hospital, and the grandmother suggested that Mrs. Andros inquire as to whether the counseling service could be useful to her. Lois Andros reluctantly made inquiry in order to placate her grandmother, who persistently urged her to proceed.

When Mrs. Andros came to my office, she seemed quite uneasy and had difficulty articulating her problem. She apparently had only scattered bits of information pertaining to the subject of her concern. I learned from our initial meeting that a number of her husband's relatives—including his twin sister, mother, several aunts, two female cousins, and his maternal grandfather—were affected with a condition that had caused gradual weakening of their leg muscles. Mrs. Andros explained that paradoxically the condition was known to have originated with her husband's maternal grandfather but had only affected females. She did not know the name of the disorder, and stated that the family was reluctant to discuss the problem.

It is very common for families having such an incidence of presumptively hereditary disease to deny its import through excluding it as a subject for conversation, as though it did not exist.

Her concern was whether the disabling condition was, in fact, hereditary, and whether her future children would be affected. I responded that our first task in seeking answers to her important questions was to establish the specific diagnosis of her husband's relatives. We agreed that Mrs. Andros would telephone us to arrange an appointment for a genetic counseling session for herself and her husband. During one of the phone conversations needed to select an appointment time Mrs. Andros mentioned that her husband's twin sister, Nancy, had said she was diagnosed by a neurologist as having Charcot-Marie-Tooth disease. Other remarks tended to convince our department that in the Andros family the inheritance of this disorder was in accordance with a dominant pattern. Further, Mr. Andros expressed his belief that because he was male he could never develop CMT disease. Confronted by this firm belief and the obvious dominant pattern of transmission, our department elected to discuss with Mr. and Mrs. Andros at their first counseling session *only* the dominant pattern of CMT transmission.

The meeting with Lois and Michael Andros took place approximately one month after the original inquiry. They were a young, attractive couple, married for three years. Michael was 31, Lois 24, and both were high school graduates. Michael was employed as a New York City bus repairman, Lois was a homemaker. At the time of counseling, Mrs. Andros was not yet pregnant, although the couple was trying to conceive a child.

In preliminary conversation, I tried to ascertain just how much the Andros' understood their problem and its genetic implications. From previous discussion it was apparent that this couple's fears concerned future children, whereas the more immediate concern, from our point of view, was whether Mr. Andros himself was likely to develop the disorder. A sampling of our dialogue follows:

G.C. [in order to elicit the couple's expectations]: Why don't the two of you give me some idea of what you would like to get out of our meeting today.

MR. ANDROS: Two boys!

G.C.: All at once?

MR. ANDROS: Yes! [I went along with Mr. Andros' attempt to be humorous in order to break the ice and create an atmosphere of ease. However, it was also important to direct the session to a more serious level.]

G.C.: I think, more than just having two boys, the reason why you've really come for genetic counseling is that you are interested in having a healthy child.

MR. ANDROS: Yes, I joke around a lot. The main reason we're here is to find out about the disease that my family has.

MRS. ANDROS: Maybe they can do something if I have a baby, so that it can be healthy.

MR. ANDROS: What she means is: Let's say they test my genes and it shows up. Usually it hits the female and passes the male. Let's say she has a girl, and it's already been detected in my genes, and you detect it in the baby. The main thing is: How would you go about taking care of the matter after the baby's born?

G.C.: So what you want to know is whether we can prevent the condition in the baby, or treat it in some way?

MR. ANDROS: Yes.

G.C.: You did say on the phone that the name of the disease was Charcot-Marie-Tooth disease.

MR. ANDROS: Yes. From what my sister and my cousins tell me, the doctors say it's a Mediterranean disease, from the southern part of Italy and Greece. It's usually caused by some distant relative's marrying another member of the family. And like I told you, some members of my great-grandmother's generation married a cousin. [Although this was obvious misinformation, I didn't want to intrude with a disagreement so early along. I thought that by correcting the information at this point, I might inhibit the conveyance of other information to me. It was evident that although their understanding of genetic facts was somewhat confused, the Andros' had received genetic information somewhere along the way.]

The counselor is behaving with careful regard for the necessity to establish rapport above all. There is no better way to do this than by attentive listening and by permitting counselees to tell their story in their own way. This approach rapidly permits assessment of the limits of counselee knowledge, and of the distortions and misinformation included.

G.C.: Let's get the family history information down on paper. What we will get by doing this is a "pattern" of how the disorder is transmitted from generation to generation. We will be able to see who is at risk. Have you ever thought that *you* might be at risk? Did you ever worry about that? [Rather than stating "You are at risk," the use of the question form, I believe, draws the thought into the interview focus without necessarily eliciting a defensive reaction.]

The counselor knows that the early declarative statement "You are at risk" might very well have such distressing impact as to compromise the usefulness of the balance of the interview. There has as yet been very little opportunity to develop rapport, without which the task of helping counselees contend with distressing emotion is difficult or impossible. As Mr. Andros' response will inform us, there will be considerable spontaneous denial of the painful truth, bolstered by earlier medical contacts, which may have been misinterpreted along the lines of the counselee's wishes.

MR. ANDROS: No. I've been checked by doctors as a kid and they never found anything wrong with my legs. I never gave it much thought because it never hit the male, only the female.

G.C.: Did you ever worry about your husband, Mrs. Andros?

MRS. ANDROS: No.

G.C.: What do you know about the severity of this condition? [I continued my effort to assess the range and boundaries of this couple's knowledge and misinformation.]

MR. ANDROS: Well, it gets worse as you get older. It hit some of my family members in their teens, and it hit my mother when she was in her thirties. In four or five years she'll be in a wheelchair like my aunts.

G.C.: I think you understand the problem well. It is a progressive situation, but it doesn't shorten the life span in any way.

MR. ANDROS: My sister told me that in this disease, the good genes dominate the bad genes. . . . In the older generations these bad genes are all there, but in later generations they are slacking off. No one has the disease anymore. [He was referring to the last two generations in the pedigree. This is an easily understandable misconception about a late-onset disorder.]

G.C.: We don't really know if it's slacking off. CMT disease is a genetic disease in that you're born with the gene for it. But the disease doesn't show up until the teenage years or even the thirties. You've told me this yourself. As far as these younger generations are concerned, it's too early to know.

MR. ANDROS: Then why didn't the disease affect me, my brother, or my sister's son? [Mr. Andros' persistence in this train of thought about sex linkage may have helped him to deny his own vulnerability to the disease.]

G.C.: You're right in assuming that some diseases affect one sex and not the other. [Hemophilia was used as an example to illustrate this.] This is not true here. Your family shows a different pattern. [I pointed out the pattern on the pedigree, illustrating that many males in his family had not survived to adulthood, and the preponderance of females in the family made the disease *appear* to affect only females.]

MR. ANDROS: But you're taking a shot in the dark! My sister has a boy and he doesn't have it.

G.C.: Well, your nephew is only 8 years old. We can't know at this time if he has the disease.

MR. ANDROS: Oh!

[At that moment the concept I was trying to convey appeared to have registered. For a while he changed the conversation back to the consanguineous marriages many generations before. During this conversation Dr. S., the medical geneticist, entered the room and was introduced. I took up the conversation regarding consanguinity and explained why it had no significance in the Andros family. Then I went on to explain autosomal dominant inheritance, in due course emphasizing the 50 percent probability of transmitting the faulty dominant gene in every pregnancy.]

MR. ANDROS: Let's say I have two children; you're saying one of them is bound to get the disease?

DR. S: No. I'm saying that both may have the disease; or neither may have it; or one may have it and one may not.

G.C.: It's like flipping a coin. There is a 50 percent chance of getting heads on the first two flips. However, it is possible on only two flips to get heads twice, or tails twice.

MR. ANDROS: Then, if we have a child, we would have to wait until it's in its teens to find out.

DR. S.: Do you have Charcot-Marie-Tooth disease? How old are you?

MR. ANDROS: Thirty-one.

DR. S.: As you get older the chance that you will get the disease becomes smaller and smaller. The central question here is, Will you get the disease? If you don't have the faulty gene, you will not become affected with the disease and there is no way that you could pass it on to *any* of your children.

Notions of probability are part of the everyday thinking of all who work in the health professions. Genetic counselors must keep in mind that many people are less sophisticated about this branch of mathematics than they are. In the clinic setting, indeed, we encounter counselees who have not the slightest notion of what "a chance" described mathematically is all about.

With Mr. and Mrs. Andros, the counselor and the geneticist are taking the necessary time for clarifying dominant pattern inheritance, with particular emphasis on the fact that the probability of giving birth to an affected infant is the *same* with every new conception. It is natural for counselees to fall into the "gambler's fallacy" thought pattern ("If the chance of a sick child is one in two, and we've already had one who is sick, then the next will be all right.") Such a thought pattern, after all, accords with the powerful wish for a healthy infant. Not to disabuse counselees of this fallacy deprives them of making full use, for family planning, of the balance of the information being conveyed.

MR. ANDROS [apparently having understood]: And, I don't know if I have it or not.

G.C.: I think that is what we have to find out.

DR. S.: Have you ever been hospitalized, or tested for the disorder?

MR. ANDROS: Every year and a half I develop sand, or stones in my kidneys and I have pain in my side. They tested me and that's what they found. [There is some question here as to whether these symptoms might be related to gastrointestinal manifestations of CMT disease.]

DR. S.: The chances with you are that you *won't* get the disease because you are already 31 and you don't have it. Why don't we check you and then talk more about what we find.

[While Dr. S. and Mr. Andros were out of the office, I tried to learn more about Mrs. Andros' feelings. She had remained quiet during most of the previous interview. I found my conversation with Mrs. Andros somewhat strained. She was less articulate than her husband, and though she appeared to be willing to answer questions, she never conveyed any deep feelings to me.]

G.C.: You never thought about Michael's being affected with the condition before this?

MRS. ANDROS: When I married him, I knew his family had the problem. My family said I shouldn't marry him. [Perhaps at this point I might have explored her response more deeply.]

G.C.: Do you ever discuss the problem with your husband's family?

MRS. ANDROS: Well, his twin sister, Nancy [who is affected], will talk about it, but you can't say anything to his mother. She wants to go places with us, but she can't keep up. She gets depressed because she can't go anywhere and won't go into a wheelchair. Do other people have this disease? Can it be picked up easily? [Mrs. Andros' response continued on a superficial level, never referring directly to how *she* felt about the family situation.]

G.C.: Neurologists are the doctors who usually see this problem. Unfortunately, it is not one of those conditions where we are able to test a pregnancy to see if the baby is affected. It is a matter of "Do I want to take the risk, the 50 percent chance?"

Mrs. Andros: What about treatment?

G.C.: My understanding is that perhaps things can be done to delay the progress of the disorder, but that there is no cure at present. We can check this with the doctor when he returns. Did you ever think in terms of risk? That is, what risk would be an acceptable risk for you? For example, what if we said there was a 25 percent risk for the baby—or 10 percent—or 50 percent? What risk would be acceptable for you to take?

Mrs. Andros: I don't know.

[Since we are always dealing with probabilities in genetics, I will often pose the above question to a counselee to try to assess his or her ability to deal with the risk figure and to encourage private thought on this troubling issue.]

G.C.: This is something you should discuss with your husband. Just what chance are the two of you willing to take, and what chance is *too* high? It's not an easy decision or one you can make overnight. We usually have patients come back one or two months later to discuss things like this again.

[At this point Mr. Andros and Dr. S. returned to the office. The doctor explained that no conclusions could be drawn from Mr. Andros' examination and suggested that a nerve conduction test be performed at a subsequent visit. It was also suggested that, if possible, Mr. Andros bring his sister and/or mother with him on the return visit. The Andros' willingly agreed to return. (Dr. S. later told me that there appeared to be some muscle weakness in Mr. Andros' lower extremities. However, a conclusion could not be drawn without definitive testing.)]

G.C.: That still leaves us up in the air about the problem of trying to have a baby now.

Mr. Andros: Well, I think we should wait, but if she wants a baby now, I guess we would go ahead.

Dr. S.: Perhaps it would be best to wait the few weeks till your next appointment. If Mr. Andros has the disorder there are different possibilities we could discuss.

[Assuming that Mr. Andros is affected, we would discuss these alternatives with the couple: (1) to proceed to have children, taking the 50 percent risk; (2) to make the decision not to have children; (3) to adopt children; (4) to have children by artificial insemination by a donor.]

From the counselor's point of view I was relatively satisfied with the course of this ninety-minute first session. I telephoned the Andros' one month later and learned that Mrs. Andros had already collected some medical records from affected relatives. She read some excerpts from them. Her excuse for not having called for an appointment was rather weak, having to do with bad weather.

Eight months have passed since the session described, and I feel it would be inappropriate to call again. The inability to have further opportunity to counsel the couple leaves me understandably frustrated. The summary letter which was sent to the Andros' soon after their meeting with us may in time help to stimulate their return. It is a tangible link between us.

Further Comment

In this case we encounter yet another variation of the manner in which the psychological need to deny painful information may operate for individuals involved not only with family planning but with questions about their own health. CMT disease is a late-onset neurological disorder with characteristics quite different from Huntington's disease, mentioned in discussion in the previous report. Yet the inheritance pattern is likewise autosomal dominant; and one may attain adult years—family-planning years—and not yet know with assurance that one is free of the disease and cannot transmit it.

The Andros family was aware that the disease is heritable. It was the facts and figures of the precise pattern that they did not know. Judging from their reluctance to participate in the counseling experience, it is possible that they preferred their homemade theory about the inheritance pattern to the actual facts, which did not exempt from possible affliction male members of the family, including Mr. Andros.

The fact that Mrs. Andros said so little when asked about the warning she had received prior to marriage suggests that this was an extremely touchy subject, with much potential for causing marital friction.

When the counselor employed percentages in her discussion, she was not just playing with numbers, but was trying to learn what constituted, for this couple, an acceptable risk. Acceptability can, of course, only be judged in terms of the idiosyncratic meaning of the illness to Mr. and Mrs. Andros. In turn, this meaning depends upon their closeness to the clinical progression of various affected family members. Each family's experience being somewhat different, what is acceptable to the Andros' may not be so to another couple, and can be quite at variance with what the counselor believes she could accept if she were in their shoes.

Why didn't the Andros' return in response to the invitation to Mr. Andros to undergo further testing of his own clinical status and participate in additional discussion of family-planning options? The thrust of the final remarks of the clinic team was that the couple should await further evaluation of Mr. Andros before planning to have children. We may presume that this is precisely what they did not desire to do. More to the point, Mr. Andros may have been quite alarmed at not already receiving a clean bill of health. To proceed with conception as if he were in fact all right would be to deny through action a scary possibility.

One cannot estimate the later impact of the single counseling session. We may agree with the counselor about further telephone approaches. The couple already have the valuable summary of their counseling interview. But, rather than a phone call, what of another letter of invitation to return? A phone call may put a counselee "on the spot." A letter can be read and reread, thrown away, recovered from the wastebasket, reflected upon, and reconsidered; and perhaps a delayed affirmative response will be made, whereas the prompt one might have been negative. The further show of counselor interest may eliminate any impression that the counselor was angered by the delayed response.

References

BRUST, J.; LOVELACE, R.; and DEVI, S. (1978). Clinical and electrodiagnostic features of Charcot-Marie-Tooth syndrome. *Acta Neurologica Scandinavica* 58 (no. 68): 1–42.

DYCK, P., and LAMBERT, E. (1968). Lower motor and primary sensory neuron disease with peroneal muscular atrophy. Part 1: Neurologic, genetic, and electrophysiologic findings in hereditary polyneuropathies. *Arch. Neurology* 18:603–618.

DYCK, P. (1975). Inherited neuronal degeneration and atrophy affecting peripheral motor, sensory, and autonomic neurons. In P. Dyck; P. Thomas; and E. Lambert, eds., *Peripheral neuropathy,* pp. 825–864. Philadelphia: W. B. Saunders.

THOMAS, P.; CALNE, D.; and STEWART, G. (1974). Hereditary motor and sensory polyneuropathy (peroneal muscular atrophy). *Annals Human Genetics* 38:111–153.

6

Neonatal Death and Counseling Error: Potter Syndrome

The counseling experience of the Jeromes was selected primarily because it included a demonstrated error in the advice offered at the time of the initial counseling. That advice was based on the information available at the time, and later observations were needed in order to correct it. Human beings being "human," this sequence is not unique. The narrative indicates that professionals can acknowledge a good-faith error without subverting further counseling. Style, in this regard, is everything.

Certain additional observations are included of the different ways in which professional staff react to a neonatal fatality, and how such responses impinge upon counselees.

Potter syndrome, or oligohydramnios anomalad, is a disorder characterized by peculiar facies and ears, clubbed feet, underdevelopment of the lungs, and a deficiency of amniotic fluid. Possible causes suggested for this syndrome include bilateral malformations of the kidneys, bladder or urethral obstruction which would limit urinary flow, and chronic leakage of amniotic fluid.

Normally the fetal kidneys produce urine, which is the major component of amniotic fluid. If the kidneys have not developed in the fetus, urine is not formed, causing a lack of amniotic fluid. The deficit permits servere external compression of the fetus, resulting in a host of secondary defects, including flattened facies, low-set ears, hand and foot position anomalies, and underdevelopment of the lungs. The child usually dies within the first few hours of life as a result of respiratory insufficiency.

Bilateral absence of kidney development may occur as a single malformation or may be part of a pattern of malformations. Most cases appear to be sporadic, but autosomal recessive inheritance has been documented in several families. An autosomal dominant form in which

53

some family members are missing a kidney on one or both sides of the body has been described. It is often very difficult to distinguish between the sporadic and the inherited types of kidney absence, which complicates genetic counseling.

The mother who received counseling in the report presented below, Marge Jerome, was adopted as an infant and knows nothing about her biological family. Raised as an only child, she spent her childhood in a large city until she was 12, when her adoptive mother died. Her father then decided to move to the small rural town where she and her husband, Bill, now live. Bill Jerome, one of three children, was born and raised in this same community, and most of his relatives live nearby.

Bill and Marge met soon after her move to the community, dated throughout high school, and were married shortly after graduation. Marge went on to nursing school and has worked in the local hospital since graduating. She rotates both shifts and services and has particularly enjoyed working on the maternity floor. Bill worked for the town maintenance department until after the birth of their second child. He then changed jobs to work as a carpenter in a small shop, which he enjoys doing and which offers opportunity for advancement.

Both Marge and Bill wanted children very much and had chosen names well before their first child was even conceived. When Marge became pregnant about two years after their marriage, they were very excited and immediately began making plans for the new baby. At about three months' gestation Marge became moody and expressed concern that something was going to be wrong. Although her obstetrician assured her that she was overanxious because this was her first pregnancy, the facts that she gained very little weight or girth and that the baby rarely moved caused her to worry. When she went into labor at full term, she said she knew the child would die.

Labor lasted twenty-four hours. When the doctor ruptured her membranes, Marge noticed the lack of amniotic fluid and said, "See, I knew something was wrong." The doctor did not respond and walked out of the delivery room. From that point on, Marge reports, no one spoke to her, and she was drugged very shortly after delivery. The baby was immediately transported the forty miles from the local hospital to the Neonatal Intensive Care Unit at our Medical Center, where he died shortly thereafter. The baby's death was reported to the local hospital and then to Marge by a floor nurse.

This behavior by professionals is tending to become less common. Reproductive catastrophe has most impact on the mother, but to some extent is experienced as catastrophe also by the professionals. Too often the emotional coping mechanism employed is to break off all contact with the mother for a while.

For the mother this compounds the problem, and that was especially true for Marge Jerome, herself a professional maternity nurse. In the absence of certain news — even depressing news — the mother is left to fill the vacuum with her own unavoidable musings. One's private fantasies in such circumstances are usually much worse than reality.

The Jeromes wanted to have another baby as soon as possible, but decided to wait at least until they had gotten more information about their baby's problems. The Medical Center neonatologist who had cared for their infant referred them to our Medical Genetics Unit. The genetic counselor arranged an appointment for two months later, hoping that this time interval would allow the parents to begin working through their grief. At the same time the Genetics Unit was obtaining and studying the baby's postmortem examination report. Examination of the baby revealed bilateral renal underdevelopment, imperforate anus, ambiguous genitalia, low-set ears, and midfacial maldevelopment.

To allow for some private working-through of grief by counselees is one approach to this crisis. Another is to establish an initial relationship during the period of acute grief (1) to assess its severity and possibly facilitate its accomplishment; (2) to seek to forestall precipitate efforts to get pregnant again while acute grief is still a burden; (3) to have a workable rapport already developed when mourning has progressed sufficiently for the hard work of exploring genetic issues to begin.

At the counseling session Bill's family history was found to be non-contributory regarding the baby's syndrome, and we had no family history for Marge. We discussed the pathogenesis of Potter syndrome. It was emphasized that the unborn child's lungs, ears, and face had been developing normally, but had become malformed because of external compression. The Jeromes were told that although absence or underdevelopment of kidneys was known to have recurred in some families, the findings about their son were not consistent with those cases. The finding of the imperforate anus and ambiguous genitalia led us to believe that this had been a sporadic event with little, if any, increase in recurrence risk.

During the visit Marge mentioned that she did not like the way the obstetrician had handled the delivery, and that she intended to change doctors.

Because Marge seemed calm, I decided not to question her about her feelings regarding the pregnancy and its outcome. Bill was quiet throughout the visit, letting Marge do most of the talking since she had the medical knowledge. They both seemed to understand what was discussed and no further appointment was made. The hour-long visit was followed by a letter reviewing what had been discussed.

> A counselor may feel reluctant to risk revivifying sad feelings when counselees present themselves in a calm, composed mood. For many counselees, however, it is only at the point of having achieved some composure that they may be able to usefully speak of the details of their grief. Suitable questioning at such a point can help the counselor ascertain their current emotional status.

Marge became pregnant six months after the birth of that first child. She felt hopeful because of the counseling that had been offered. But this hope was not to last, since Marge's uterus was not expanding as expected. At twenty-four weeks' gestation her obstetrician referred her to the Medical Center for ultrasound studies. The studies were inconclusive, and the possibility of error in the estimate of gestation time was suggested. Marge was asked to return one month later to have the ultrasound studies repeated. From that time on, Marge said, she knew the baby would not be normal.

Bill and Marge, one month later, were on their way to the Medical Center for the second ultrasound survey when Marge began to have uterine contractions. Premature labor was followed by the birth of a daughter at the Medical Center. The baby was taken immediately to the Neonatal Intensive Care Unit, where she died an hour later. Since Marge had no complications following delivery, she chose to be discharged from the Center the same day she had given birth.

Postmortem examination revealed bilateral absence of kidneys, congenital heart disease, brain abnormalities, and two umbilical vessels.

At the Medical Center, a Perinatal Mortality Counseling Team has been organized to help couples whose baby dies soon after birth. Couples are visited by the special perinatal nurse as soon as there is knowledge of a fetal or neonatal death. Usually the nurse meets with couples during the mother's hospital stay and when the mother is examined four weeks later. When the baby has malformations or a suspected genetic disorder, a Genetics Unit staff member also makes a postpartum visit. A genetic counseling session is planned, if needed, for three or four months later. The perinatal nurse meets with the family for a third time approximately six months following the initial visit in the hospital. Throughout this period contact is maintained among members of the medical teams involved, as well as between medical personnel and the family.

Owing to Marge's prompt departure from the hospital, the perinatal nurse was able to have only a very brief visit within a few hours of the baby girl's death.

At Marge's four-week checkup she was seen again by the perinatal nurse. Marge requested additional genetic counseling, which was arranged for her and Bill three months later. We used the time interval to review the postmortem findings, to search the literature further, and to allow Marge a chance to try to unearth some information about her original biological family. During these three months I telephoned the Jeromes several times.

The second genetic counseling session was altogether different from the first. The physical setting was the same, but all other circumstances had vastly changed. More than a year had elapsed, and a *second* defective child had been born and died. Our original counseling (still regarded to be appropriate under the circumstances prevailing at the time) that the Jeromes' first loss was not likely to be repeated had obviously been incorrect. The Jeromes had left that first session filled with hope for a normal child, and now they returned disconsolate.

The session began with a review of the events since we had last met. I volunteered that our staff had previously presented information which had proved not to hold true. I felt it important to discuss this at the very beginning of the session for two reasons. First, I knew I would feel uncomfortable until I did so. Second, I hoped this acknowledgment of our staff's fallibility would shed light on the Jeromes' current feelings toward us. This was essential for evaluating how receptive they would be for counseling that very day.

This step and its timing were absolutely essential. To have omitted it would have been to risk trying to work with covertly hostile counselees. Under such conditions advice tends to be "written on water," since the counselor's authoritative position has been undermined. The repair of that undermined condition is the first item on the agenda.

Marge did most of the talking, as previously. She commented that they understood we were dealing with a rare situation, and that errors were easily made with so little to go on. Such freely given, wholehearted acceptance had not been anticipated, and it meant that we had every opportunity to make this counseling session valuable. After we had all become more at ease, we began speaking of the second pregnancy and loss.

G.C.: When did you think something would be wrong with the baby? Had you expected it ahead of time?

MARGE: There was a mix-up on my dates. I thought I was seven months pregnant but I was only twenty-four weeks. That was when I started having problems. My doctor didn't know what was going on, but he could tell the uterus wasn't expanding as it should. In my mind from that time on, I knew.

G.C.: I was surprised that this baby was born here at the Medical Center. Did you plan this because you expected problems?

MARGE: No, we were on our way to the Center for the second ultrasound test when I went into premature labor. By the time we got there my contractions were very hard. I was very frightened. Labor was natural; I didn't have anything for pain.

G.C.: Although I wasn't here when your baby was born, I did get to see pictures of her. She had such delicate features. Did you get to see her?

MARGE: Right after she was born, they had a team working on her. I caught glimpses of her before they took her to the Intensive Care Nursery. When I was back in my room, nobody asked "Do you want to see your baby?" They just brought her to me and I was really glad. I had told my husband "I'm going to see this baby." When they brought her, she was dead. They let me hold her, and that helped a lot. To me she was really pretty. She was really small. It was good.

G.C.: After they took her away to Intensive Care, who told you the baby had died?

In some hospitals a mother's viewing her dead baby is discouraged one way or another as institutional policy. Some articulate mothers have expressed the wish that they could have seen their dead baby and held it, and some would have liked to give it a proper ritual burial. Not to have done so, they consider, is to have left the experience of the pregnancy and birth somehow "incomplete." To have contact with one's dead infant is not an experience for everyone, but why not make the experience available to those who feel up to it? Attitudes toward the dead vary; and professionals, if they abhor such contacts, ought not to assume that their counselees share that attitude.

For Marge—though she was not asked if she wished it—the experience turned out well. Perhaps the baby's prettiness ameliorated the painful impact of her lethal defectiveness.

MARGE: Nobody, really. When I delivered, I started crying. They didn't come out and say the baby was dead. It was kind of an understood thing, because I had told the doctor so many times the baby wasn't going to make it. He just said "I'm sorry," and that was a clarification. Then a little later they just brought the baby to me and I held her for about fifteen minutes. Afterward the nurse came in and spoke to me and Bill for a little while. [The R.N. referred to here is a member of the Perinatal Mortality Counseling Team.] Then we went home.

G.C.: You mentioned that you wanted to see this baby. Did you get to see the other one when he was born?

MARGE: No. When he was born and he didn't cry, I said "Something's wrong, the baby's not crying," so the doctor zonked me. Later the nurses were there, but they were very close-mouthed. A nurse did ask if I wanted to see the baby. When I said yes, she said, "The baby is terribly deformed." I said, "No. I don't want to see it." I had the feeling everybody was laughing at me—well, not really laughing, but acting strange, not normal. The baby was taken to the Medical Center. Later a nurse told us that the baby had died. I have very bitter feelings because my doctor didn't try to help me at all. I saw the baby at the funeral and I thought, "To you he may be deformed, but this is still my baby." It wasn't so terrible seeing him, but I felt really bad—like he died alone.

It is precisely when a baby appears hideous that parents may opt not to view it. On the other hand, if the mother's emotional status permits, she can be *prepared* by a professional for what she can expect to see. As Marge afterward asserted, whatever its condition, it was still her baby.

G.C.: Bill, were you asked if you wanted to see the baby? Who talked to you?

BILL: When our first baby was born, Dr. W. came out of the delivery room holding his hands up. He had on gloves with powder and blood all over them. This was before I knew anything was wrong. I'll never forget them—those bloody gloves he was holding up while he was telling me that something was wrong. He was telling me all the stuff about the baby and all I could focus on were those bloody gloves. To him it was an everyday thing; to me it is something I will never forget. It's a ghost in my mind.

Another lesson for us—never to assume that what is "routine" for us will register quite the same way to nonprofessionals personally involved in a tragedy. Bill was twice assaulted: once by the doctor's appearance, and then again by his news.

G.C.: Did you see the baby then or did they just tell you that he was deformed?

BILL: I saw the baby at the funeral. The doctor had mentioned his ears being deformed and this, that and the other, but I never would have seen it. The professional may have seen it, but I would never have known.

G.C.: Looking back over the second birth, were there some things that the doctors and nurses did that were helpful?

MARGE: They were open, and that's what mattered the most. They didn't try to make my decisions about my child. The doctor talked with me about how he was sorry that things happened the way they did. Let me compare the differences: With my first, the doctor was very uncaring, like I was just another patient. This time the staff seemed to be more caring. My doctor before didn't come to the room to see me; he came as far as the door. Here they didn't avoid me.

Here we have an excellent illustration of the good consequences that may accrue from staff and patient openly sharing bad news: The staff need not feel individually fearful that they may disclose the dreaded secret, a fear that tends to make them avoid the patient altogether. Marge describes having had ample contact with the nurses precisely when she most needed them.

[At this point in the session Dr. K., the medical geneticist, joined us. During the next few minutes he also acknowledged the fact that our staff had been in error in our previous counseling.]

DR. K.: I was called in to see your daughter when she was born. Since that time I have reviewed both autopsy reports. As this is an unusual situation, I have discussed it with several other doctors to see if they have had any similar cases. Putting everything together, we feel that the Potter syndrome, or oligohydramnios anomalad, is in your case inherited in a manner we call "autosomal recessive." [Dr. K. proceeded to explain in detail the mechanism of autosomal recessive inheritance, including emphasis on the 25 percent risk of recurrence in each pregnancy.]

MARGE: Can this problem be detected by amniocentesis?

DR. K.: No. In an amniocentesis, some of the fluid surrounding the baby is withdrawn so specific studies can be done on it. There is no specific amniotic fluid test which would be indicated to detect this problem. However, there is a way possibly to identify the problem through the use of ultrasound examinations. As you know, normally the baby's kidneys produce urine, which is the major component of amniotic fluid. This fluid can be detected through ultrasound examination from about the fifteenth or sixteenth weeks of pregnancy. Should you decide to have another pregnancy, you could have a series of ultrasound exams to determine whether or not the amniotic fluid appears to be accumulating normally. If everything appears normal, we can be reasonably sure the baby is okay. If there is doubt, we can try to visualize the baby's bladder. To do this, we give the mother a diuretic. Some of this would cross the placenta and cause the baby's kidneys to form urine in the same way it would in the mother's kidneys. Then we would try to identify, by ultrasound, the baby's bladder filling and emptying. This last test requires a very sensitive ultrasound machine. We would possibly have to send you to another center for this.

[After answering several questions, Dr. K. left. We then reviewed and expanded upon his discussion. The session ended shortly thereafter. A follow-up letter was sent to the Jeromes, and a copy to Marge's obstetrician, Dr. O.]

Two months later (six months after their child's death), the Jeromes met again with the perinatal nurse. This visit was at the couple's home and was arranged by the nurse specifically to determine how they were coping with their grief. The following is a portion of the dialogue of that meeting.

R.N.: When people found that you had lost a baby, how did they react? What kind of responses did you get at work?

MARGE: They let me know they were sorry for me. They didn't question me about it.

R.N.: How about you, Bill?

BILL: Some people tried to give advice or ask questions like ''Are you going to try again?'' That gets me upset because when you lose one, that one is the most important.

R.N.: How helpful were your relatives?

BILL: I wasn't really interested in anything they were saying.

MARGE: I felt relatives were cool this time. They said things like ''I would never have another child if my baby were abnormal.'' I felt very angry. I feel angry even now, and it's been six months. When someone is drowning, you don't pull away their last lifeline. People would say we could always adopt children. I don't think I will, and I don't like people trying to tell me what I should do.

R.N.: Has the death changed your relationship with any of your friends?

MARGE: With friends, no. More with relatives.

R.N.: Has this brought you two closer together?

BILL: Yes and no. At the beginning we were closer than we'll ever be. Then we went to the counseling doctor. He explained that out of thousands of genes it so happens that we both have the same one that's weak. This is what causes the problem. Then one thinks, ''Will she be happier or better off married to somebody else?'' Then I can turn to myself and ask if I would be happier or better off with someone else. Would she be happier with me or with some kids?

R.N.: Have you said that to her?

MARGE: Yes, we talk about it. To me, children are important, but not unless I can have his children, because he's the person I love. But I feel guilty because he wants a family as much as or more than I do. But one could talk about it a million years and it would just be talking. There's no answer.

This talking is more than "just talking." While it is true that talking over what happened does not undo the two neonatal deaths, or replace the dead infants with healthy ones, or eliminate the estimated probability of recurrence, it does accomplish a good deal for this couple. Talking is their way of sharing the most painful emotions and reflections, some of which threaten to wrench them apart. Doing this painful sharing requires courage, and is quite valuable.

R.N.: What has been the hardest thing to understand about losing the babies?

MARGE: Why me? Why do so many people who really don't want to have children have them and they're fine. Why couldn't I have at least one?

R.N.: What have the doctors recommended to you for the future?

MARGE: It's a one-in-four chance that this could happen again to our children. I wanted a tubal ligation immediately after the second baby. Dr. O. wouldn't do one. He wanted me to think about it first. They left the final decision up to me. It's so hard, because it would be easier for someone to make my decision for me.

R.N.: Is there any way to detect this through amniocentesis?

MARGE: No, because there's no amniotic fluid. They recommended serial ultrasound so they could tell beforehand if the baby would have these problems. They could also give me a diuretic and the baby's bladder would fill up and empty, which would tell if the baby would be normal. If not, talking about abortion, I don't think I could do that.

R.N.: We were trying to feel you out about whether you had discussed having children or whether to adopt.

BILL: I don't think we've waited long enough to decide. One week we'll feel "up" and think we can try again. The next week we think, "It happened to one and it happened to the other, and it might be the same thing again." I'm trying not to make that decision now.

These circumstances demonstrate the limitation of the bare statement of a one-in-four probability of recurrence with each pregnancy. In their very small series of two, the Jeromes were on the wrong side of the ratio both times, which is quite shocking. The human experience of losing two babies at birth, and the impact on the parents of such losses, counts far more than the mathematical statement. Not every couple can decide to try again, but some can.

R.N.: Is there any particular decision you're faced with now?

BILL: As far as big decisions, I associate them with if we try again and they run the tests. If they find something wrong, would we abort? That would be a big decision. Even if we did decide to abort, I would wonder, "What if there isn't anything wrong?"

MARGE: I could never do that and live with myself afterward.

R.N.: That is a decision that may someday have to be made.

BILL: It would be easier for me, because she is the one who would be carrying the baby. The only thing she would be concerned with is the baby. I would be as much concerned for her. I'd rather abort than know it's just not going to turn out.

R.N.: How are you doing right now? You're both working, and, Bill, you're in a brand-new job.

BILL: I don't associate our kids at all with it. For a long time I wanted to give it up. What's there to work for? I don't have that feeling anymore. If I did have kids, it would give me a stronger will to go forward, or it would have a couple of months ago. Now I can think I still have a wife to take care of.

R.N.: How about your work, Marge?

MARGE: It has helped me because it keeps me busy. The hardest thing is working maternity. The first day I was in the delivery room, a baby girl was delivered. I had a terrible time controlling myself. When I came home, I cried and cried and felt better. It gets better each time, but there is still pain. If I have to work in labor and delivery four or five days a week, I get depressed.

R.N.: Have you been able to tell anybody?

MARGE: I love labor and delivery. I had feelings of resentment at first. I told myself I can't go on this way throughout life so it's time I tried to do something about it. After my first baby I didn't try at all and things got worse. Now it's not easy, but it's getting better.

[In the closing minutes of the interview, the nurse asked if there was anything they wished to discuss further. She then asked if they had any advice for other couples in their situation.]

BILL: I would tell them they've got to go on living and taking care of each other. They may get depressed, but they have to do it.

MARGE: Also, it really matters what one believes in. Every religion is different, but when you have a child that dies, that religion becomes very vivid to you. It can help you get through.

R.N.: How has this discussion been for you? I know I am opening up old wounds.

BILL: It has been helpful to have somebody to talk to who can understand how we're feeling; somebody who is trying to make things better for couples like us. It's a good feeling to know we may be able to say something that will help someone else.

The nurse left them with the understanding that they were welcome to contact her or the genetic counselor whenever they had questions or just wanted to talk.

The cooperative efforts of the Medical Genetics and Perinatal Mortality units enable families such as the Jeromes to understand their problems and feel continuously supported in the hard work of making family-planning decisions.

Further Comment

Marge, we are promptly informed, is herself an adopted child. This so-briefly stated historical item is of the greatest moment, and not only in terms of her own developmental years. With adoptive parents she doubt-less had special experiences, both good and bad, that contributed to the shaping of her wishes and thoughts about the kind of marriage she would seek and the family she would raise. The fact of adoption does add an ex-tra stimulus to the wish for a person's own, non-adoptive, biologically natural family. It would be no surprise if this factor enhanced the traumatic impact of the Jeromes' losses, and in the long run reenergized their desire to try again.

The occurrence of worrisome anticipations or fantasies concerning the course or outcome of pregnancy is extremely common. Such thoughts are almost never taken as truly predictive of actual future events, and are most often forgotten unless followed by obstetrical misfortune. Some women will become consciously aware of such worries only when finally presented with their newborn infant, whom they hasten to examine and whose fingers and toes they eagerly count. Any symptomatic occurrence during pregnancy other than what is entirely expected will stimulate uneasy anticipations.

If one has the opportunity to learn from women with such anxieties many details of their earlier emotional and psychological life, one usually encounters inner conflicts, guilt, and fears of punishment for past urges, thoughts, or deeds considered by the subject to be blameworthy. Fre-quently the latter are of a sexual nature, but not necessarily so.

This was a first pregnancy. Until a woman has delivered a healthy in-fant, as we note many times in this casebook, she does not know with cer-tainty that she can. Reproductive success pretty much cures such worries. Reproductive failure underscores the doubt expressed in the sentiment "Something is wrong with me."

Living through the period of acute grief is most difficult. Meddlesome relatives, as recorded here, may make irresponsible comments, albeit sometimes with the intent to be helpful. Outsiders can only speculate as to how they would behave with the same dilemma. Until one is actually in it, there is simply no way to know. Solutions to the same dilemma vary somewhat, depending upon the unique situation of those who are in it.

When tubal ligation was first requested, the gynecologist deferred consideration, prudently taking the position that acute grief is no time for rational reflection about sterilization. Only the Jeromes live with the consequences of that decision, either way. It is also made clear to us that for this couple the options of adoption or amniocentesis/abortion present difficulties, too.

Through all this turmoil both of the Jeromes appear to be actively working to cope with their loss. Marge presses toward active mastery of her distress by returning to nursing assignments. Not every bereaved mother is a nurse, and not every nurse is up to working in the maternity area, especially under such painful circumstances.

References

BAIN, A.; SMITH, I.; and GAULD, I. (1964). Newborn after prolonged leakage of liquor amnii. *Brit. Med. J.* 2:598–599.

POTTER, E. (1946). Facial characteristics of infants with bilateral renal agenesis. *Amer. J. Obstet. Gynec.* 51:885–888.

7

Multiple Miscarriage and Translocation

Mr. and Mrs. Andrews have been unable to start their family because Mrs. Andrews is a habitual aborter. Naturally, they are both anxious to learn why this occurs and whether anything can be done about it. The counselor's approach to this couple presupposes that both husband and wife will be jointly involved in the counseling interaction. To her surprise, she discovers that the husband participates very little, and only much later does she learn that in this marriage it is the wife who is "the strong one," and rather protective of her husband. That this is the case does shape somewhat the tone of the counseling, in that Mrs. Andrews works very diligently to assimilate as much as possible of the proffered information.

A great deal of technical information has to be conveyed to an anxious couple, and the counselor must also deal with inability to provide a definitive answer to the all-important question "Why?" Although this answer is not available, a great deal of potentially useful information is, and something can be done to monitor future pregnancies.

Mrs. Andrews, a habitual aborter, had three spontaneous, first-trimester abortions in less than three years, and she has no living children. Her third miscarriage occurred in the hospital, and her obstetrician sent fetal and placental tissues to our genetics laboratory for cytogenetic study. Mr. and Mrs. Andrews were aware that these studies were being done, as the procedure had been explained to them by Dr. G., the obstetrician. During the next few weeks, Mrs. Andrews called the laboratory three times. Although we hadn't yet met the Andrews', the laboratory technicians transferred all the calls to my office. Mrs. Andrews was told that as the genetic counselor I would be able to answer her questions. The telephone conversations were all more or less the same.

MRS. ANDREWS: I'm sorry to bother you. I know I'm being a pest, but it's very important for me to know the test results. I just lost a baby and I need to know. Are you going to tell Dr. G. or call me?

G.C.: Please try to be patient, Mrs. Andrews. I will call you as soon as I have anything to tell you one way or the other. If it is necessary, we will have you and your husband come in to go over the results with you and answer all your questions.

The studies took three weeks to complete, and the chromosomal results indicated a female fetus with a very unusual balanced translocation: 46, XX t(1q+;2p-). A small piece of the short arm of chromosome #2 had broken off and become attached to the long arm of chromosome #1. Whether it was a *de novo* or familial translocation, we could not yet know. As promised, I telephoned the couple, and I spoke to Mrs. Andrews:

G.C.: Mrs. Andrews, this is Mrs. Y., the genetic counselor. I have called to tell you that the test results are now available.
MRS. ANDREWS: Are they all right?
G.C.: We found that the baby had a very unusual—what we call "chromosome rearrangement." There were the correct number of chromosomes, but a piece of one had become attached to another. We don't know if this was the cause of the miscarriage or if the other miscarriages involved similar problems. In order to know more we have to see if this rearrangement runs in your family: that is, if either you or your husband has the same balanced rearrangement.
MRS. ANDREWS: What do we have to do?

The counselor's placement of the term "chromosome rearrangement" in quotation marks reflects her impression that she is saying a rather large mouthful to a woman for whom the terminology may have little or no meaning. Terminology of everyday currency to the professional would be utterly bewildering to a counselee ignorant of the biology of reproduction.

I asked her to come to the laboratory with her husband so that we could take some blood for their chromosome studies. We made an appointment for the following day, and another for a consultation in four weeks' time to discuss the results in relation to their reproductive problem. I was not present when the blood samples were drawn. The technicians reported that Mrs. Andrews had wandered around the laboratory, looking over the work in progress, asking to see and being shown chromosomes under a microscope. Mrs. Andrews telephoned twice prior to our counseling appointment, asking for results. It seemed urgent for her to have answers; she seemed unable to tolerate the four-week waiting period. I do not know if the calls were made to alleviate her own anxiety, her husband's, that of their families, or some combination of all.

The day of the Andrews' scheduled counseling session our area was in the midst of a major snowstorm. Patients had been phoning the Genetics Unit all morning to cancel appointments. Undaunted, Mr. and Mrs. Andrews arrived for their appointment exactly on time. Mr. Andrews, a 25-year-old of Irish descent, is tall and thin with a pale complexion. He works for the post office as a clerk and is in good general health. Mrs. Andrews is 24, of German-Irish descent, of average height but considerably overweight. She holds a "desk job," which she declines to define further.

The initial portion of the session included a family history, so that we would have a frame of reference regarding the reproductive experiences of other family members. We hoped also to gain some indication of the degree of importance this family placed on childbearing. Mrs. Andrews' pedigree was discussed first. As she answered questions regarding her family, she exhibited twitches of her neck, shoulder, and eyebrow, and an increasingly wide-eyed gaze. She knew of no other habitual aborters in her family, but her mother had had one miscarriage. She was unable to provide information about her grandparents or their siblings and children. Her only aunt is retarded and has been institutionalized almost all of her life. A difficult delivery was thought to be responsible for this aunt's brain damage and for the stillbirth of a twin. Of Mrs. Andrews' three siblings, her only sister, Roberta, is single; one married brother has no children and is having difficulty starting a pregnancy; and the other brother, divorced, has two children, both of whom have confirmed diagnoses of cystic fibrosis. This niece and nephew live with their mother in Florida.

At this point Mrs. Andrews leaned quite close, looked directly into my eyes, and said, "Is anything wrong with us?" Assuming that she was referring to cystic fibrosis, which we were still discussing, I went into a detailed description of that disorder: "CF is a recessively inherited disease, and in your brother's marriage each pregnancy carried a 25 percent risk of resulting in a child with that disorder. You *could* be a *carrier* of the gene for CF since it is obviously in your family. However, since a test for detection of a CF carrier is not yet available, there is no way for us to know. In any case, this information is unrelated to the cause of your miscarriages." Mrs. Andrews listened politely to this explanation. She did not correct my assumption that her question had been about CF, nor did she repeat her question. It was only when I was reviewing the case file for the preparation of the summary letter that I understood the lack of communication at this point.

The counselor's experience here underscores the usefulness of getting counselee clarification of such an ambiguous question as "Is anything wrong with us?" Such clarification can be obtained by responding to the first question with another: "What do you mean?" Reply to the latter will usually supply the true context out of which the ambiguous question springs. In the present instance that true context was apparently not worry about cystic fibrosis.

The discussion then turned to the family of Mr. Andrews. His only sibling, a sister, is newly married and as yet not pregnant. There is no history of multiple miscarriage in his large extended family. Mr. Andrews replied to all questions directed specifically to him with single-word answers. No information was volunteered, nor did he elaborate on any of his answers. He gave the distinct impression of being withdrawn. Whether he was shy, embarrassed, depressed, or indifferent was not at all apparent to me. Mrs. Andrews attempted to include him in discussions several times by turning to him for confirmation of her responses, but in general, Mr. Andrews seemed to be uninvolved in the conversation.

I indicated that the family histories had not provided specific evidence to explain the miscarriages. (In my mind I did not discount Mrs. Andrews' retarded aunt and that aunt's stillborn twin, and Mrs. Andrews' brother who was having difficulty in starting a pregnancy.) We moved on to a discussion of the cytogenetic laboratory results. Since neither counselee was familiar with chromosomes, I explained that normal people have 46 chromosomes in each of their cells, and that too little or too much chromosome material is not good for a fetus. Sometimes the *correct* amount of chromosome material becomes rearranged, or translocated, and this rearrangement is referred to as a "balanced translocation." A person whose cells carry a balanced translocation can develop normally. An illustration of a normal karyotype was used to demonstrate a typical chromosome complement, and the fetal karyotype of the lost infant was used to point out the characteristics of a balanced translocation. I went on to explain that in order to tell if the fetus's translocation had been an accident or had been inherited, we had studied the Andrews' chromosomes. Mrs. Andrews' karyotype had revealed the identical balanced translocation found in the fetus. Mr. Andrews' karyotype was normal. We looked at all three karyotypes to confirm these facts. I reminded Mrs. Andrews that although she carried a balanced translocation, she had been unaffected by it. She would never have known about it if we had not had the opportunity of studying the fetal cells. Mrs. Andrews then asked if these findings were responsible for her repeated miscarriages.

This question is, of course, very loaded emotionally. Great tact is called for to avert the counselee's leaping to the conclusion that she is altogether to blame for her unsuccessful pregnancies. The available facts in this case do not warrant that conclusion.

I told her that we did not know the specific reason for this last loss, since the fetus's translocation was a balanced one presumably like her own and *un*balanced chromosome arrangements were a definite possibility in explaining the loss of the two previous pregnancies.

The four possible chromosome arrangements which any of the couple's unborn children could have were discussed and diagrammed. The risk probabilities for *each* future pregnancy were specified as follows: a 25 percent chance of a balanced translocation arrangement; a 50 percent chance of an unbalanced translocation arrangement (likely to result in miscarriage); and a 25 percent chance of a normal chromosome arrangement. As the explanation progressed, Mrs. Andrews would stop and summarize each new piece of information to make sure that her understanding was correct.

This is a large chunk of new information for a biologically unsophisticated counselee. Not everyone would have the temerity to interrupt for confirmatory feedback. A good rapport is necessary for this to occur. In part, counselee anxiety fuels the process.

The availability of prenatal diagnosis by amniocentesis for any future pregnancy maintained to sixteen weeks was presented to the couple for their consideration.

Mrs. Andrews then suggested that hormone levels could be the underlying cause for the miscarriages, adding that Dr. G. had proposed to conduct hormone tests. It seems that she had not fully comprehended all that had just been discussed, and was trying to find an answer that was easier to accept. After a pause she asked about chromosome rearrangements found in other families, and the statistics for miscarriage resulting from the amniocentesis procedure. Factual information seemed to satisfy her, and she concluded that her most recent miscarriage was due to some fault in her body rather than an abnormality in the fetus.

We discussed other possible causes for miscarriage, including hormone abnormalities, gynecologic problems, and subclinical infection. We also discussed the possibility that Mrs. Andrews had inherited the balanced translocation from one of her parents, and if this was so, what the implications would be for her sister and brother. It was suggested that Mrs. Andrews' parents come in for chromosome analysis.

Before the end of the ninety-minute session, Mrs. Andrews summarized the future steps to be taken: (1) She would ask her parents if they would come for testing. (2) She would call Dr. G. for any other necessary investigation. (3) She would consider the possibility of amniocentesis should a future pregnancy last for sixteen weeks. Then she reviewed the risk probabilities for chromosome rearrangements in future pregnancies.

In a follow-up phone call one week later, Mrs. Andrews admitted that she remembered very little of what was said during the session. She did, however, report leaving the session with a feeling of relief. When I encouraged her to explain this feeling further, she said that she and her husband had come to the session expecting to be told that they would never be able to carry a pregnancy to term, that they would never have their own children. The idea of abnormality in future pregnancies seemed not to have been absorbed. She felt that part of the sense of relief was due to the fact that the translocation was found in her chromosomes, not her husband's. It was her opinion that he would not be able to ''take it'' if he were implicated as a contributor to the miscarriages; he would ''flip out.'' On the other hand, she felt that she could deal with the situation, and would call if she wanted further counseling or was ready for amniocentesis. She did not mention the possibility of bringing her parents in for cytogenetic studies, and it was my impression that she would not, or could not, follow through with this proposed plan.

A letter summarizing the counseling session was sent to Mr. and Mrs. Andrews. As I reviewed this case, I realized that it had been a difficult one for me personally. I have interviewed couples many times when the man has been reluctant to participate. In these cases the circumstances have usually been such that he opposed his partner's decision to have testing or counseling. Occasionally, not being married to his partner, he was uncomfortable in the situation. Attending under protest, his input was limited. In cases like that of the Andrews family, however, the husband is concerned about his wife's emotional stress and thus is usually eager to cooperate in the investigation and evaluation. My error regarding this couple was to have a preconceived idea of how the session would proceed, and what interactions we would experience.

In contrast to my expectations, Mr. Andrews took little part, and I found myself guided by his wife's overt impatience and anxiety, her urgent need for definitive answers to her questions. Once beyond my discomfort at realizing the session would not be genuinely a joint experience for husband and wife, I could focus more effectively upon Mrs. Andrews alone. There was no way I could have known in advance her private agenda: to be able to protect her husband. The tilt in the situation toward Mrs. Andrews heightened my desire to give her the needed answers, and I felt tense and frustrated at not having all those answers.

Within a year of our last contact Mrs. Andrews called to announce that she was fifteen weeks pregnant and wished to arrange for an amniocentesis. Her sister, Roberta, accompanied her when she came in for the procedure and had her blood drawn for chromosome studies. Both the fetus and Roberta carry balanced translocations. We are now awaiting the birth of the baby. My self-confidence rises.

Further Comment

A counseling interaction such as this helps to keep us humble when it comes to deciding that we "know" precisely what is happening, on the basis of inferences drawn from limited observation. The counselor had an impression of Mrs. Andrews as the more active and articulate spouse. That was plain from her interview behavior. But it could hardly be guessed that she regarded her husband to be so fragile emotionally as to be unable to tolerate any sense of biological complicity in unsuccessful pregnancies. Mrs. Andrews knew many things about her husband that the counselor could not know, and willingly shouldered the burden, albeit with great anxiety pending diagnosis.

In keeping with her sense of herself as the strong one, Mrs. Andrews diligently attempted to maximize her benefit from each conversation by making certain she had grasped and remembered all essential information and advice. Later she acknowledged over the telephone that she recalled very little. Such a sequel is not at all uncommon, given the emotional overloading of the counseling experience. Having the other spouse or another close family member present simultaneously may somewhat reduce this problem with direct recall. The post-counseling summarizing letter is a further measure designed to combat expectable defects and distortions in recall.

This narrative also demonstrates how counselees may distort recall in keeping with private wishes and fears. At the same time, as Mrs. Andrews' later contact for amniocentesis informs us, she did manage to properly note the use of prenatal diagnosis for her situation. One cannot know very promptly all the items that counselees silently assimilate and later act upon.

References

CHAO, Y. (1977). An habitual aborter's self-concept during the course of a successful pregnancy. *Maternal-Child Nursing J.* 6 (no. 3):165–175.

NEU, R.; ENTES, K.; and BANNERMAN, R. (1979). Chromosome analysis in cases with repeated spontaneous abortions. *Obstet. Gynecol.* 53:373–375.

PEPPERS, L., and KNAPP, R. (1980). Maternal reactions to involuntary fetal/infant death. *Psychiatry* 43:155–159.

STOLL, C. (1981). Cytogenetic findings in 122 couples with recurrent abortions. *Human Genetics* 57:101–103.

8

Resisting Counselee Pressure for Decision by Others: Duchenne Muscular Dystrophy

The two case reports that follow (Chapters 8 and 9) present counselors' reactions to encounters with counselees whose value systems vary, in different ways, from those of the counselors. In each instance a different pathway out of the dilemma is found. In both instances there is strong pressure upon the counselor to go along with the objective—the private agenda—of the counselee.

In the first, the counselees press the counselor to adopt the stance of supreme authority and tell them just what to do—something the counselor resists, ceding the authority to someone else accustomed to doing just that, the couple's rabbi.

The Iranian-Jewish parents of Ron Cohen, 13 years old and confined to a wheelchair since the age of 11 due to Duchenne muscular dystrophy (DMD), were referred to our clinic for genetic counseling by a children's rehabilitation center. Mrs. Cohen was fifteen weeks pregnant and 40 years of age; Mr. Cohen was 43. The couple had one other child, Rena, a 9-year-old. The father, who had received only three years of formal education (in Iran), worked as a diamond polisher. The mother, a housewife, had learned to read and write Persian but had no formal education. The Cohens had emigrated fifteen years before to Israel, the locale for this report.

The fact that this son is confined to a wheelchair tells us immediately that this family's experience of the reality of DMD must be profound.

Although the counseling clinic staff and the counselees are all coreligionists and Israelis, they are vastly different in educational and cultural background. To overlook these differences would court counseling failure at the very outset.

In view of the fact that conception had already occurred, the genetic counseling team could only inform the family of the chances of having another child with DMD and advise them to choose between two alternatives: either to do nothing, carrying the pregnancy to term and accepting the implied risks, or to undergo amniocentesis for fetal sex determination. If the fetus proved to be male, they could then decide whether or not to terminate the pregnancy.

The genetic counseling interaction with this family spanned a period of about five months, involving at least eight patient contacts until the problem was resolved. Early in this period our unit established that the affected son, Ron, had marked elevations of his levels of serum aldolase (four times the upper normal limit) and serum creatine phosphokinase (six times the upper normal limit). Despite her being pregnant, when serum creatine phosphokinase level is elevated, Mrs. Cohen's titre was at the upper limit of normal. For the healthy daughter, Rena, the creatine phosphokinase level was well within normal limits.

Creatine phosphokinase studies can identify approximately 70 percent of the carriers of Duchenne muscular dystrophy. Bayesian analysis of this family indicated that the likelihood that Mrs. Cohen was a carrier was two chances in three. The possibility that the disorder was caused by a mutation could not be ruled out.

The maternal age of 40 raised, as well, the increased risk for Down syndrome, specified as a minimum of one chance in a hundred at this age.

Mrs. Cohen arrived unexpectedly for her first visit to our clinic. She appeared bewildered, and with considerable difficulty blurted out that she had come for a test because she was pregnant. When asked who sent her and why, she answered, ''The doctor at the Children's Rehabilitation Center where my son goes to school.'' Further questioning revealed that although Mrs. Cohen did not know the name of her child's disease, she knew it was a ''muscle disease'' and that he would die in early adulthood. Gentle probing about her family background revealed that she was an unsophisticated woman who wanted more children desperately, especially ''a healthy son to care, in later years, for the sick one, and also to be of support to our daughter, since my husband and I are elderly.'' It was clear that the nine years of infertility had weighed heavily on her, making this unexpected pregnancy exceedingly joyous and desirable to her, her husband, and the extended family. As we pieced her story together, we surmised that Ron had a genetic disorder, and this factor plus her pregnancy and age were the reasons for the referral to our clinic. We contacted the Rehabilitation Center and were informed that Ron did indeed have DMD. This disorder has an X-linked recessive pattern of inheritance.

The intense yearning for a healthy son is bolstered by cultural factors, such as the desire for a male to continue the family name in the community; by economic factors, such as the need for a son to help care for the rest of the family; and by longings to undo the wound to self-esteem produced by Mrs. Cohen's long period of infertility.

Having learned these facts, we explained to Mrs. Cohen in simple language that families who have a child suffering from DMD are at risk for having more children with the same disease. We emphasized that this risk applies to male children only. Female children will not be born with the disease, but about half of them may give birth to sons who have it. We took pains to make clear that the chance that a newborn son would be affected would be about 50 percent. Practically speaking, this meant that if the baby she was carrying was a male, there would be a 50 percent chance that he would be healthy and a 50 percent chance that he would have DMD. In addition, we explained that it was also possible that her son's disease was due to a new mutation. In this case the chance that she would have another affected child would be very small.

Whereupon Mrs. Cohen asked, "How can I know if I'm carrying a boy or a girl?" We explained that her physicians had referred her to us because we were able to determine the sex of the baby by using a fairly safe test. Visibly shaken by this revelation, she asked, "Will you also tell me if the child will be healthy?" We replied that unfortunately we could not; the only thing we could tell was the sex of the baby. As to whether or not the baby would be healthy, one simply had to wait until the child was born in order to make that determination. "Then what good is the test if you can't tell me if the baby will be healthy or sick?" she asked. We explained that if the sex of the fetus could be determined, she would then be in a position to make a decision whether to continue or terminate the pregnancy. "Yes, but how can I make a decision to have an abortion? Maybe the boy would be born healthy." We replied that this was a very difficult decision to make because of the uncertainty involved, and that perhaps she would like to think about it and talk it over with her husband.

We gently inquired about her relationship with her husband, about the ways in which she was accustomed to make difficult decisions, about her religious beliefs and her feelings concerning possibly undergoing abortion. She described her relationship with her husband as very good: "He's a good man, works very hard, he understands me, and always tries to help me as much as he can." She added that she usually tended to leave major decisions to him. They were not strict religious observers and did not belong to an organized congregation. They were, however, steeped in the traditional beliefs common to people of their background. Mrs. Cohen was against abortions, but her objections seemed to be based less on religious or moral principles than on fear of punishment from God.

We suggested that she return later in the week with Mr. Cohen so they could make a joint decision about what to do. After further discussion about amniocentesis, however, she decided to undergo the procedure and explain the problem to her husband herself. An appointment was arranged for her that very day. A genetic counselor would accompany her through the entire procedure to provide her with needed emotional support.

The staff of the clinic reviewed this situation at conference, at which the following major issues were identified:

1. This was a 40-year-old woman in her fifteenth week of a much-wanted pregnancy, occurring after a long period of infertility.
2. In view of the fact that this family came from a background which placed a premium on large families and on male children in particular, we anticipated that having to consider termination of the pregnancy might provoke a great deal of inner conflict.
3. It was our impression that Mrs. Cohen could not resolve this conflict by herself, and that she expected her husband to make the major decisions that affected their lives. Because the relationship between the couple was apparently a good one, we felt safe in advising them to deal with this problem jointly.
4. This case presented us with a medical-ethical dilemma: whether to discuss with the couple, explicitly, the genetic transmission of an X-linked disease. On the one hand, we considered their right to be informed of all aspects of the problem, including the mode of genetic transmission of the disease. On the other hand, we were concerned about the possible negative effects such a disclosure might have on these unsophisticated people once they understood that Mrs. Cohen might be the carrier and transmitter of the defective gene. We were acquainted with the fact that in such a male-dominated cultural background, infertility or known hereditary disease in the wife's family can cause marital stress and may even result in divorce. After long deliberation we decided to omit discussion of the carrier issue with this family, and concentrate solely on the practical choices facing them if Mrs. Cohen were carrying a male fetus.

The discussion with Mrs. Cohen has already indicated the mode of genetic transmission in sufficient detail to clarify the need for amniocentesis. But it has not been made explicit that it is Mrs. Cohen who transmits the defect if it is not caused by a mutation. Strictly speaking, one could say the Cohens did not learn "the whole truth." There is, however, no treatment for Mrs. Cohen that requires her to know her own genetic status more precisely. What can be done in this situation is being done already, and the clinic staff believes that specific information about the mother would be a harmful addition to a seriously burdened situation. Clinical considerations take precedence over any others.

Mrs. Cohen was extremely anxious during the amniocentesis, and was greatly relieved by the presence of one of the genetic counselors. Unfortunately, the amniocentesis had to be repeated two weeks later because of poor cell culture growth. The three-week waiting period for the results of the second test proved to be understandably difficult for Mrs. Cohen, who was agitated and depressed and slept very poorly.

The meeting with Mr. and Mrs. Cohen for discussion of the test results was dramatic and emotionally charged. Mrs. Cohen was now twenty weeks pregnant. As luck would have it, the test indicated a chromosomally normal male fetus. The doctor informed the couple of the results in a calm, matter-of-fact tone, and briefly reviewed the implications for them. He reemphasized that while the sex of the fetus was certain, there was no way to judge whether the child would be born healthy or affected with DMD. It was, therefore, for the Cohens to decide whether to terminate the pregnancy in the light of this dreadful uncertainty. Both Mr. and Mrs. Cohen were visibly upset by the news, and Mrs. Cohen wept. Her husband gently cradled her in his arms and comforted her. Mr. Cohen turned to the team, saying, "You must tell her what to do; she can't decide!" We explained that we were sympathetic with the Cohens' position. However, a decision of this sort could not be made by us, since they alone had the responsibility of deciding and having to live with the consequences of their decision. We then addressed ourselves to Mr. Cohen: "Maybe you can help your wife, since from what she told us you are always helping her make difficult decisions. What are your feelings, Mr. Cohen?" Obviously "on the spot," Mr. Cohen answered, "If it were up to me, I would go ahead and have the baby. But I can't tell her [pointing to his wife] to do so, because she will have to take care of the child. I'll be at work." Clearly we were at an impasse. Mrs. Cohen, growing increasingly more agitated, demanded (to us) "Tell me what to do!" while her husband continued to maintain his neutral posture.

The situation has become compounded because of the husband's own conflict. Were he concerned only about the potential burden on his wife in caring for another handicapped child, he would decide for abortion. His equivocation signals that he, too, is torn by his desire for a child, and perhaps by ambivalence about abortion.

After some additional attempts to mobilize this couple's decision making, we suggested that perhaps it would be best if they returned home and discussed it further between themselves. We invited them to meet with us in a week's time and added, "Our experience shows that when people have to make difficult decisions, it is good for them to spend a little time with each other alone and let their true feelings come out. Usually, after a while, people resolve their doubts and make the right decision." At this point Mrs. Cohen asked us, "In America they can give you a test to tell if the baby will be sick or healthy?" We reassured her that such a test was not yet available anywhere in the world. (That was 1975.) We reiterated that as painful as it seemed, the decision rested solely with her and her husband. "No matter what decision you will come to by the end of this week, you should consider it the 'right decision' for you." Mrs. Cohen was obviously not yet satisfied. With renewed vigor she demanded, "Why should I have an abortion? Maybe I will kill a healthy baby. Wouldn't it be better to let the baby be born, and if it is sick, then the doctor could kill it." We patiently explained, "When a doctor performs an abortion, he does not consider that he is killing a 'baby.' A fetus is not so fully developed as a baby, which has grown during nine months of pregnancy. The doctor does not consider the fetus to be a person like you or me. An abortion, when it is performed for medical reasons, as it would be in your case, is just another procedure to the doctor. But the killing of a child already born, even if it is very sick, and even if we are sure that it will die, is definitely considered murder. No doctor has the right to take the life of any other person, be it baby, child, or adult, no matter how ill it is." We returned to our initial proposal that the couple think the entire matter over in the privacy of their home for a few days, and return to meet with us again.

Two days later we received a phone call from a Mrs. Mizrachi, who identified herself as a neighbor and close friend of the Cohens. Mrs. Mizrachi called to tell us that the Cohen family was unable to resolve their dilemma, that they were extremely frustrated and needed our help to decide "what to do in this case." Mrs. Mizrachi bluntly told us, "These people simply are unable to make such a difficult decision; you must decide for them and tell them what to do. You must help them out of their predicament."

Realizing that the neighbor's call probably represented an indirect message to us from the Cohens to assume an authoritarian role and decide for them the course of action they should follow, we decided to deal with the call as an extension of our previous counseling session with the Cohens. We explained to Mrs. Mizrachi, "We have given the Cohens all the relevant medical facts. Their inability to decide whether to continue or terminate the pregnancy is due to their fear of accepting responsibility for their actions. Apparently they don't want to risk having another sick child, but they are also afraid to decide on abortion because the child might be a perfectly healthy son. There is also their fear of punishment from God. So, you see, by asking us to decide for them, they really would like us to assume responsibility. That we cannot do, since we would not have to live with the guilt feelings that might follow a decision to abort, nor would we have the burden of caring for another sick child if the newborn were to have the same disease.'' Thus, we explained further, ''Our refusal to make the final decision in this case is not because we are unwilling to help or are afraid of decision making. It is simply that no one has the right to make decisions which will affect the lives and feelings of other people.'' We concluded our conversation by commenting that it was obvious how much Mrs. Mizrachi cared for the Cohens; it was fortunate, we said, that the Cohen family felt free to discuss their problems with her. We hoped that she would explain to them our reasons for insisting that they make their own final decision.

The clinic staff is being subjected to the greatest pressure to decide. Considering that the time for performing an elective abortion is now running late, the seduction "to play God" is indeed strong. The staff is, however, imbued with the overview that the privilege/obligation of decision *must* remain in the hands of those who will bear its consequences indefinitely. To succumb to such pressure would soon subject the staff to unbearable guilt and anxiety about the fate of their counselees.

Mr. and Mrs. Cohen arrived promptly for their second appointment. This time Mr. Cohen opened the discussion: ''We could not decide what to do, and we want to ask you to tell us.'' While empathizing with their feelings, we felt compelled to review the reasons for our inability to relieve them of this responsibility. Tension was very high. At this point we all felt trapped and frustrated, so we decided to resort to psychodrama with the hope that it would break the deadlock. We asked Mrs. Cohen to cooperate with us in a little ''play-acting,'' which, we hoped, would help resolve the conflict. We asked her to imagine that she had already had the abortion and had just returned home from the hospital. ''How do you feel now?'' we said. ''I feel terrible,'' she responded. ''I killed my baby and God is going to punish me for my sins. From now on, anything bad that happens to me—I will know that it is God's punishment for what I have done to my baby.'' Her tone of voice and body gestures confirmed the depth of her feelings. Her husband also appeared very tense. Although he did not utter a word, it was plain that he concurred with his wife's feelings. We then said, ''Mrs. Cohen, now imagine that you have decided to go through with the pregnancy and you have just given birth. The doctor informs you that the baby has the same illness as Ron. How do you feel?'' After a long, painful silence Mrs. Cohen said in a near whisper, ''I feel total despair. I can't take having another child like my Ron, I just have no more energy left.'' We were all drained by the impact of her responses.

The play-acting, we explained, had revealed once again why it was impossible for them to make a decision. "You see, you feel trapped; you can't bear the thought that you may have another sick child, and most likely you would like to have the abortion, but you want us to tell you to do so because you are afraid that if you decide on abortion, you will feel guilty and be punished by God. So you can't decide at all. Unfortunately we cannot make things easier for you, because you will be stuck with the consequences of any decision that we make. We cannot even tell you which decision will prove to be more painful for you. People who face difficult choices in life must make the choices on their own, because when one decides to take a risk and the worst happens, at least one is comforted by the knowledge that it was he who made the decision. That knowledge will help the person to live with his decision more easily than he would if someone else decided for him."

This comment by the counseling staff reflects their steadfast conviction that they cannot employ hunches about how they might react in this dilemma. Such speculations may readily be erroneous predictions.

After some reflection, Mrs. Cohen suddenly turned to her husband and said, "Let's go to the rabbi and ask him what to do!" Instinctively we realized that she had come up with a viable solution to their dilemma. If we, the representatives of the medical world, would not take an authoritative stand and decide, the rabbi (particularly one of a Middle Eastern fundamentalist background) might. We supported Mrs. Cohen in her decision and expressed our readiness to supply the rabbi with the medical facts if he should want them. The meeting was adjourned, to everyone's obvious relief. The Cohens left, promising to call and let us know their decision following the meeting with the rabbi.

Several days passed without news. Then Mrs. Cohen phoned to tell us that she had decided "to keep the baby." The rabbi had deliberated and had decided that "the signs were in their favor." He assured them that the baby would be healthy. Mrs. Cohen sounded positively elated. We, too, felt relieved.

Four months later Mrs. Cohen was delivered of a healthy son whose CPK level was normal. The baby was examined twice more after delivery and was found each time to be in perfect health.

We would be so pleased to know what the "favorable signs" were that the rabbi referred to. As the man closer to God than the clinic staff was, the rabbi sanctified the choice to retain the fetus — a benediction that met the counselees' apparently primary need to remain on good terms with the Lord.

How would it have been if the rabbi's assurance, however well-intended, had not been borne out in fact?

Despite the fact that the genetic counseling team had resorted to a variety of techniques to help the Cohens resolve their conflict about elective abortion (supportive therapy; encouraging the couple to take "time out" for private deliberation; "social network" therapy through counseling a "significant other," the friend; and psychodrama, the actual resolution was obtained through an altogether different route. This family could not but find our response inadequate for them, and so sought help from the rabbi, who assumed full responsibility for the outcome and gave them assurance that the baby would be born healthy. For the Cohens this was the "right" course of action, and so we buttressed their plan to consult the rabbi.

Further Comment

From Mrs. Cohen's viewpoint, all abortion was equated with murder, whether the fetus was healthy or defective. For a brief period, during the inquiry as to possible prenatal diagnosis, there was an implication that the abortion issue might have been less problematic if the clinic had been able to state with certainty that Mrs. Cohen was bearing an afflicted fetus.

Nor will we ever be in a position to comprehend what cues or clues led the rabbi to his reported advice that the "signs were favorable." In the latter context we are perhaps crossing the boundary from what can be known with rational certainty to matters of religious belief and mysticism. While the clinic staff welcomed this avenue of possible successful exit from a stalemate, neither they nor the Cohens could know initially whether this recourse would turn out to be useful.

This summarized counseling experience also draws into the spotlight a general question that is simultaneously clinical and ethical, namely, how much of "the whole truth" needs to be conveyed to the counselee. The counselor notes in her summary that Mrs. Cohen was not told she was the likely carrier. Granted that this information could not be validated with absolute certainty, the question persists. It is a question that physicians deal with in every specialty in their discourse with patients; and just as the psychotherapist is concerned in his statements to patients with issues of dosage, timing, and tact, so is every counselor and physician.

References

APPEL, S., and ROSES, A. (1978). The muscular dystrophies. In J. Stanbury, J. Wyngaarden and D. Fredrickson, eds., *The metabolic basis of inherited disease*, 4th ed. New York: McGraw-Hill.

Golbus, M.; Stephens, J.; Mahoney, M.; et al. (1979). Failure of fetal creatine phosphokinase as a diagnostic indicator of Duchenne muscular dystrophy. *New England J. Med.* 300:860–861.

Mahoney, M.; Haseltine, F.; Hobbins, J.; Banker, B.; Caskey, T.; and Golbus, M. (1977). Prenatal diagnosis of Duchenne muscular dystrophy. *New England J. Med.* 297:968–973.

9

Hazardous Pathways in Nondirective Counseling

The following report is the second in which there is strong pressure by counselees to have the counselor support their privately determined objective, without exploratory questioning. The desire of the Reids and their family is to have immediate buttressing by the counselor for their intention to arrange prompt placement of their newborn with Down syndrome.

The counselor resists, and again alternative authority figures take over the situation, a transfer that is facilitated by attenuation of the link to the counselor.

As noted in the Introduction, counselees' objectives usually prevail when there is a disparity between their agenda and that of the counselor.

Elaine Reid, a 24-year-old woman, gave birth to her second child, a daughter with Down syndrome. Her first daughter, Linda, was a normal toddler three and a half years old. Stephen, her husband, was 28 and engaged in the practice of podiatry. This couple had been reared and currently was living in a closely knit, religiously orthodox community. They were people of considerable financial means, with a wide network of close family and community ties.

I was asked by the attending pediatrician, along with the medical geneticist, to see the baby in the newborns' nursery two hours after her birth. (The parents had seen the infant immediately after the delivery, prior to the pediatric examination. The obstetrician, noting the stigmata of Down syndrome, had requested pediatric consultation, but said nothing to the parents.) As we examined the baby, Stephen, now aware that something was amiss, watched anxiously through the nursery window. There was no doubt about the diagnosis. We joined Steve in the corridor.

PEDIATRICIAN: Steve, I'm afraid that the geneticists share my belief that the baby has Down syndrome. I think we had better sit down and talk. The genetic counselor, Mrs. W., and Dr. D. will explain everything to you.

STEVE: I can't believe it. It seems impossible. Are you sure? The baby looks perfectly normal to me.

G.C.: The baby does look quite normal. It is very difficult for parents to detect anything unusual about the appearance of a baby with Down syndrome. Some babies are not readily identified at birth even by a physician. If you wish, we will explain to you what it is about the baby that makes us suspicious.

STEVE: I still can't believe it. Can I ask my father-in-law to join us? He's in the solarium with my mother-in-law.

G.C.: Of course, but what your mother-in-law?

STEVE: No, not now.

The three of us accompanied Steve and his father-in-law, Mr. Post, into a small consultation room. Mrs. Post was left waiting in the solarium, having been told by Steve, "The doctor wants to talk to us; don't worry." At the pediatrician's request I reiterated our impression that the baby had Down syndrome.

G.C.: Would you like me to describe to you the physical signs that we noted which make us suspect this diagnosis?

STEVE and MR. POST: Please.

G.C.: As I tell you about these signs, remember that these are minor physical findings which serve as clues to suggest a particular diagnosis. Individuals who do not have Down syndrome may have one or two of these signs, but ordinarily not a cluster of them.

STEVE: Please go on.

[At this point I detailed for them the physical findings that alert professionals to the possible or probable diagnosis of Down syndrome.]

STEVE: You said earlier you weren't absolutely sure that the baby has this. [He couldn't bring himself to say "Down syndrome."] You're telling us about the shape of her ears. Our other daughter has ears like that, and my father has small hands, too.

G.C.: You're right in noting that many physical characteristics which run in families are just benign familial traits. Sometimes we have difficulty deciding what is a "something" and what is a "nothing." As far as your baby is concerned, although it's quite possible that other family members have some similar traits, when we look at her as a "whole baby," it seems quite likely that she does have Down syndrome.

STEVE: I know that babies who have this . . . are retarded. Is that for sure? I've heard that some are normal.

G.C.: You will hear stories of children with Down syndrome who have near-normal intelligence, but realistically you have to expect that the baby will experience some degree of mental retardation. There are Down syndrome children who are mildly to moderately retarded, and others who are more severely affected.

Mr. Post: How do we find out for sure?

G.C.: We have to do a special test, which I will explain. Are you familiar with the concept of chromosomes?

Steve: Yes.

Mr. Post: A little.

[I now explained the role of chromosomes in transmission of hereditary material. With the help of an illustration of the karyotype for a child with Down syndrome I explained that in that instance the cause of the disorder was the presence of an extra #21 chromosome in all the baby's cells.]

G.C.: In order to look at your baby's chromosomes we will need a small amount of her blood. Cells in the blood, when analyzed, will reveal the number of chromosomes.

Steve [after a pause]: I just can't believe this is happening. [He wept and Mr. Post patted his shoulder.]

Mr. Post: When can you do this test, and when will we get the results?

G.C.: We can start today, and expect preliminary results in four to seven days.

Steve: I can't believe it! It seems impossible. Nothing went wrong in the pregnancy!

G.C.: Other parents frequently say that. You can't predict how the baby will be from the way the pregnancy is going. When a baby with a problem is born following a "perfect" pregnancy, it is even more of a shock. It's important that you understand that this could happen to anyone, and it doesn't mean that there is anything wrong with either of you, or that you did anything to cause this to happen. What happened to your baby was "programmed" at the time of conception, and was not influenced by events later in the pregnancy.

Steve: Right now I don't want Elaine to know anything. Let's wait for the results of the chromosome test. Why tell her and make her crazy with worry if the test shows there is nothing wrong?

Mr. Post: I agree. Let's not tell my daughter or my wife until it's necessary.

G.C.: Your wish to protect Elaine is understandable, but it does seem likely that the baby has Down syndrome, and I think it is very important that we tell Elaine as soon as possible for these reasons:

First, anxiety can serve some beneficial purpose. It can provide preparation for the bad news she is almost certain to hear. Secondly, how do you imagine Elaine might feel if you allow her to think she has a "perfect" baby and later tell her that the baby has Down syndrome, which you were aware of from the beginning? Don't you think the disillusionment would be greater if you wait? Do you think you can successfully hide your own anxiety and depression from her? And lastly, it seems likely that Elaine will sense something is wrong from the behavior of the hospital personnel. You know, their discomfort will be difficult to conceal, too. She would be deprived of their support when she most needs it. Waiting may seem the right course, but a delay may result in more long-lasting repercussions.

[After hearing this, Mr. Post seemed to have a change of heart. He suggested that we tell first Mrs. Post, then Elaine. Steve acceded without further discussion. After Mrs. Post was told, she said, "Don't tell Elaine now. Let's wait until we are sure."]

MR. POST: Mrs. W. has explained to us why it is important to tell Elaine now. After all, she is bound to realize something is wrong. I think Mrs. W. is right.

MRS. POST [sighing]: I guess that's probably best. But what about Linda [Steve and Elaine's three-and-a-half-year-old daughter]? How is this going to affect her? Who will "stand up" for her when she marries? And who will marry her at all?

G.C.: I don't understand.

MRS. POST: We come from a very close community, and we live according to very traditional customs. Many marriages are arranged, and before the marital agreement is reached there is a thorough investigation of each family. If it gets out that Linda has a retarded sister, she will not be able to make a good match. Even if she does, it is our custom to have the sister who is "next in line" as the maid of honor at the wedding. How can we have a retarded girl standing up for her sister?

G.C: You should understand that it is most likely that this condition has *not* been inherited. Linda's chances for having a similarly affected child are probably no greater than those of anyone else in the population. Therefore her marital prospects should not be affected.

MRS. POST: *We* might understand this but people in our community will not. They are ignorant. No, they'll never accept it.

STEVE: Let's not talk any more about this now. I would like to tell Elaine.

The counselor has given advice to inform Elaine of her daughter's probable diagnosis in keeping with a principle elaborated in many case reports in this book: A "prepared" subject tolerates bad news better than one who has not been prepared.

It is worth noting that the husband and father are focused upon the needs of Elaine, who is as yet uninformed. The worries of Elaine's mother are immediate and then future-oriented in rapid succession.

As regards the anticipated impact of the news in the larger community, Elaine's mother is closer to the mark than the counselor. The latter addresses matters as they should ideally be, not as they are.

G.C.: Would you like to tell her first and then have one of the staff explain, or would you prefer that one of us tell her?

STEVE: Please, you tell her. I don't think I can. Let's all go together.

[The entire group—Steve, the Posts, the medical geneticist, the pediatrician, and I—entered Elaine's room. Elaine immediately looked alarmed. Steve looked down at her tenderly, sat on the bed, and took her hand.]

STEVE: Elaine, there's a problem with the baby. [He choked up.]

[Elaine flushed, looked at us expectantly, and asked what was wrong.]

G.C.: I'm afraid that the baby has Down syndrome. You may be more familiar with the term "mongolism." Do you know what I am talking about?

ELAINE: No—I mean yes, but I can't believe it. [She started to weep.]

STEVE: It's true. The baby is going to be retarded.

G.C. [after a pause]: Would you like me to explain what this diagnosis means?

ELAINE: Yes.

[I explained Down syndrome as I had earlier. No one interrupted.]

ELAINE [looking at Steve]: What are we going to do?

STEVE: We're going to take her home, of course. She's ours.

[At this point both Steve and Elaine were tearful.]

G.C.: Perhaps you need to be by yourselves. If you like, we will wait outside for a while in case you have some questions.

STEVE AND ELAINE: Yes, yes, please wait.

It is common during the initial phase of explanation of the diagnosis for family members to remain silent. This outward composure results from the intense effort to maintain control, to avoid at all costs "falling apart." Expecting my counselees' internal emotional response to be an overwhelming mélange of anger, guilt, shock, disappointment, and sadness, I anxiously waited. In view of the fact that we had just met, it would be especially difficult for them to allow themselves to show their real feelings. Usually more than one session is needed for counselees to feel sufficiently trusting to be less inhibited. Couples do not know what questions to ask when they are first confronted with a diagnosis. Since their primary response is disbelief, questions do not yet seem relevant to them.

Giving couples an opportunity to be alone, to talk together, to cry together, to ''collapse'' together, allows them to begin to believe and ultimately to accept the diagnosis. After such an interlude tension is somewhat lessened, and counselees are able to participate by asking questions.

> The counselor underscores with these remarks her awareness of one of the special dimensions of her particular form of crisis intervention: She has had to proceed as if she had a leisurely opportunity to develop a rapport with Elaine in several spaced-apart visits. In fact, the nature of the crisis has precluded this. The counselor therefore waits in order to be available to aid the process of "after-digestion" of the shocking news.

[Fifteen minutes later Steve asked us to return to Elaine's room. both seemed more in control, though obviously distraught.]

ELAINE: How could this happen? What is the cause? Steve said you were going to do blood tests.

G.C.: Yes, we will do chromosome studies, although we are relatively sure the baby has Down syndrome. [I repeated my earlier explanations regarding Down syndrome and chromosome analysis. Steve expressed his gratitude to us for waiting and explaining further.]

ELAINE: Can you tell how the baby will . . . what she'll be able to . . . how retarded she'll be?

G.C.: A baby with Down syndrome is a lot like any baby in that she will do all the things that babies do in their first year or so, but with a longer timetable. When Linda was born, you couldn't predict when *she* would sit, walk, talk, etc., and the same is true for this baby. It's a ''wait and see'' proposition. Of course, it will be difficult for you as you wait. [They nodded.] Your expectations will not be what they were for Linda, but you should be open. Let this baby *show* you just how much she can do.

MRS. POST: How will she be when she grows up?

G.C.: What exactly do you want to know—whether she will be able to marry and have children?

MRS. POST: Yes—will she be able to live a normal life? Will she get better as she gets older?

G.C.: As she gets older, she will continue to learn. She will be able to do more things independently, but it is likely that she will not be able to live a completely independent, adult life. Some sort of care will be needed. Many individuals who have Down syndrome work and earn money, but usually they do better in a protected environment. Some individuals marry, but again they do better with some help. It is possible for a woman with Down syndrome to conceive, but *she* has a 50 percent risk of having a child with Down syndrome.

ELAINE: You mean I'm going to be taking care of this baby for the rest of my life?

G.C.: That *is* a pretty frightening thought.

ELAINE: Yes.

Elaine's question draws attention to a weighty aspect of the losses sustained with the birth of this infant: In addition to the current disappointment and the diminished future marital prospects, the usual anticipation of an independent, emancipated youngster some twenty years later must also be relinquished.

G.C.: I can't tell you that it's not a difficult problem, but try and remember that there are other parents like yourselves, special programs to help you almost immediately—infant programs, parent support groups, etc. You do not have to feel alone.

ELAINE: When will we know for sure?

G.C.: Well, today is Monday. Probably by Friday we'll know something.

MR. POST: How many people who have a child with Down syndrome get another one?

G.C.: The risk is not more than one percent. You may find it easier to think of it this way: If 100 such families had another child, 99 would be free of Down syndrome. Also, it is unlikely that Linda or other family members would run an increased risk of having an affected baby. A test called amniocentesis done during pregnancy can effectively rule out or confirm this condition.

MRS. POST: Elaine didn't have this test

G.C.: That's right. Amniocentesis is not offered to patients routinely until they are 35 years old. Although the test is quite safe, the small amount of risk it carries would have been greater at Elaine's age than the risk of having a child with Down syndrome. [Pause.] If there are no other questions, perhaps we should stop for now. You have had quite enough for today, and there will be other opportunities for us to meet. I will stop by early tomorrow morning.

Steve agreed, adding that they were going to call the baby "Susan" and were definitely planning to take her home. Mr. Post nodded in seeming agreement; Mrs. Post had a set look on her face, and I felt that she had reservations about the decision. I remarked that decisions were difficult to make, and did not have to be made that moment. My last suggestion was that they not consider any decision to be irrevocable. Elaine asked to see the baby. I volunteered to ask the head nurse to bring Susan in. Steve and Elaine thanked me.

The following morning I found Elaine newly transferred to a private room, which was filled with flowers. She was sitting up in bed looking much better. Her hair was combed, and she was wearing makeup. She greeted me cheerfully and appeared composed. I asked her how she was feeling.

ELAINE: All right. We've decided that we are definitely *not* going to take the baby home.

G.C.: Have you and Steve made this decision together?

ELAINE: Yes. Last night Steve wasn't looking ahead to what it would be like if we took her home. He definitely agrees with me.

G.C.: What has happened since last night to make you change your minds?

ELAINE: After you left, our obstetrician came by. He thought we should place the baby immediately so that we wouldn't become attached to her. He thought that we would probably have to place her within a year anyway, and it would be easier now than later.

G.C.: Why did he tell you that you would have to place her?

ELAINE: He said we wouldn't know how retarded she would be until much later, and that we shouldn't take a chance.

G.C.: As I told you yesterday, babies with Down syndrome may be quite mildly retarded. She doesn't have to be severely retarded. Usually children with Down syndrome do better at home than they do in institutions.

ELAINE: I talked to my parents last night, too. Mrs. W., we have to consider our other daughter. She's beautiful and smart—everything we could want. If we take this baby home, our lives will be terrible. We have a happy home. Everything has gone the way we have wanted until now. And what about Linda? Bringing this baby home will ruin her future. No one will marry her. You don't understand. There's no one in our community who has an abnormal baby. Everyone would know and talk and think that something is wrong with us. They would pity us. I can't go through with it. We are getting ready to go to the beach for the summer. Many families from our community will be there. It would ruin our summer. I want to place the baby and get it over with!

G.C.: Again, please keep in mind that you needn't make a final decision now. You can place the baby temporarily and give yourselves more time to consider all the implications. [Pause.] Did you see Susan last night?

ELAINE: No . . . well, I sort of wanted to, but Steve didn't think it was a good idea if we were going to place her. He told the nurses not to bring her in again.

G.C.: How do you feel about that?

ELAINE: Well, I would have liked to see her, but I guess Steve is right. It would make things harder.

I asked Elaine what they were planning to tell Linda, their friends, and their family. She said they would tell them that the baby had died of a heart defect or "something like that," adding that Steve had already told his brother the truth and a few others that the baby was in danger because it was having breathing difficulties. I raised the possibility that there was a small chance the chromosome studies would reveal an unbalanced translocation. I explained this, and the implication that Elaine's own sister or Steve's brother might be balanced translocation carriers and therefore at increased risk to have a child with Down syndrome. Steve and Elaine would then be in a difficult position.

ELAINE: That's no problem. If my sister was at risk, she wouldn't have to be told. My mother would just tell her to have an amniocentesis. She'll do anything my mother tells her without asking questions. [No mention of how Steve would deal with his brother if he was a possible translocation carrier.]

[I cautioned Elaine to rethink what they were going to tell people so that they didn't back themselves into a corner.]

G.C.: Have you thought about the difficulty of keeping this secret? Your brother-in-law and parents already know the truth. Are you sure that no one else will find out?

ELAINE: They would never tell.

G.C.: What if Linda somehow later discovers that she has a sister who is living?

ELAINE: She probably won't, and if she does, we will tell her we didn't think the baby would live, and thought it was for her own good not to know. She'll accept this. My mother and I talked about this and the baby's placement. She made me see how hard it would be to raise a retarded child, and how it would also affect Linda's life. I agree with her. Placement is the answer.

During this conversation Elaine seemed unswerving in her decision. She was decisive and assertive; there was little about her to suggest tragedy or even sadness. She remarked that Steve was taking it harder than she, but was trying "to be the strong one." My impression of Elaine was that she had experienced a relatively trouble-free life, that she had been privileged and indulged and protected from emotional disharmony and pain. These factors would make her ill-prepared to deal with her current circumstance. She and her family had very close ties, and she fitted easily and willingly into the cultural life of the community. Although she assumed a somewhat passive family role, she was in reality a determined and aggressive young woman. The family accepted the grandparents' right to participate in important decisions. This contrasts markedly with the majority of other families we have met, in which the young parents act unilaterally in decision making rather than in concert with their own parents. Within Steve and Elaine's community it is traditional for grandparents to have as much stake in their grandchildren as do parents. Success in rearing a daughter is measured by her "making a good match" and bearing children. Parents' primary responsibility toward a daughter is to effect this goal. Failure to achieve this would constitute an unacceptable injury to parental self-esteem.

How can we understand what occurred overnight?

Why does the obstetrician advise immediate placement? Does he in fact know the family so thoroughly as to be in a position to select the "best" option for them? The report does not clarify this. It is known that some obstetricians assume that all new parents will react to a defective infant just as they do. The newborn child has promptly been transferred from the category "baby" to the category "defective," and removal of the living assault to self-esteem is the answer.

Lest we leap to the conclusion that the obstetrician has taken the decision out of the parents' hands by virtue of his authoritative position, I must add that differently disposed parents may react to such professional efforts at guidance with outrage. As one mother responded to the same professional advice, "But it's *my baby!*" For this mother, it was unthinkable not to take her baby home.

Plainly, the counselor is troubled by what has occurred, and her remarks are initially slanted in the direction of what she considers are the best interests of the child. Her suggestions, from the beginning, to proceed without haste in making such an important decision take into account that decisions made with reflection and deliberation rather than at a time of acute shock and dismay may not be the same.

The narrative emphasizes the consonance of the family's decision with strong cultural group pressures. To put it another way, this couple is not sufficiently emancipated to be capable of making a decision contrary to group sentiments. One may, incidentally, encounter the same rationalizations with altered phraseology from individuals in other cultural subgroups. The point is that if a couple cannot envision contending with the problems of the new situation, any usable aspect of social concern or authoritative pronouncement will be drawn upon to rationalize a decision for placement.

The counselor assessed the inflexibility of the decision in short order, and thereafter lent her energies to trying to help the Reids accomplish what they had decided to do.

Later that afternoon, we all met again. Steve dominated the conversation while Elaine remained silent. It was almost impossible to elicit any response from her, although I intentionally addressed questions to her directly. Her behavior was remarkably changed from that of a woman "in control" to that of a childlike adult. We began the session by talking about their decision to place the baby. To what Elaine had already told me Steve added the information that the social worker thought it would be possible to find a foster family of similar religion. He expressed relief that the placement would be in a family rather than an institution, and guilt that a family would want to care for Susan when they couldn't. I reassured him that there is a considerable difference between *choosing* to care for such a child and having one born to you. Again, Linda's future was discussed.

STEVE: Since Dr. G. said that we would probably have to place the baby in a year or so, we can avoid the problem of what to tell Linda at that point by doing it now. If we brought the baby home, *she* [looking toward Elaine] would "fall apart." I think Elaine would have a nervous breakdown!

[Elaine bowed her head and said nothing. I had the thought that Steve might be projecting his own fear of "falling apart" onto Elaine; that it might be he who suffered more intensely. I asked Steve if he had told his parents. He said he couldn't think of telling them the truth since they had never fully recovered from the death of *their* young daughter when Steve was 12.]

G.C.: You know the decision to place or take a baby home is very personal. What is "right" for one family may not be "right" for another. But please, keep in mind that *no* decision is irrevocable. [Pause.] Let's talk about what you are going to tell friends and family, and, most importantly, Linda.

Again, the counselor indicates her view of this family-planning dilemma as having a much longer time dimension than the immediate decision for placement tends to suggest. It is expectable that in most instances considerable afterthought will occur. When tension is highest, one yearns for relief as quickly as possible. The counselor is mindful that such decisions as these must be lived with by the Reids for the balance of their lives. To whatever degree she can, the counselor is trying to legitimize any latent disposition toward leisurely reconsideration. Still, she maintains rapport with this family by offering them assistance with their currently perceived major problem: what to tell whom.

> [In addition to repeating what Elaine had told me earlier, Steve said that Linda would be told that the baby needed to stay in the hospital.]

G.C.: As Elaine and I discussed this morning, there are other problems that crop up when you begin to weave a fabric of untruth. For example, you may forget what you've told to whom and be caught in a lie.

STEVE: Maybe.

G.C.: Regarding Linda, you might want to reconsider the story about the hospital. If she ever requires hospitalization, she might fantasize that you don't come out once you go in. You can imagine how frightening that would be.

STEVE: What would you tell her?

G.C.: I think I would tell her that Susan needs special care which you are unable to give her and which others are better able to provide. Also, leave the door open and tell her that you aren't sure whether this will change in the future. Reassure Linda that she is fine and will never develop similar problems. Tell her that you are sad and allow her to share your grief. Continue to discuss the baby over a period of months and even years, and from time to time remind her that she has no responsibility for the baby's problems. [Steve nodded.] Let me caution you *not* to say Susan is in a "special school," as Linda may associate going to school with not coming home.

These pieces of advice about what to tell various people are excellent, and it is instructive to observe the different degrees of resistance with which the different items are received. The scope of the advice may be, for some readers, rather more extensive than expected from a genetic counselor. This counselor is very direct in conveying her definition of her professional role as capable of being useful to the family concerning all features of their genetic problem.

What to tell Linda is clearly suggested, and the basis for those suggestions alluded to. How to explain difficult realities to children is always a problem, and the reasons offered by the counselor for her proposals are drawn from vast experience by many professionals. The Reids appreciate this.

What to tell other adults is quite another story. In this context the couple's reluctance to be truthful, emanating from their fears of community reverberations, is very strong. Here the counselor's reasoning has no influence, since the Reids feel quite convinced that they know what it is necessary to do in their community.

G.C.: Regarding other people: If you tell them the baby has died, you are precluding the possibility of changing your minds. I wonder if you realize that keeping the truth to yourselves tends to isolate you from friends and family who might support you in your grief. And then, you must always be on guard not to let your secret leak out.

MRS. POST: You still don't understand! Telling the truth will ruin Linda's life, and Steve's, and Elaine's—and ours, too!

STEVE: Yes, that's true. We will be tied down for the rest of our lives.

G.C.: Look, it does seem best for you to place the baby now, at least temporarily. Again, let me urge you to leave all your options open.

During the course of this session, which went on for two hours, Steve looked increasingly depressed. Elaine continued to be unresponsive, Mrs. Post was assertive and supportive of placing Susan, and Mr. Post said little. He had a softened look about his face, suggesting that although he agreed with the decision intellectually, he mourned it emotionally. It was my impression that although the men of this family assumed the role of articulating the family's position and appeared to be the decision makers, in fact it was the women who were less conflicted and stronger in their resolve to place the baby.

The counselor has persisted in her efforts to persuade the Reids to adopt attitudes that her experience has indicated to be in the best interests of both infant and family in the long run. For many reasons, however, the contrary currents are too strong. Apart from the different cultural reference points, the Posts, who in their way are the representatives of the community on the scene, have endless opportunity to reinforce their pressure for immediate placement. The counselor's contacts with the couple are, by contrast, very limited. Mrs. Post is quite candid in her assertion that taking the baby home will ruin everyone's life, including her own. There is clearly no support for the Reids' taking a contrary position.

I saw Elaine briefly several more times during her hospital stay. By Wednesday the social worker was able to find a family of the same faith who would take Susan. Steve and Elaine were greatly relieved. Elaine stayed in the hospital an extra two days (a total of five days) to await the results of the chromosome studies (which confirmed trisomy 21) and the completion of the placement arrangements. The last time I saw Elaine and Steve together was on the fourth day. We spoke again about what they were going to tell people. Steve admitted that he was already confused as to what had been said to whom. I was left with the impression that they were going to tell everyone the truth. On the day that Elaine was discharged Steve stopped in to congratulate and thank me and the other staff members for the quality of the services they had received. "We couldn't have made it without you," he said. "I can't thank you enough. I would be willing to be interviewed by medical students if you think it would help them to understand what we went through." I recommended that we meet and talk again in two to three weeks, when they would have settled down somewhat and would perhaps have new questions.

When I still hadn't heard from them in three weeks, I telephoned. Steve answered and was a bit curt, saying that they were not ready to come in, but were still planning to do so. I inquired about the baby's placement. Steve said he was extremely pleased. He whispered that he had seen the baby twice, and the family was "crazy" about her. He hadn't told Elaine about these visits. I wondered if he was having second thoughts about the placement. He asked me not to call him at home in order not to upset Elaine.

I spoke to him several times after that. Each time he told me they weren't ready to come in. He seemed reluctant to converse and I didn't press him. The last time I called, he told me they were leaving for a European vacation and would call me when they returned. I suggested an appointment. He let that pass. He did not call.

By consistently presenting options for action other than placement, the counselor has made the Reids aware of at least some of the expectable content of any follow-up visit with her. It is no surprise that they do not come in—behavior heralded by their not having telephoned spontaneously after the suggested two-to-three-week interval.

Also, it is very striking that despite that family's apparently monolithic determination to place the infant promptly lest any sense of attachment develop, Steve has surreptitiously visited the baby twice. This is in keeping with his early, spontaneous statement that of course they would be taking the baby home, since it was theirs.

Six weeks later, an evaluation of the genetic service the family had received, which is routinely requested of counselees, was sent in by Steve. Patients are asked to rate the service and explain their rating. Because of Steve's earlier glowing compliments, I was stunned by the evaluation. Although rated "satisfactory," the service was angrily criticized. "When I met with the staff at the nursery," Steve wrote, "they informed me of the problems. I was later quite turned off by them when they strongly made recommendations. They made me feel as if I was obliged to accept these recommendations without considering any alternatives. The choices were theirs. At times I felt embarrassed to voice my decision, and my wife felt harassed by the staff's coercion in the attempt to influence her."

My first impulse was to telephone Steve, but then I decided to write, thinking that a phone call would be too threatening. I expressed my concern, and my desire for an opportunity to discuss the comments with them in person. "Since my intention was to be nondirective, I am especially disturbed that you felt I was coercive," I wrote. I asked them to call me. When I had all but given up hope of hearing from them, Steve called. He apologized for the tenor of the letter and said he would call again for an appointment. Again, months passed.

I spent a considerable amount of time speculating about the ways in which I might have been seen as coercive. It occurred to me that although I had intellectually understood the considerable social pressure felt by this family in a community such as theirs, I had not fully believed in the reality of the bases for their anxieties. Their concerns for Linda's future were *not* speculative; the barriers to her well-being *were* insurmountable! These concepts were truly foreign to my experience.

In retrospect I realized that Elaine and Steve had decided well *before* other alternatives were offered that their baby could not be taken home. Consequently, they perceived the counseling as being nonsupportive and interfering. The obstetrician who urged them to place Susan was not seen as coercive, but as supportive.

Furthermore, "truth telling," I realized, need not be an absolute. I had assumed that everyone would be uncomfortable keeping a secret. Obviously, not everyone handles such a situation in the same way. My bias is to share the truth, to "clear the air," but it was presumptuous of me to assume that this would be the proper path for *them*. Because there was no familial translocation, only Steve and Elaine were at increased risk. No important information was being withheld from their relatives. No harm was being done.

Before I met with Steve again, there was an opportunity to counsel a second family from this same community who had also given birth to a Down syndrome baby. They, too, immediately expressed concern for the marital prospects of their daughters. They decided to place the baby, at least temporarily. I suggested that they tell people a partial truth to give themselves leeway for whatever was to be their final decision. Their alternatives were offered in a somewhat different way. "Look," I said, "you have two difficult and anxiety-provoking situations. You have to consider the ostracism which would affect your daughters' futures and the very difficult course of possibly placing your baby permanently in either foster or institutional care. Your decision would be made even harder by the difficulty of keeping everything secret. Both options are extremely upsetting, but we will support you in whichever path you think is best for you." This family was extremely grateful that their concerns were recognized and appreciated in spite of the differences in our values.

A third family from this community, whose infant had a different but serious genetic disorder, indicated that they could not reveal the true nature of the disorder to anyone. In trying to confirm my understanding of the mores of this community, I asked them if they had ever heard about any baby in their community with a problem.

MR. COLE: No—wait a minute. I think Steve Reid had a baby that died. In fact it was here in this hospital. Maybe you know them.
G.C.: Did you know what the problem was?
MR. COLE: No, not really. I think Steve mentioned a serious heart or lung problem. They decided not to take the baby home, as it wasn't expected to live very long. I think I heard that the baby died.

Not long after this incident, approximately a year and a half after Susan's birth, Steve popped into my office without an appointment. Fortunately, I was free.

STEVE [joyously]: Elaine is upstairs and ready to go home. We've had a beautiful baby girl. She's perfect!
G.C.: I'm so happy for you. Congratulations. [I hadn't known of the pregnancy.] Did Elaine have an amniocentesis?
STEVE: Yes, at another hospital. I only have a few minutes; we're getting ready to leave.
G.C.: Please sit down a moment. You know, I thought a long time about what you wrote in the evaluation.
STEVE: Yes, well I'm sorry it sounded so bad. I didn't mean to hurt your feelings.
G.C.: Frankly, you did me a favor. I've learned from your honesty. I certainly never meant to be coercive, but I understand how you saw it that way.

We discussed my idea that my suggestions had followed a decision which had already been made and had thus been seen as coercive. I added that if I had fully understood the Reids' concerns for Linda's future I would have handled the counseling differently. In fact, I had done so with two subsequent families. Steve expressed his pleasure that his criticism had been helpful, and agreed with my analysis of why my suggestions had been perceived as being nonsupportive and directive whereas the obstetrician's view was welcomed.

In retrospect it appears that Elaine was avoiding any contact with me from the time of her original discharge from the hospital. She had her amniocentesis done elsewhere, even though the same obstetrician was retained and the delivery was at our hospital. Perhaps this was additional evidence of Steve's desire to protect her and Elaine's willingness to have him do so. In most instances Steve took on the responsibility of being spokesperson and confronter. Elaine, by comparison, seemed to experience less overall distress and ambivalence than Steve. Her involvement in the counseling seemed more reluctant, being restricted to ascertaining answers to the questions ''Will the baby be retarded? and ''Will she be able to lead a normal life?'' I think Elaine, in reality, was very angry. I do not know whether her firm belief in and adherence to the mores of her society will afford her lasting peace of mind. Her sense of comfort may be illusory if she is not able to psychologically ''work'' at the confrontation of painful emotions. Steve, I felt, because of his more active role as spokesperson, arranger, and confronter, had been less able to avoid his true feelings and as a result was more likely to resolve his conflicts; he was probably less angry.

The majority of returned evaluations are complimentary. Seldom can one learn from them. Having the opportunity to become aware of counselees' dissatisfaction—and to follow-up, further discuss and reflect on this dissatisfaction—presented a rare opportunity for learning.

Further Comment

Although we can understand the counselor's distress at receiving a less than complimentary appraisal of her work with the Reids, how should we try to develop a perspective on what took place in this complicated interaction?

That the couple was angry, and thereafter sought to avoid the agent who seemed to them to be the cause of their anger, seems clear. To a counselor seeking to be "nondirective," to be called "coercive" is more than unwelcome.

We were not there, and must allow for artifacts of summarization in the preparation of this report. Taking what we have at face value, we can say that the counselor wished the clients to take time for more leisurely reflection on a decision of long-term importance. In the face of the strong push toward placement, she certainly posed alternative routes, and probably did so in a style conveying her private perspectives. Whether this can be viewed as truly "coercive" is moot; but we should note that the account never suggests the counselor felt that she would sever all further contact with the family if her proposed options were rejected. Quite the contrary.

It is a truism of psychotherapeutic interactions that when one disturbs a psychological "defense," the interviewee does not thank us for this. The reason is that defenses evolve spontaneously in order to protect the subject against the conscious experience of anxiety, depression, or some other unpleasant emotion. When the defense is disturbed, the unpleasant emotion threatens to emerge into conscious awareness, and who likes that?

In the situation of the Reids, the counselor's energetic suggestions of alternatives to placement opened a vista of all manner of problems, not the least of which was probable open conflict with Mr. and Mrs. Post if the baby was taken home. For such a possibility the Reids could not be expected to be grateful to the counselor.

Does this make the counseling "coercive"? I think not—but it was rather scary and therefore unwelcome.

Steve indicated that he regarded Elaine to be psychologically very fragile. Although at first he stated plainly that they would take their baby home, he could not stand against the combined forces arrayed against him. His own attachment to their daughter was reflected in his surreptitious visits. His continuing regard for Elaine's fragility was reflected in his inability to tell her of them.

In her work with subsequent counselees of the same cultural subgroup the counselor altered her style, but not necessarily the content of what she felt obliged to broach. And her stylistic alterations involved ways of presentation that were less disruptive of rapport, less likely to provoke such strong resistance. The Reids dealt with the anxiety-arousing counselor as they had dealt with the anxiety-arousing infant: by avoidance.

This report emphasizes the complex interaction between private dilemma and cultural context, and how the genetic counselor must become sensitive to a very large field of powerful factors in a very short time in order to be maximally useful.

References

Burgio, G.; Fraccaro, M.; Tiepolo, L.; and Wolf, U., eds. (1981). *Trisomy 21*. New York: Springer-Verlag.

De la Cruz, F., and Gerald, P., eds. (1981). *Trisomy 21*. Baltimore: University Park Press.

10

A Child with 47, XYY and Fetal Alcohol Syndrome: Not Being Allowed to Help

The Taft family's problem with their son, Andy, underscores a number of counseling issues. Because the counseling in this particular case occurs in the setting of an outreach clinic, visited by a "circuit riding" team of professionals, there is even greater than usual time constraint for getting at important issues. The fact that the staff is thus pressured means nothing to Mrs. Taft. Her conflicts over revealing many aspects of her family life and her abuse of alcohol require evasiveness no matter what.

Although the staff is frustrated in their desire to offer more in the way of counseling than the counselee will tolerate, Mrs. Taft does gain freedom from an erroneous prior diagnosis and takes with her recommendations which at some point she may be able to act upon.

While the diagnosis of Down syndrome is often made on the basis of clinical presentation, it is essential that it be confirmed by cytogenetic analysis for genetic counseling purposes. Frequently the diagnosis may be assigned to a patient despite incompatible physical findings. In these cases, a banded chromosome analysis becomes extremely important.

This is a report of a child referred to the Outreach Genetic Counseling Program with a diagnosis of Down syndrome that was subsequently found to be incorrect. Cytogenetic analysis in the newborn period was said to reveal 47,XY, + G compatible with Down syndrome. While the child did later prove to have a chromosome aneuploidy, 47,XYY, this disorder was in addition to the developmental problems resulting from fetal alcohol syndrome.

The Outreach Genetic Counseling Program (serving several states) is provided by a Genetics Center located at a university medical complex. This program was developed to provide genetic counseling services to individuals in outlying areas. A genetic counseling team, consisting of a medical geneticist and a genetic associate, travels to each of several distant clinics on a periodic basis. The clinics are reached by plane or car, and frequently the visiting team needs overnight accommodations. Clinics are usually held in the local public health facilities where a public health nurse serves as the clinic coordinator. The coordinator is responsible for handling referrals, gathering medical records, and scheduling families for consultation. Approximately two weeks prior to each clinic session, a schedule and any available information is sent by this local coordinator to the Genetics Center, where it is reviewed by the genetic associate. Five to seven families are seen during the clinic session for initial diagnostic evaluation and counseling or for follow-up counseling. Specimens obtained for diagnostic testing are brought back to the Genetics Center. Whenever possible, arrangements are made to perform tests locally (e.g., X-rays). When indicated, additional medical records are obtained. The genetic associate is responsible for coordinating the needs of patients seen at the clinic; i.e., arranging for follow-up testing, counseling, and referral.

The case history of each family seen in an outreach clinic is presented to a group of medical geneticists and genetic associates during a conference held at the Genetics Center. This conference enables each family to have the input from the outreach genetics team augmented by other genetics professionals. The genetic associate is responsible for seeing that recommendations made by this group are carried out. Upon completion of all testing and/or recommendations, the family is scheduled for a return visit to the outreach clinic. Many families require multiple genetic counseling sessions over a long period of time. After the final counseling sessions, a letter is sent by the genetic associate to the family. This letter summarizes the counseling (the diagnosis, genetics, and recommendations) in layperson's terms. Copies of the formal evaluation are sent to the family's primary care and/or referring physician.

At the age of 3 years, Andy Taft was referred to the Outreach Genetics Program by Dr. R., who was concerned about both the child's growth and his diagnosis of Down syndrome. Andy's case was one of seven scheduled for the clinic that day. The local coordinator had sent Andy's medical records, which revealed the following:

1. A skeletal survey, performed when Andy was one day old, was interpreted to be "probably diagnostic of trisomy 21."
2. The question of achondroplasia, a growth disturbance, was raised.
3. Two blood samples for cytogenetic analysis had been drawn. The first

was lost in transport and the second was reported as "47,XY, + G consistent with the diagnosis of Down syndrome."

There was neither an obstetrical history nor a specific physical description included with the records.

When the family was informed that the chromosome analysis confirmed the diagnosis of Down syndrome, they were quite upset and immediately changed to their current pediatrician, Dr. R. Throughout Andy's records, there were comments on the disparity between Andy's physical appearance and the chromosomal diagnosis. When Andy was seen in our Genetics Clinic three years later, he nonetheless still carried the diagnosis of Down syndrome. No one had pursued the investigation further.

Promptly at 1:00 P.M., Andy and his mother arrived at the public health department for the Genetics Clinic. Mrs. Taft was an attractive woman and very neatly dressed. Andy clutched her hand and stood quietly by her side. I introduced myself, describing the relationship of the Genetics Center with the Outreach Genetics Program, and my role as a member of the genetics team. It was explained to Mrs. Taft that Dr. G. (the medical geneticist) would join us after I had obtained some background information.

Andy was extremely shy, staying close to his mother as we talked. I found some toys for him to play with in one of the cupboards. It was immediately apparent to me that Andy did not have any of the typical features of a child with Down syndrome. He was an extremely short child with a square face, blonde hair, and deep-set blue eyes that had an *anti*mongoloid slant. He had a long philtrum and down-turned corners of the mouth. Despite several attempts to get him to smile or laugh, he would not.

I attempted to determine Mrs. Taft's understanding of Andy's problems, what she and her husband had been told, and what specific concerns she had. It was immediately apparent that Mrs. Taft did not believe her son had Down syndrome. She emphatically stated, "I know that Andy doesn't have it. He doesn't look like any other children I've seen who do. What I'm most concerned about is how short he is. I'd also like to know why his stomach is so big." Throughout this discussion, she was extremely bitter about her experience with the medical profession and her original pediatrician's insensitivity to her continued questioning regarding the diagnosis of Down syndrome. "Since the first chromosome test didn't work out," she said, "we had to wait until Andy was one month old to find out he had Down syndrome." Dissatisfied and still skeptical of the results of the chromosome analysis, Mrs. Taft decided to change pediatricians and began seeing Dr. R. But a very close family friend (in the medical field) was the only person in whom she seemed to have any confidence. According to Mrs. Taft, he did not feel that Andy had Down syndrome either. Mrs. Taft spent the first fifteen minutes of the session voicing these concerns, frustrations, and angry feelings.

It is very important that the genetics team be fully aware of the counselee's bad earlier experience with the first pediatrician. The residual bitterness will most probably produce some anxious speculation that she might experience with the new group of professionals a repetition of the earlier frustration. The good interaction with Dr. R., the referring physician, has doubtless tempered the bitterness sufficiently to permit a diagnostic reevaluation.

To know the details of prior frustrating medical experience aids the counselor in circumventing pitfalls. (This is true for all health care interactions that patients have with professionals.)

Mrs. Taft insisted that many people had told her that Andy did not look like a typical child with Down syndrome, even though "that may be what the chromosomes showed." I agreed and openly stated, "Andy's appearance is not typical of children with Down syndrome, and I think it is very important to check this diagnosis. This would require that we repeat the chromosome analysis in our laboratory."

Not wanting to continue at this clinical level, I commented on how reserved and shy Andy was. Mrs. Taft replied, "He's just shy with new people. I think he's probably shy because he's so short. That's what I'm worried about. Why is he so short?" (Although he was three years old, Andy appeared to be approximately one.) This seemed to be an appropriate time to begin the family history. Although Mrs. Taft needed time to voice her feelings, the constraints of the outreach program (e.g., airline flight schedules) impose a time limit on the sessions. Since I sensed that Mrs. Taft could continue talking indefinitely about her frustrations and dissatisfactions with hospitals, physicians, nurses, and so on, it was necessary to direct the conversation toward the family.

In most information-gathering interviews we regularly learn some of the most helpful, important items by permitting the interviewee to proceed conversationally in his or her own way. In the present instance this preferable path had to be compromised in deference to an appointment schedule involving air travel. One way—not the only one—for constructing such a compromise is to inform the counselee politely that there are certain questions you *must* ask. At the end of the inquiry, if anything of importance has not come out, the counselee may add it then.

Andy was Mrs. Taft's second child. She had had one spontaneous abortion (not documented) and a daughter by a previous marriage. At the age of 6, her daughter was doing well both developmentally and physically. Andy was born in a small community hospital when Mrs. Taft was 23 years old. Mr. Taft was 25 at the time of Andy's birth. While she never openly stated that there were problems with this marriage, her comments implied that it was not going smoothly. According to Mrs. Taft, "I hoped that he'd be able to come today. We made this appointment thinking he'd be in town, but another job came up." Mr. Taft was a truck driver and was frequently on the road.

Andy was the result of an unplanned pregnancy. During the first three months of gestation, Mrs. Taft had remained in bed because of severe back pain and bleeding. Although she was given pain medication, it was quickly discontinued because of a possible allergic reaction. Andy was born at term following an uncomplicated labor and delivery. His birth weight was 6 pounds, 1 ounce and he was approximately 16 inches long. He did not breathe immediately and required oxygen for forty-eight hours. "When he was born," Mrs. Taft explained, "they told us he'd be retarded and that he'd be a dwarf or a mongoloid. But Andy is *not* retarded; he's only shy when he meets new people."

During these consultations we routinely ask about drugs taken during pregnancy, including alcohol specifically. Regarding alcohol consumption, Mrs. Taft blushed, saying, "I only drank a few beers now and then." After Andy was born, she admitted, she began drinking more heavily, and, in fact, she had recently joined a group similar to Alcoholics Anonymous.

Alcohol abusers frequently minimize their consumption. That Mrs. Taft sought an AA-type group tells us that the problem was serious and eluding her control. Marital tensions are most probably implicated.

She was quite emphatic about her recent "reformation" and appeared to feel it was necessary to clarify this further. "Now I'm a reformed alcoholic. Since joining, I haven't had a single drink in two months." She was proud to have acknowledged her addiction, because "that's the first step in getting away from the bottle." She described her therapy group and was pleased that there were several people she could talk to who had successfully conquered alcoholism. Mrs. Taft was adamant about her abstinence from all alcohol since joining the group two months before. We talked briefly about her past alcohol consumption, and she also mentioned that Mr. Taft drinks quite heavily. "When he returns from a cross-country trek, he's ready for a drink and sometimes he has already had a few," she admitted. She was annoyed that her husband had not joined her therapy group and was upset that he was not at all supportive of her recent reformation. When discussing her husband, Mrs. Taft's tone was noticeably sharp. She described her husband's reaction to Andy's diagnosis of Down syndrome as being very negative. ''He's not taking this well at all.''

With her first husband, Mrs. Taft had produced a normal daughter. With her present husband she gave birth to Andy, who is defective. The contrast may make Mr. Taft feel a sense of special responsibility for Andy's problems—rightly or wrongly.

This is plainly a troubled family with several problems. When a spouse brings with her (or him) a child of a former marriage, the new marriage is instantly more complicated: The other spouse becomes not only a new husband (or wife) but at the same time a stepparent, a demanding challenge. Often women like Mrs. Taft who enter a second marriage ''encumbered'' with a child take upon themselves an impossibly large share of the burden of making everything ''nice'' at home. It is not unthinkable that such worries are among the factors fueling her need to deny retardation in Andy, and adding to the burden of anxiety behind her alchoholic excesses.

Throughout my discussion with Mrs. Taft, Andy would periodically interrupt us by handing a toy to his mother or to me. We would briefly stop our conversation to talk to him. Andy did not verbalize while playing, nor did he do so when interacting with either his mother or myself. From observing Andy, I felt that his development was more delayed than his mother acknowledged.

As we continued with the family history, I found no one else with learning problems, mental retardation, or extremely short stature. One first cousin had a congenital heart defect. I had already spent more time with Mrs. Taft than was usual. Because there were still three families to be seen, there would not be time for as thorough an evaluation and examination of the child as we like to give. However, given the social history and diagnostic complications in this family, I felt that the additional time spent with Mrs. Taft had been necessary.

Mrs. Taft undressed Andy so that Dr. G. could examine him. While she was doing so, I talked with Dr. G. in a separate room. We discussed Andy's behavior and appearance, the family history, Mrs. Taft's hostility about Andy's past diagnosis, and her history of alcohol consumption. I suspected that Mrs. Taft could easily have consumed more alcohol during her pregnancy than she admitted, and I discussed this with Dr. G. This was an area which Dr. G. and I agreed should be carefully explored.

We then joined Mrs. Taft and Andy in the examining room. In the interim, the clinic coordinator had recorded Andy's height and weight. While I plotted these figures, Dr. G. began examining the child. Dr. G. and I talked freely with Mrs. Taft during the physical exam, explaining what we were looking for and asking more questions regarding Andy's development. "Dr. G. and I are seeing if Andy has any of the subtle findings seen in children with Down syndrome." We learned that Andy did not enjoy playing with other children and seldom talked to himself, nor did he talk as much as his sister had. Mrs. Taft did not think he had a hearing loss. She could not remember the timing of his developmental milestones but thought, "He was pretty much like his sister, so he must have been okay."

Andy's sister was described as normal, so this characterization of Andy's development is plainly defensive. Considering the heavy maternal alcohol consumption that presumably occurred during the pregnancy, the need to respond in a self-protective style is altogether understandable. Considering that Mr. Taft works as a driver and therefore must be absent fairly often, we can imagine what a troubled time it has been for Mrs. Taft ever since the early days of her unplanned pregnancy.

After the exam, Dr. G., Mrs. J. (the local clinic coordinator), and I sat down to review our findings and discuss some possible diagnoses with Mrs. Taft. First Dr. G. explained that the physical exam showed Andy did not have Down syndrome. It was necessary, however, to repeat the chromosome analysis using banding technique to confirm this. On the exam, Andy's height plotted well below the third percentile, which was appropriate for a child of 7 months! His weight, also well below the third percentile, would have been appropriate for a 9-month-old. Mrs. Taft was extremely relieved that we supported her feeling about Andy not having Down syndrome. Although we did not discuss specific diagnoses with her, we were considering several alternatives which would require further investigation. We expressed our concern about Andy's development: specifically his lack of speech and his delayed motor milestones. In order to determine the exact level at which Andy was functioning, a developmental evaluation would be performed prior to our next genetic counseling visit. The physical findings and our suspicion of maternal alcohol consumption during pregnancy strongly suggested the possibility of fetal alcohol syndrome. However, we did not discuss this impression with Mrs. Taft. We did make and discuss with her the following recommendations:

1. Chromosome analysis utilizing G-banding.
2. A metabolic screen (routine for patients with developmental delay).
3. Developmental evaluation.

4. Review of previous skeletal survey to assess the possibility of skeletal dysplasia.
5. Requests for previous endocrine evaluation results.

The initial session with Mrs. Taft lasted about two hours. Normally a return visit lasts about forty minutes, but Dr. G. and I both agreed that Mrs. Taft should be scheduled for at least an hour to allow enough time for discussion.

Prior to our next session, a banded chromosome analysis was completed at our cytogenetics lab. The results revealed a 47,XYY karyotype, thus ruling out Down syndrome. Banding was critical for identifying the extra G-group chromosome. Since the original chromosome analysis had been performed without banding, the extra G chromosome was assumed to have been a #21, when in fact it was a Y chromosome. The pediatric radiologist at our university center felt that Andy's skeletal X-rays did not reveal any abnormalities characteristic of skeletal dysplasia. On his recommendation, a repeat thyroid screen test was obtained, and the results fell within normal limits (the prior thyroid screen had also been normal). The results of the metabolic screen were also within normal limits. Andy's developmental evaluation had been performed at the local public health department, and the results had been forwarded to the Genetics Center. Andy's overall score on the Bailey Mental Scale at a chronological age of 37 months was appropriate for a 20-month-old child. His most significant delays were in the area of verbal skills. The evaluator noted that Andy did not speak, was reluctant to perform, and displayed a lack of emotional response during the evaluation.

Andy's case was reviewed and discussed at the genetics conference. In addition to the cytogenetic finding of XYY, Andy's phenotype was generally felt to be compatible with the fetal alcohol syndrome. Since its initial description, fetal alcohol syndrome has come to represent a widely accepted entity. The diagnosis is dependent on the history of alcohol consumption during pregnancy in association with specific clinical findings. As in this case, an accurate history of maternal alcohol use during pregnancy is frequently difficult to obtain. A considerable amount of time was spent discussing how to broach the diagnosis of fetal alcohol syndrome, how and what to explain about the XYY aneuploidy, and what recommendations to make to the parents.

Two months later, the Tafts were scheduled for a second visit to the outreach clinic. Mrs. Taft arrived almost an hour late for the 9:00 A.M. appointment. Her clothes were wrinkled, and she reeked of alcohol. Her speech was quite slurred as she explained that her husband wouldn't be able to attend this session either. We immediately realized how difficult the counseling was going to be. Originally, we had planned to explain that Andy did not have Down syndrome, to discuss the possibility of fetal alcohol syndrome, and to introduce the cytogenetic finding of XYY. Given the situation, we knew that very little progress would be made during this session and that a third session would be necessary.

Genetic counseling is difficult enough under optimal circumstances. With the counselee obviously intoxicated, it is probably almost impossible. It matters little that the counselee is able to sit still through the interview: Grasp of difficult facts and memory for what is discussed are usually much impaired.
  We can hardly help wondering what led Mrs. Taft to arrive in this condition, considering the importance of the counseling. Did she have an argument with her husband about their jointly participating in the counseling? Did she feel she needed to "fortify" herself for an interview that she feared would overwhelm her with its fresh disclosures? Later in the interview Mrs. Taft denies the latter possibility.

When the local coordinator returned with coffee, we began the second session by discussing with Mrs. Taft the results of the chromosome analysis. We explained that Andy did not have Down syndrome; he did have an extra chromosome, Dr. G. pointed out, but not the one associated with that disorder. Copies of Andy's karyotype were used to illustrate this. Mrs. Taft was extremely relieved that we could provide "proof." (The presence of an extra chromosome, as long as it wasn't the one involved with Down syndrome, did not seem to bother her.) She had heard what she wanted to know and did not appear to absorb the rest of what was said. Given that she was drunk, and that the clinical significance of the 47,XYY aneuploidy is not well understood, we decided not to dwell on this during this session. Mrs. Taft's only request was for a letter stating that Andy did not have Down syndrome, because their insurance company refused to cover children with this condition. We readily agreed to provide the letter.
  Mrs. Taft acknowledged that she had had a few drinks before coming to the clinic, so she really "couldn't think that well." We asked if she had been worried about what she might hear today and if this was why she had been drinking. She vehemently denied that this was the case, explaining that she and her husband were not getting along. At this point, the secretary let me know that the next family had arrived. It was an appropriate time for me to excuse myself; so Dr. G. continued the session alone.
  In an attempt to explain Andy's short stature and developmental delay, the importance of environmental factors during pregnancy was discussed. Rather than specifically point to Mrs. Taft's alcohol consumption during pregnancy, Dr. G. carefully explained that many en-

vironmental agents—e.g., infections, drugs, X-rays, and alcohol—can be harmful to the unborn baby. If Mrs. Taft were to become pregnant again, she should be aware of this relationship and avoid alcohol. Dr. G. was worried about the impact this discussion would have on Mrs. Taft. She had been relatively quiet, thus making it difficult to determine her reactions to the counseling. Despite Dr. G.'s attempts to elicit Mrs. Taft's feelings, she mumbled only brief answers. This was in extreme contrast to the first session, where she had been quite talkative and opinionated.

It is hard to imagine that this information, however tactfully phrased, can be absorbed without the counselee's experiencing an increase in her burden of guilt. The bad consequences of alcohol abuse have been underscored. Even if Mrs. Taft succeeds in reforming herself, she will be forever reminded of her prior overindulgence in the person of her son. Had she been altogether sober during the interview, we would expect the impact to have been even more profound.

Plans were made to have the local coordinator make a home visit. Mrs. Taft agreed to return for a third visit when she would be "feeling better" and there would be time to complete the counseling.

During lunch, Dr. G. and I were able to review the morning's families with the local coordinator. When it came time to discuss our sessions with Mrs. Taft, it was obvious that there were still a number of issues that had not been dealt with. The only thing we had definitely accomplished was to reassure Mrs. Taft that Andy did not have Down syndrome. During her home visits, we asked the local coordinator to try to determine what Mrs. Taft's feelings were about our discussion; what she had understood; and whether this had raised additional guilt feelings. Since the family lived in the community, the local coordinator felt she would be able to maintain close contact with Mrs. Taft.

The staff may well have been correct in its impression that the only definite outcome of the counseling interviews, so far as Mrs. Taft was concerned, was her learning that Andy definitely did not have Down syndrome. They intended to try to achieve considerably more for the Tafts, but have discovered that the couple are not able to collaborate further.

The staff are understandably frustrated, since the help that they are able to offer cannot be usefully dealt with by the Tafts at this time. Mrs. Taft's own agenda, to "disprove" the diagnosis of Down syndrome, has been achieved. Why she limits herself to this one particular counseling outcome, we cannot explain.

There are so many aspects of a counselee's private situation that we know little or nothing about. It is very impressive how much we can

achieve in surprisingly many instances even when we are in ignorance of
the full details of the counselees' private lives.

We have not had another opportunity to meet with the Tafts. A third appointment was scheduled, but the family cancelled for "personal"
reasons. The local coordinator did report that on our recommendation
Mrs. Taft had enrolled Andy in a special education program; but his attendance was not regular. The Tafts subsequently moved from the area,
and this case remains lost to follow-up.

Dr. G. and I were dissatisfied and personally frustrated with our inability to provide further support and information to the family. Even
under optimum conditions, discussing a diagnosis of fetal alcohol syndrome proves difficult. We suspected that Mrs. Taft felt very guilty
about Andy's problems and that she was not receiving emotional support from her husband. Unfortunately, we have never had any contact
with Mr. Taft to assess his feelings and his understanding of Andy's
problems.

The family's lack of response to attempts to have Andy become involved in specific programs made it difficult to provide any continuity of
care for them. When it became obvious that the family would not return
to the clinic, a summary letter was sent to the Tafts. At least one positive
outcome of the genetic counseling was the fact that we were able to docu-
ment that Andy did not have Down syndrome—something that should
have been done when he was much younger. Unfortunately, we will be
unable to follow the effects that the XYY aneuploidy and fetal alcohol
syndrome may have on Andy's future development.

Further Comment

This report is more than an account of staff frustration in the face of a
situation that they had only limited power to change.

It is a very vivid illustration of the fact that we have no choice but to
deal with our counselees as we find them, rather than in a particular frame
of mind optimal for the counseling interaction. In usual parlance Mr. and
Mrs. Taft would be regarded as especially "resistant" counselees. But
however energetic their inner reluctance to involve themselves in the
counseling—he obviously more than she—that resistance did not preclude Mrs. Taft's circumscribed participation. She did get something out
of it all right away. The report of Andy's being brought to a special educational program, however briefly, suggests that she assimilated more of the
recommendations than was at first apparent. A period of delay before a
recommendation can be acted upon is by no means rare. Everyone has her
or his own timetable for digestion of painful realities.

There is no way to know whether the counseling team would have been more successful if they had had additional time to spend with the Tafts. But they did not. Availability of counseling staff time is another of the factors that can detract from the optimal counseling situation.

References

IosuB, S.; BINGOL, N.; and GROMISCH, D. (1981). Fetal alcohol syndrome revisited. *Pediatrics* 68 (no. 4): 475–478.

ROBINSON, A.; LUBS, H.; and BERGSMA, D., eds. (1979). Sex chromosome aneuploidy: prospective studies on children. In *Birth defects, original article series,* vol. 15, no. 1. The National Foundation–March of Dimes. New York: Allan R. Liss.

ROSETT, H.; WEINER, L.; and EDELIN, K. (1981). Strategies for prevention of fetal alcohol effects. *Obstetrics and Gynecology* 57 (no. 1): 1–7.

11

Helping the Counselee to Focus Her Feelings: Chondroectodermal Dysplasia

Mrs. Donaldson's dilemma about whether or not to proceed with recommended fetoscopy to evaluate her developing fetus is rather instructive for us. This intelligent lady has had the procedure carefully explained to her in all details by a knowledgeable professional, yet she still equivocates. In her conversation she is specially focused on the medication necessary for the procedure, rather than any other detail.

The counselor did not belittle Mrs. Donaldson's reluctance, but inquired interestedly about it, and discovered that the counselee's focus upon the medication was very likely displaced from a much more important issue: whether she would be prepared to abort a fetus found to be affected. Once this displacement of focus had been communicated to her, she promptly found a way out of her dilemma.

This example demonstrates what may be regarded as an "analytic" approach to dealing with a conflictual issue impeding decision making.

The situation involves a family with a history of three children: one normal girl and two full-term boys who were both diagnosed as having Ellis–van Creveld syndrome (EVC). This syndrome is also known as "chondroectodermal dysplasia," and is inherited as an autosomal recessive disorder. The disease is characterized by shortened distal portions of the extremities, dwarfism, polydactyly, nail dysplasia, dental problems, a short puckered upper lip bound by frenula to the alveolar ridge, and in 50 percent of cases, cardiac defects.

I initially learned about the patient, Mrs. Donaldson, when her obstetrician, Dr. B., telephoned to inform me that he had a 42-year-old pregnant patient who had had two children with EVC disease. He intended to refer her for amniocentesis because of her age. He also mentioned that one of the EVC children had died in infancy. Mrs. Donald-

son had told Dr. B. that she intended to have a fetoscopy in order to see if
the fetus was affected with EVC.

Referral for amniocentesis would be in order on the basis of the mother's
age. The obstetrician's brief history reminds the reader that the 25% percent probability of giving birth to a child with autosomal recessive disease
is no comfort to parents for whom the probability has not "worked out"
well. The patient's expressed desire to undergo fetoscopy highlights her
concern about possible repetition of the misfortune.

Dr. B. also told me that the living son, Michael, was now a teenager
and seemed well adjusted to his short stature, was very bright, and did
very well in school. He had been born with an extra finger, which had
been removed surgically. I inquired about the family attitude toward
Michael, and he explained that the Donaldsons were very proud of him;
he was "tops in his class and popular." Mr. Donaldson was a successful
lawyer.

That afternoon Mrs. Donaldson called for an appointment, which
was arranged for the following week (at which time she would be ten
weeks pregnant). While chatting on the phone, Mrs. Donaldson asked if
Dr. B. had mentioned her history. I said that he had. She went on to say
that she was going to have a fetoscopy at one of the large medical centers
on the East Coast. I suggested that she consider having the amniocentesis for chromosome analysis at the same time she was having the
fetoscopy. Her response to this suggestion was that she would like to
discuss the fetoscopy with me, since she had not fully decided to go
ahead with it.

The following Wednesday Mrs. Donaldson came in. She was a very
attractive woman who seemed markedly agitated and a little depressed.
At the beginning of the counseling session she discussed having had two
boys with EVC, one of whom, Edward, had died at age two and a half
months at home, following surgery for a serious heart defect. This baby
had been born nine years after the birth of Michael. A second child,
Mary, was then three years old. The family had been extremely anxious
about the sick baby. Edward had not been well since birth, and although
Mrs. Donaldson felt that the baby's death was probably for the best,
that judgment did not make his passing any less painful. The surgery
had been performed at a large New York City medical center, and the
family had had genetic counseling at the time. Mrs. Donaldson understood the inheritance pattern for EVC.

She explained that when she had discovered her pregnancy several
weeks earlier, she had called the New York City center which had
previously counseled the family to ask whether they had discovered any
new information about EVC in the prior four years. In response to her

query the availability of the fetoscopy procedure was mentioned, and she was told where the procedure could be performed.

As Mrs. Donaldson recounted her narrative, she interjected that she was ambivalent about going ahead with the procedure. She said she had learned the name of the physician who performed it and had called him long-distance. He had spent one hour explaining fetsocopy to her with patient attention to all details. She was to let him know her decision about undergoing the procedure so that he might make a suitable appointment for her.

(Fetoscopy gains a direct view of the developing fetus by inserting an optical instrument through the abdominal and uterine walls into the uterine cavity. The position of the fetus is determined first by sonography, and it is then temporarily immobilized with medication to ensure maximum opportunity for locating the body parts of greatest interest. In this instance the physician would be seeking evidence of polydactyly.)

Mrs. Donaldson told me that she understood the fetoscopy procedure carries a high risk of miscarriage, but that this risk did not worry her nearly so much as the effects of the immobilizing medication on the baby. Her feeling of trust in this physician and in his reassurances regarding the procedure did not alter her fear of drugging the fetus. I asked, ''If the doctor stated that the drug would not hurt the fetus, would you then go ahead?'' She answered, ''I cannot believe that it would be safe. Suppose that there was an aftereffect, or that this was an exception?'' She commented that this test was relatively new and had not been done many times. She tried to convince me that the medication was a genuine threat to the pregnancy.

As Mrs. Donaldson talked, it seemed that she vacillated between going ahead with the procedure and abandoning any plan to do so. She wanted me to decide for her. It is not my practice to make decisions for any patient, as I believe a patient has to make such important judgments from the reference point of her own experience. I considered it would be wiser to have Mrs. Donaldson discuss the technicalities and pros and cons of this procedure with a medical geneticist.

By this point in the interview it was obvious that Mrs. Donaldson was agonizing over a decision. I began to suspect that she did not really want to have the fetoscopy but had not yet come to an understanding of the underlying reason for rejecting it. Her behavior was marked by a great deal of fidgeting and she looked very sad.

I felt that we had reached an impasse. It occurred to me to ask her if she would have the procedure if the fetus would not be given medication. She said she had not thought of that as a possibility because of the need to view the fetus in a special way. I then asked her why she had bothered to consider the procedure at all. Was she prepared to terminate the pregnancy if the fetus proved to have EVC? This question struck a chord!

Mrs. Donaldson began to cry. She avoided my eyes and seemed excited. She claimed she was too confused to know what to do. I asked her why, but she did not answer. After a five-minute silence she volunteered that she could not verbalize a reason. She and her husband had discussed having the fetoscopy but had not actually discussed the possibility of abortion! In retrospect, she said, the possibility had of course been understood, but it had not been mentioned. In her talk with her husband, they had only stressed their concern about the drug's effects on the fetus. I said, "Are you upset about this pregnancy?" She said, "No, just surprised." Mrs. Donaldson is Catholic, but would consider an abortion in certain instances, as she revealed shortly by the following:

I said, "You have come here today to discuss having an amniocentesis for the purpose of ruling out chromosome abnormality in your baby. What would you do if you found you were carrying a chromosomally damaged child?" She said, "When Dr. B. suggested I come to you for amniocentesis counseling, and I called you, I guess I made my decision then regarding a chromosome abnormality. Yes, I think I could at least consider termination, but I just don't know what I would do if they discovered my child had EVC. I try not to worry or think about it. Michael is such a wonderful kid! He's doing so well in school, and has made such a fine adjustment. He has brought such pleasure and happiness to the family."

Privately I speculated as to the nature of her further thoughts, and next asked her if she were avoiding the fetoscopy because she was unable to consider terminating a pregnancy that would result in the birth of a baby with EVC—one that would represent for her the son that she loved so dearly.

The drop in her anxiety was dramatic. She suddenly realized that since she loved her affected son so much, she could never entertain the thought of aborting a child like him. Mrs. Donaldson now realized that this was the heart of her perplexing dilemma.

Faithful to her concern to have the patient arrive at an independent judgment, the genetic counselor has energetically investigated her counselee's conflict. It is very striking that the counselee links the notion of a possible EVC fetus with her successfully adjusted teenage son, and not with the boy who died at two and half months of age. In terms of the genetic "facts," another affected infant might just as readily be like the nonviable son as like the hardy survivor.

Although Mrs. Donaldson was concerned about having another child with EVC because of her previous experience with two affected children, she stated with great feeling, "I could never in a million years consider destroying a child that represents Michael."

At once her mind was made up not to have the fetoscopy. She was obviously in a better frame of mind, and we went on to discuss amniocentesis. She seemed to be able to cope with the concept of aborting because of chromosome anomaly. Arrangements were made for the amniocentesis. (The test reported a chromosomally normal male.)

The session with Mrs. Donaldson lasted for two and half hours. By the end of our meeting her behavior was markedly changed. She left comparatively unburdened, promising to let me know when the new baby had arrived. I felt that this was a successful counseling interview. The client was able to come to a serious decision by herself, one that seemed "right" for her.

At a later date, Mrs. Donaldson telephoned elatedly to report the birth of a nine-pound, nine-ounce son, completely free of EVC syndrome.

Further Comment

This brief report underscores the degree to which genetic counseling is *not* a simple matter of conveying statistical probabilities. Although EVC syndrome is an autosomal recessive disorder, it is quite striking how differently this disorder affects family life as compared with any number of other recessively inherited problems, such as cystic fibrosis. Polydactyly, for example, is relatively simple to contend with. Also, it is notable that for the Donaldsons the relatively good experience with Michael has more than counterbalanced the desolate experience with Edward, and supports the Donaldsons' desire to enlarge their family.

It is precisely such very personal meanings of a given diagnosis that regularly complicate what to the outsider may appear to be a "simple" choice. Had the counselor been less energetic in clarifying the history with regard to the decision at issue, the counselee would have departed as troubled as she had been on arrival. Nor should we overlook the fact that this clarification made the fetoscopy, with its irreducible risk to the pregnancy, unnecessary.

References

DeVore, G.; Venus, I.; Hobbins, J.; and Mahoney, M. (1981). Fetoscopy: general clinical approach. In Rocker, I.; and Laurence, K., eds., *Fetoscopy*, pp. 51–64. Amsterdam: Elsevier/North Holland.

Ellis, R., and van Creveld, S. (1940). A syndrome characterized by ectodermal dysplasia, polydactyly, chondrodysplasia, and congenital morbus cordis. *Arch. Diseases of Children* 15: 65–84.

McKusick, V.; Egeland, J.; Eldridge, R.; and Krusen, D. (1964). Dwarfism in the Amish: the Ellis–van Creveld syndrome. *Johns Hopkins Med. J.* 115: 306–336.

Walgrigues, A.; Grohmann, L.; Takahashi, T.; and Reis, H. (1977). Ellis–van Creveld syndrome: an inbred kindred with five cases. *Revista Brasileira de Pesquisas Medicas e Biologicas* 10: 193–198.

12

Dealing with the Specifics of Amniocentesis and Elective Abortion

Amniocentesis for prenatal diagnosis of high-risk pregnancies has become an ever more common experience. Lest the procedure's frequency lead to an impression that it's "hardly anything," the report that follows details both the preparation for it and the steps of the procedure itself.

Nor is it necessarily a simple matter, once the indication for an elective abortion has been discovered, to move ahead and have the abortion. In the situation of Mrs. Janet Williams, the issue at the time of this counseling was whether to abort a male fetus with a 50 percent chance of suffering from hemophilia. The possiblity that one may be aborting a normal fetus renders the decision not so simple.

Janet Williams, age 30, married two years to Ron, age 32, was about fifteen weeks pregnant when she came to our center for amniocentesis. She was known to our Genetics Department from the contact she had made three years before with our Hemophilia Clinic. At that time, shortly after the death of her father, a hemophiliac, she came to the clinic for genetic counseling. According to the clinic's records, she was seen by a member of its staff, who obtained a pedigree and explained her obligate carrier status and the availability of amniocentesis to determine the sex of the fetus. Since then she had married, become pregnant, and made contact by telephone with our department in order to arrange for prenatal sex determination.

In response to a referral, the standard scheduling procedure in the Prenatal Diagnosis Clinic is for the secretary to phone the patient and arrange an appointment for testing during the estimated fifteenth or sixteenth week of the pregnancy. Often there is not sufficient time to schedule a previous counseling appointment, or such an appointment may be impractical if the patient resides far from our center. Janet and Ron Williams lived in a small resort town four hours from the center, so there were no plans to see them before the date set for the amniocentesis. On the designated day Ron, an industrial executive, was not able to postpone a last-minute business conference and so was unable to come with his wife. Janet drove up by herself a day ahead and spent the night with her mother, Mrs. Long. When they arrived at our center, Janet checked in with the clinic secretary, who then directed them to our cafeteria, where I soon joined them for my first contact with Janet. I introduced myself as the genetic counselor and was introduced to Mrs. Long. We chatted casually for a few minutes about the long drive and the absence of Janet's husband. My initial impression of Janet was of an intelligent, confident, attractive young woman who was well educated, outgoing, and friendly. I had noticed in her records that she had an M.S. in art history, and asked her what type of work she did. She explained that she was self-employed as an interior designer.

G.C.: I'd like to spend some time this morning going over with you just what amniocentesis is and how we go about getting results for you. I have a room set aside where we can go and talk—or would you prefer to stay here and finish your coffee?

JANET: Why don't we just stay here? It seems pretty quiet and we won't have to move all of our things.

G.C.: That's fine; at this time of day it's very peaceful here. Let's first talk a little about why you came. As I understand it, your father had hemophilia. Is that correct?

JANET: Yes, and now I have a chance of having a baby with the same disease.

G.C.: I see in your folder that you have spoken with the people in our Hemophilia Clinic, but that was several years ago. Do you recall what they told you about how hemophilia is inherited?

Although the counselor is aware that Janet has been told enough, and has seen enough, concerning hemophilia to be motivated for prenatal diagnosis, she makes no assumption about the degree of Janet's actual sophistication. The counselor's inquiry will clue her as to the status of Janet's useful, integrated knowledge, and thereby permit all further communications to be precisely tailored for her.

JANET: Well, I know I could have a child with the disease and I am quite concerned.

G.C.: Would you like to review how it all works?

JANET: Yes, please. I sort of remember from when I was here at the Hemophilia Clinic, but I think it would help to hear it again.

G.C.: You see, the genetic information that causes a person to have hemophilia is located on the X sex chromosome, which is one of the two kinds of sex chromsomes. This is what chromosomes actually look like [she is shown a male and female karyotype], and these two chromosomes are the sex chromosomes. The karyotype represents the chromosome complement of one of our body cells, but remember that each body cell has the same chromosome complement as the one in the karyotype. Hemophilia is a heritable disorder, and to understand how it can be inherited we need to be concerned only with the sex chromosomes, the X and the Y. [While I am speaking I start to diagram on paper what I am trying to explain.] Males have an X and a Y chromosome in all of their body cells, while females have two X chromosomes in all their cells. When a child is conceived, each parent has contributed only *one* of their sex chromosomes. Females can only contribute an X. A male, however, having an X and a Y, can contribute either. If by chance his X is contributed, the child will be female (XX); if the Y is given, the child will be male (XY).

JANET: Yes, now I remember!

G.C.: Now, let's relate this to hemophilia and your particular situation. We know that your father had hemophilia; therefore we know that he carried that information on his X chromosome. [I draw a dot on the X chromosome on the diagram.] We know that you, Janet, since you are female, have two X chromosomes—one of which you received from your mother and the other from your father. Since your father's X chromosome carried the genetic information for hemophilia, we know that one of your X chromosomes in all of your cells carries that information too. The difference is that you *carry* the trait for hemophilia but are not affected by the disorder because you are protected by your *normal* X chromosome, contributed by your mother. We call you a "carrier." I hope I am not confusing you.

JANET: No, not at all. Now I see how they knew for sure that I could pass on the trait for hemophilia.

The counselor has offered a plain explanation of sex determination through chromosomal pairing to a concerned counselee; she cannot know whether Janet ever took a biology course and makes no assumptions about her knowledge. Without doubt she was offered a similar explanation of X-linked recessive inheritance a few years previously. Janet's response, "*Now* I see how they knew for sure [italics mine]" strongly implies that the earlier explanation was only partially absorbed.

G.C.: Yes—they also tested your blood for the clotting factor levels, so there is no doubt that you are at risk for having a son with the disease.

JANET: I understand how only a son could have it; but even so, it's a fifty-fifty chance, isn't it?

G.C.: Let me show you [I returned to the diagram]. To each of your children you will pass on one of your X chromosomes. Now, if your husband passes on his X chromosome you will have a girl. Depending on which X chromosome you have given, the girl will either be totally free of the hemophilia information or be a carrier like yourself. But suppose your husband passes on his Y chromosome; then the child will be male. This time the X which you pass on is crucial. If you contribute your normal X, then your son will be free of the disorder, and, of course, not having the trait, will not possibly be able to pass it on. However, if he inherits your X chromosome which carries the gene for hemophilia, he will have hemophilia as your father did. The risk for a male child of yours to have hemophilia is 50 percent.

Up to this point the counselor has not used the term "gene," but rather "genetic information" or "trait." The careful selection of terms indicates how it is possible to convey the essentials of what to a novice can be quite complicated without employing burdensome technical terminology.

JANET: Now it all seems clear, and I see that my cousin Susan is at risk, too! [This is said with some surprise.]

G.C.: Let's take a look at your family pedigree and see what's what. [We do this and note that Janet's father, his brother, and their first cousin all had hemophilia.]

JANET: I see that my father's cousins' children are at risk, too. My father's brother died before he had children. His sister decided not to risk having her own children and has adopted a son.

G.C.: Have you and your husband discussed your feelings about this pregnancy?

JANET: Oh, yes. We decided long before I became pregnant that we would abort a male child.

For Janet and her husband to have decided this in advance of this consultation meant that (1) she already understood that the prenatal diagnosis then available could not distinguish an affected from an unaffected male fetus; and (2) the disease, in human terms, was for her altogether unacceptable.

As of 1982 in the United States there were two medical centers with the skill and equipment to utilize ultrasound and fetoscopy to obtain the fetal blood necessary for an assay to determine the presence of hemophilia in a male fetus. Placental or cord blood vessels are used. The reliability of this procedure is 100 percent provided that (1) a 100 percent pure fetal blood sample is obtained, and (2) a blood sample from a relative affected with hemophilia is available. At one of these centers the fetal loss risk with this procedure is 4 to 5 percent. There is also the risk of premature birth, which is reported as 6 percent at one center and as 9 to 10 percent at the other.

G.C.: Does your husband feel as strongly as you do about this decision?

JANET: Yes, because he realizes that it was I who had lived with this problem, and he understands the enormous difficulty and sadness involved. He respects my feelings on this. My father was only 50 when he died. He had been a musician, and for the last several years before his death was unable to work because of the pain in his hands.

MRS. LONG: What about Janet's brother—my son? Will he have to be concerned about this?

G.C.: No, he cannot be a carrier of the hemophilia gene. The fact that he is male means he received the Y chromosome from his father and therefore cannot have the trait for hemophilia. Are there any other questions you have thought of?

JANET: Could you tell me what the amniocentesis will be like?

G.C.: Did your obstetrician tell you anything about it?

JANET: Not really; he said you would explain it all when I got here. I have read a little about it, though.

G.C.: The amniocentesis involves taking a sample of the amniotic fluid which surrounds the fetus. Before the procedure begins, you will have some ultrasound pictures taken. Have you heard of ultrasound?

JANET: No, what's that?

G.C.: It's a simple, safe procedure that uses high-frequency sound waves, not X-rays, passed through the uterus. The resulting visualized image of these sound waves bouncing off the fetus gives us important information about the pregnancy. What will happen is: You'll have to change into a hospital gown, then lie on your back, and the technician will put some mineral oil on your stomach area. They have a piece of equipment that looks like a microphone attached to a long metal arm. They will rub this ''microphone'' across your abdomen, and as they do, you will see a picture appear on a TV-like screen in front of you. The picture will look something like this. [I show an ultrasound picture.] This is the fetal head, the placenta, and the fluid.

JANET: It certainly isn't a very clear picture.

G.C.: Well, it's not a picture in the normal sense. One thing to remember is that it is only in one dimension. That is, each picture just shows one section of your body. If you think of your body as a loaf of bread, each ultrasound picture would be like looking at one slice. Many ultrasound pictures will be taken so the technician gets a good idea how things are in three dimensions, but you will never see one single picture that shows the whole of the fetus.

JANET: That's really amazing! Can you see if there are any defects in the fetus, like if a hand is missing?

In the context of this dialogue Janet's question reads as simple intellectual curiosity about the capabilities of diagnostic ultrasonography. We should not, however, glide over the content of the question without noting that it reflects the virtually universal concern of mothers-to-be that they may give birth to deformed babies.

G.C.: It is easy to imagine that ultrasound could show such things, but actually that isn't possible. At this point in time, as you saw in the picture, the ultrasound image is not that well defined, and the fetus is still quite small. Also, because the ultrasound picture is only of one section at a time it is almost impossible to say whether or not a hand is absent or just not in the right place at the right time to be able to be seen. Still, the procedure is very helpful to us. It allows us to tell how far along you are in the pregnancy; if there is enough amniotic fluid available for us to remove some for the amniocentesis; where the placenta is located on the uterine wall; *and* if you are carrying twins!

JANET: Twins! I never even thought of that. I sure hope not. What would we do if there are twins?

G.C.: It is possible to sample the fluids from the twins' two amniotic sacs, but I think that we needn't discuss that now. Let's wait and see.

JANET: A good idea: We'll worry later if we have to. Will the amniocentesis be done in the Ultrasound Department?

G.C.: Yes. This is how it will take place: First, when you arrive at Ultrasound, they will take their pictures. By the way, is your bladder getting full?

JANET: Yes, as a matter of fact it is.

G.C.: Good. Even if you are a little uncomfortable, it is better that way. A full bladder pushes the uterus up and allows better ultrasound pictures. Immediately after these are done, you will be able to empty your bladder. Then you will go into another ultrasound room where the studies will be repeated. *This* time they will look for the exact spot which is best for introducing the needle; in fact, the technician will mark your abdomen for the doctor's convenience. The amniocentesis will then be done.

JANET: Does that take a lot of time—to get the fluid, I mean?

G.C.: Not very long, usually ten or fifteen minutes; and most of that time is spent in preparation. First the doctor will listen to the fetal heartbeat. Then the area on your abdomen will be washed with some iodine solution and a sterile sheet will be draped across. Then a little bit of local anesthetic will be injected right on the spot the technician marked, and that will sting. It does take effect right away, so after that it shouldn't be too uncomfortable. As the amniocentesis needle is introduced, you will probably feel a sensation of pressure and maybe even a mild cramp. It varies, though. Some women feel absolutely nothing once the anesthetic is given, and some feel cramping throughout the whole process, so it's hard to say exactly how it will be for you. One of the most frequent comments I hear from women after amniocentesis is that if they had known it would be that simple, they wouldn't have been so anxious.

JANET: Well, I'm really not all that anxious about the test. I'm sure it won't be bad at all.

[I found Janet's composure most untypical.]

Recalling that Janet is a well-educated woman with a master's degree, the reader may wonder why the counselor is setting forth the details of ultrasonography and amniocentesis with such attention to every particular.

The counselor is aware that everyone facing such a procedure — or any unfamiliar, possibly frightening procedure — is bound to be feeling some degree of anxious expectation. To reduce and to protect against such expectable anxiety, experience shows that the most precisely detailed description is the most helpful. Surprises — any unexpected turn of events — are the most frightening feature of any such procedure. Silently, and in some hard-to-describe manner, the prepared individual "braces herself" and tolerates the encounter better. After all, the awake, alert subject of amniocentesis is slated to observe a rather large needle penetrating her gravid abdomen.

Even though, for geographical reasons, Janet is being interviewed on the very day of the amniocentesis, it is still highly preferable to take the time for this careful preparation.

G.C.: I would like to take a few minutes to talk about possible drawbacks, or risks of the procedure. Amniocentesis is essentially safe; otherwise we wouldn't do it at all. However, there are some potential risks that we want to make sure you understand. The chance that something could go wrong is small, probably less than half of one percent, or one chance in 200. This "something" could be infection, bleeding, or temporary loss of amniotic fluid. The most serious complication would be that the amniocentesis could cause a miscarriage. The chance that this would happen is small. In our clinic, about one percent of the women who have an amniocentesis later miscarry, but in most cases it is impossible to know if the miscarriage was actually a result of the amniocentesis or if it would have happened anyway.

JANET: I see what you're saying. It's hard to look back and find out the exact cause.

G.C.: Right. In fact, our miscarriage rate is not any higher than the miscarriage rate for those women who do *not* have amniocentesis.

JANET: Actually, I'm not overly concerned about the risk. I know that no matter what, I'm much more worried about the hemophilia.

For Janet's consent to be valid as "informed," these possibilities must be broached. Her response underscores the overriding impact of her earlier family experiences with hemophilia.

G.C.: I understand what you're saying. I would like to take a minute to explain how it's possible to determine the sex of the fetus. In that sample of fluid that we take are some of the fetus's skin cells. These are cells that are sloughed off as the fetus grows. These cells from the fetus are like any other cells, so they contain chromosomes. However, in order to get a look at the chromosomes the cells have to go through a process that includes getting them to multiply in number. The cells are actually put into a little container with some nutrients, and they begin to grow. When there are enough of them, then we can begin the procedure that enables us to see the chromosomes. If the two X's are present, then it's a female; an X and a Y means it is male. One point I feel I should bring up is that occasionally the cells don't grow.

JANET: What does that mean?

G.C.: It means that we would be unable to get results from that sample, and would have to ask you to come back so we could obtain a second sample. It does not mean that there is any problem with the fetus. It's not very common for the cells to fail to grow. I want to mention it so that just in case it does happen, you won't be unnecessarily concerned.

Again, in keeping with the principle of psychological prophylaxis already described, the counselor alerts Janet to a possible surprise which could alarm an unprepared counselee.

JANET: Is it possible that any other defects might show up from this testing?

G.C.: Yes. Although we are primarily interested in looking at the chromosomes to determine the sex of the fetus, all of the other chromosomes will be examined carefully to see that they look the way they are supposed to. Have you ever heard of Down syndrome, or mongolism?

JANET: That's a type of mental retardation, isn't it?

G.C.: It's one of the more common chromosome errors. There are also other things that involve chromosome changes, but usually they are quite rare. There is no reason to suspect that there is a chromosome problem with your fetus, but you will know that we check for it anyway.

JANET: That's good.

G.C.: There is one other test that is routinely done; it checks for defects of the spine or skull. We can detect this type of problem by measuring the amount of a substance called alpha-fetoprotein in the amniotic fluid. If it is present in very high amounts, it is a possible indication of a problem with the spine or skull. It's not a perfect test—we could possibly miss a defect that was really present—but it is sensitive enough that we feel it is worthwhile doing.

JANET: Oh, I want you to do everything you can. When and how will I find out about the test results for the sex?

G.C.: I will phone you directly with the results as soon as I get them, unless you would like to make some other arrangements. For example, we could phone your doctor first and he could contact you if you would prefer.

JANET: No, I'd rather have you just call me directly. How long will it take?

G.C.: It takes three to four weeks. Do you have any other questions?

JANET: No, not right now.

G.C.: We do need your permission to do the amniocentesis. I'd like you to read this consent form, and please let me know if there is anything on it that's not clear. Otherwise, go ahead and sign on the bottom line. [Janet reads it over and has no questions, so signs the form.]

I escorted Janet and her mother to the Ultrasound Department, where they were expected. After the ultrasound studies were completed, Janet commented on how interesting she had found them. She appeared calm, and we chatted a while until the doctor arrived. The measurements indicated that the pregnancy was at thirteen and a half to fourteen weeks. Although this is on the early side, there appeared to be a good pocket of fluid, so it was decided to proceed with the amniocentesis. Janet's mother was present during the procedure. Unfortunately, after two attempts no fluid was obtained.

DR. S.: I'm sorry, but it looks as though we're not going to get any fluid today. I think it's best if we wait a few weeks. By then the size of the uterus will have changed quite a bit and it will be a lot easier to do the amniocentesis.

[At this point Janet lowered her head, nodded, and began to cry softly.]

G.C. [handing her some tissues]: That's okay; there's a lot of tension that builds up. It's natural for you to feel let down after all the wondering and waiting.

JANET: Boy, I sure didn't realize how anxious I really was. I'm all right now. I just need a couple of minutes to relax.

G.C.: Take all the time you need.

What an ironic twist to encounter a dry tap, perhaps the only complication of this procedure that was not broached in the counselor's careful preparation of Janet.

In most centers amniocentesis would have been delayed until the fifteenth week of pregnancy, to minimize the possibility of what did occur. It has also been learned that amniotic cells grow more successfully after fifteen weeks. Perhaps the factor of Janet's residing so far away from the center, plus the finding of a good pocket of fluid by sonography, led to the decision to go ahead.

It was very important to indicate to Janet that the absence of fluid did not mean that something was amiss with the pregnancy, but only that further time had to elapse to permit suitable enlargement of the amniotic fluid cavity. Offering this explanation is more than common sense: It is in keeping with the knowledge that unexpected turns of events have the capacity to stimulate great anxiety.

The counselor has expressed her empathic grasp of Janet's distress, so that Janet need not suffer silently and alone. Janet's comment registering her new awareness of how anxious she was contrasts sharply to her earlier presentation of herself as calm and confident. Although she was surprised by this observation, the counselor was not.

JANET: So now I'll have to return in two weeks? In a way I'm glad because I'm sure my husband will be able to come next time. He really was disappointed not to be here today.

G.C.: That's one good thing about having to wait. Do you feel well enough to dress yet?

JANET: Yes, I feel a lot better.

G.C.: Okay, I'll come back in a few minutes. [After returning, five minutes later]: How are you doing, Janet?

JANET: Just fine. I had no idea I was going to react that way, I surprised myself.

G.C.: It's difficult to predict how you're going to react; after all, it's a totally new experience to go through.

JANET: That's for sure. Well, my mother and I are going to go out for lunch and relax for a while.

G.C.: Good idea. Here's an appointment slip with the date for you to return. You can go directly to Ultrasound, and we'll meet you there. I'm sorry we didn't get the fluid today.

JANET: So am I, but in one way I'm glad. Now my husband will be able to understand what it's all about, too.

G.C.: Yes. I'll be seeing you in two weeks then. Be sure and call me if you have any questions or concerns.

Two weeks later we met in the waiting room of the Ultrasound Department. The preliminary scans had already been taken. Janet introduced me to her husband, Ron. While we were waiting for Dr. S., we chatted about the new house they were building and about the small resort town where they live. They asked no questions about the amniocentesis. Dr. S. arrived and the procedure was performed quickly and without difficulty, while Ron was present. After Janet dressed, she expressed relief that all had gone well.

G.C.: It's too bad you had to go through this twice, but at least now I've had the chance to meet your husband.

RON: We would prefer that you call me at my office when you get the test results, especially if it's a boy.

JANET: If it is a boy, would it be possible to come up here for the abortion? You see our town is small and rather conservative [spoken in a confidential tone]. Because of my work I know a lot of townspeople, and you know how word gets around. Actually, the local hospital is a Catholic hospital, and I'm not sure they even do abortions.

RON: We'd just feel better somewhere else.

G.C.: That's understandable, and there will be no problem arranging things here if necessary.

RON: Hopefully, we won't have to go that route. Thanks for everything.

Two and a half weeks later, on a Friday afternoon, it was learned that the fetus was male. I immediately called Ron at his office, feeling somewhat apprehensive, unable to predict altogether the reaction to this bad news. I had found Ron and Janet to be calmer and more certain of their intentions than most other couples in their situation.

G.C.: Hello, Ron? This is E. B., the genetic counselor from the Prenatal Diagnosis Clinic.

RON: Hello, how are you?

G.C.: Fine, thanks, but I'm afraid I have some bad news for you; the fetus is male.

RON [sounding businesslike]: Okay, let me ask you a few questions to make sure I am correct in my understanding. It's not certain that the baby would have hemophilia, but it is a fifty-fifty chance?

G.C.: That's correct.

RON: Is the severity of the disease consistent? I mean, is it likely that the child would be affected like Janet's father, or could it be less severe or worse?

G.C.: The degree of severity may be similar within a family, but not necessarily. There is no way to predict this. If you would like, I can arrange for you to talk with someone from our Hemophilia Clinic. They would be able to answer any questions about the management of the disease.

RON: No, I don't think that will be necessary. You see, Janet and I have already discussed this eventuality, and she seems to be sure that she would want an abortion. Shouldn't we start to make arrangements for it?

The questions that Ron is posing inform us about the intensity of his own desire for a son—an intensity possibly unexpected even by Ron while the sex of the fetus was not yet known, and there was a 50 percent chance of a girl. The questions grope for a possible rationale for continuance of the pregnancy. There is an implication that Ron's and Janet's desires for an abortion are unequal. Considering that Ron did not grow up in the setting of an afflicted family, the difference is understandable.

G.C.: I have spoken with the doctor here and he can have you come in on Wednesday.

RON: Can you tell me a little about what the abortion will be like? Does Janet have to check into the hospital? I understand it might be a prolonged procedure.

G.C.: At Janet's stage of pregnancy [eighteen weeks] it would be what is called a prostaglandin abortion. It is slightly more involved than the type of procedure that is done very early in pregnancy, and Janet will have to be admitted to the hospital. What will happen is that when she arrives in the morning the doctor will do an amniocentesis, but rather than taking fluid out, he will inject in a chemical called prostaglandin. This will ultimately cause Janet to have labor-like contractions and expel the fetus.

RON: How long does this take?

G.C.: It can take anywhere from twelve to twenty-four hours.

RON: That sounds pretty tough, but I guess that's the way it has to be done. What's the next step?

G.C.: I will finalize things here with the doctor's office and get back to you, but you can plan to have that appointment on Wednesday morning.

RON: Okay, but don't call tonight. We're having company, and I think I might wait and tell Janet in the morning.

G.C.: Let me give you my phone number. I'll be home all weekend and I want you to feel free to call me. I will call you Saturday afternoon in any case.

On Saturday morning I received a call at home from Ron. He had spoken to a friend of his who is an obstetrician in another state. They had discussed the possibility of doing a D & E (dilatation and evacuation) abortion for Janet rather than the prostaglandin type. (The D & E is very similar to the way an abortion is done in early pregnancy, and it is much easier on the woman, although there is a risk of uterine perforation. This procedure still requires a stay in the hospital.) The D & E, if done by an obstetrician trained in the technique, can be done until about eighteen or nineteen weeks of pregnancy. According to ultrasound measurements, Janet would just fit in under this time restriction. I told Ron I would contact the doctor who would be doing the abortion and see if he thought this would be possible. As it turned out, this particular doctor was well experienced with D & E, and had been planning to do this as long as Janet was not too far along. I spoke with both Janet and Ron a few more times over the weekend. Janet was upset, but very determined about the correctness of her decision.

I next saw Janet and Ron on Wednesday morning when they came in for Janet to be examined by the doctor. She was still composed, but looked very tired and pale. She admitted that she hadn't slept very well the previous few nights. The doctor decided that Janet was still early enough in pregnancy to permit the D & E. She was admitted to the hospital that afternoon, the D & E planned for the following morning. I stopped in to see Janet and Ron several times during the next twenty-four hours. I waited with Ron the next day for Janet to return to her room from the recovery room. Ron asked a few questions about the genetics of hemophilia, and it seemed that he had a good understanding of the basic inheritance pattern. He explained that he didn't have strong feelings about having his own children, and would be willing to adopt or to have no children at all. Since both he and Janet had career commitments, and enjoyed their life together without children, their desire to have their own family was probably not great enough for them to go ahead and try another pregnancy. Ron acknowledged that Janet probably had stronger feelings than he about having a child but wasn't sure she would want to face the prospect of another amniocentesis and possible abortion.

Janet had not been under heavy anesthesia, and when she came down to her room, she was able to sit up and talk to us. She still looked tired and pale, but her spirits were surprisingly good as she said she felt glad the procedure was over. She even made a joke or two about how she could wear her normal clothes again, and talked about wanting to go home and get back to work.

I visited with Janet several times after that. As she regained her strength, she looked better and better. We talked about how she was feeling both physically and emotionally. While she mentioned that she was a little sore in spots, she never gave any indication that she was hurting emotionally, even when I mentioned that she should expect to feel the loss at some point. I think this was mostly a result of the type of person she was. She was not one to be brooding and introspective. Rather, she faced the situation as it was and dealt with what was happening here and now.

After a few days, she was well enough to go home. I spoke to her on the phone about a week later in order to help arrange her follow-up appointment. She said she felt a little more tired than she had thought she might be, but eager to get back to work. I made plans to see her when she came in for her appointment, but the plans got crossed and I missed her. Neither Janet nor Ron ever asked any questions about the abortus.

The absence of questions about the abortus suggests that the possibility they had aborted a healthy male fetus was more than they could bear to speculate about. This jibes with the rapidly arranged adoption mentioned below, a move simultaneously to replace the lost fetus and to eliminate a possible interrupted second pregnancy.

About five months later, I telephoned Janet. She was very glad to hear from me and apologized that she hadn't phoned first. Apparently, much had happened during this time. The first thing she told me was that they had adopted a little girl about three months before. They were extremely pleased that they were able to do this. Janet was no longer working, since she had found that caring for a baby was taking more time and energy than she expected. As the conversation continued, Janet explained how things had gone after the abortion. Three weeks later, complications related to the D & E had developed, and Janet found herself in the local hospital for ten days. A few weeks after that, she became very depressed and couldn't even talk about her experience. During this time, Ron became irritable and short-tempered. There were frequent arguments and bad feelings.

This development does not surprise us. It is striking that at the time of the abortion the counselor's effort to draw depressed or mournful feelings into the open were unavailing. We can presume that the crisis setting of the abortion required a cheerful demeanor to get through it, and that Janet had to be "in the clear" before grief could be tolerated.

Janet decided to consult a psychologist. He helped her to realize that what she had gone through was no small thing. She was finally able to admit that she had been frightened and miserable. Janet said, "Now I can look back and see what a trauma it was. All along people were saying to me 'You're so strong, so courageous.' I was being strong, at least on the outside, but I found that it doesn't pay to be a good soldier."

G.C.: I know what you're saying. You can't go on pretending nothing has happened.
JANET: That's right. I certainly found that out! Ron and I don't talk too much about it anymore, except to close friends who didn't know what had happened.
G.C.: That's probably okay, since you've done the hard part—facing it and admitting it was painful. Although the experience cannot be erased, you will gradually learn to put it behind you and find that you can survive quite well.
JANET: Surviving . . . Yes, that's the key. You accept things and go on with your life. You know what *really* bothers me? One of my relatives keeps on calling me every time she hears about some new advances in hemophilia. I don't want to hear about it! We're not going to try again, so what's the difference? I just don't want to dwell on it.

We talked for quite a while, and I generally got the feeling that Janet would be all right.

Further Comment

This interesting account of one couple's experience with amniocentesis and elective abortion simultaneously details what amniocentesis is like and how complicated the circumstances connected to this now-common prenatal diagnostic experience may be.

Hemophilia is a large, complex subject in its own right. To attempt to go into it in detail would be much beyond the scope of this book. Suffice it to note that sex-linked heritable disorders present all manner of special features. While it is true, for example, that both partners contribute to a pregnancy, and that the pregnancy would not have been interrupted had Ron contributed an X rather than a Y chromosome, still, the knowledge that Janet was the bearer of the trait that made the difficulty is a special feature that could not fail to have particular impact.

When Janet in the initial interview remarked that her husband shared her attitude concerning abortion, we had a sense of a firm bond between her and Ron in the face of difficulty. That he later became irritable in the face of her depression does not contradict this, for the latter response is quite complicated on its own.

Fortunately Janet was not obliged to undergo the prostaglandin abortion, experiencing a miniature labor without happy issue, but the later complications of the D & E had to underscore the trauma of the abortion. During Janet's immediate recovery from the D & E, the visits by the counselor were very valuable in helping the couple to live through the acute response to this distressing event.

References

DeVore, G.; Venus, I.; Hobbins, J.; and Mahoney, M. (1981). Fetoscopy: general clinical approach. In I. Rocker and K. Laurence, eds., *Fetoscopy,* pp 51–64. Amsterdam: Elsevier/North Holland.

Golbus, M. (1982). The current scope of antenatal diagnosis. *Hospital Practice* 17: 179–186.

Hilgartner, M., ed. (1976). *Progress in pediatric hematology oncology,* vol. 1. Littleton, Mass.: Publishing Sciences Group.

Venus, I. (1982). Personal communication regarding current techniques and results in detecting hemophilia by fetoscopy. Yale University School of Medicine, Department of Obstetrics and Gynecology, New Haven, Conn.

13

Counseling After Multiple Infant Deaths

Here is another situation in which the original diagnosis turned out to be erroneous. One might speculate that the professional staff who encounter a family which was previously misdiagnosed would be in for tough going, since confidence in the professionals would be undermined by the earlier experience. Further, in view of the fact that the new diagnosis carries a higher recurrence probability than the earlier diagnosis, one might speculate that the counselees would find the current counseling more distressing.

As this account will demonstrate, for the Greens this was not so. A major impact of the counseling was to enable Mrs. Green to redistribute her burden of ''responsibility'' for two infant deaths, with considerable benefit for the Greens' marital equilibrium.

Compare this situation with that of the Tafts, in the report on fetal alcohol syndrome; in that case an incorrect diagnosis (of Down syndrome) was also ruled out, but the impact of the correction was quite different.

Medically, the central issue of the report that follows was the differential diagnosis of achondroplasia versus other forms of congenital dwarfism. Infants affected with achondroplasia usually have large heads with prominent foreheads and depressed nasal bridges, disproportionately short limbs, and trident hands. It is an autosomal dominant condition, but when normal parents have an achondroplastic dwarf, it is considered to be a new mutation in the child. The parents' risk of recurrence will then be the same as that of anyone else in the general population, or about one in 12,000 births.

Achondroplasia is sometimes confused with other forms of short-limb dwarfism, one of which may be asphyxiating thoracic dystrophy. A baby so affected will have short limbs, a narrow thorax, and occasionally, polydactyly. The narrowness and immobility of the thorax usually

135

cause respiratory distress and death in early infancy, although some children do survive. Diagnosis of this condition is based upon X-ray findings, which reveal shortening of the ribs and abnormalities of the pelvis and long bones. Asphyxiating thoracic dystrophy is known to have an autosomal recessive pattern of inheritance.

Karen and David Green were a handsome couple of Jewish-American background in their mid-twenties, in excellent health. David worked as an accountant and Karen was employed as a teacher in a business school. They were not related; Karen's grandparents had come to this country from Eastern Europe, and David's family was of German extraction. When they were married six years previously, they had planned to have a large family, but their attempts to do so had been shadowed by tragedy.

Karen's first pregnancy, a year after their marriage, was normal and uneventful, but ended with a full-term, six-and-a-half-pound stillborn female. Autopsy revealed no abnormalities, and the death remained unexplained.

For a first pregnancy to conclude with a stillbirth is especially shattering to a mother. Doubt about one's capacity to carry and deliver a normal infant is not rare during girls' adolescence, and is related to all kinds of activities and inner feelings of that maturational period. Certainly such doubt is frequently encountered prior to or during a first pregnancy, when the outcome is yet to be known. The occurrence of the stillbirth underscores that variety of doubt, and leaves the mother more than slightly depressed and uneasy about her biological (reproductive) capacity. Naturally, there will be associated concern about the impact of reproductive catastrophe on husband and marriage.

When autopsy, as in this instance, fails to reveal an identifiable cause for the disaster, anxiety and doubt are compounded with expectable concern that the disaster may be repeated.

A few months later Karen conceived for the second time. The pregnancy began normally, but toward its conclusion high blood pressure and edema developed, together with a falling estriol level. For these reasons a cesarean section was done in the thirty-seventh week of gestation. The baby was a boy, whom his parents named Charles. He weighed four and a half pounds, was forty-six centimeters long, and had an Apgar score of 2–7. (A score of 9–10 would indicate a "good baby" with no problems.) He was noted to have disproportionately short limbs. By the second day the infant was in acute respiratory distress. Attempts to treat this condition failed, and he died the same day with a diagnosis of achondroplasia, respiratory distress, and cardiopulmonary arrest.

The new conception just a few months later raises the question of whether the Greens had permitted themselves opportunity to mourn the loss of their first baby before seeking the reassurance of a new, hopefully healthy infant. Although that pregnancy is reported initially to have been unremarkable, in these circumstances it is unimaginable that it could have occurred without considerable anxiety.

For the second pregnancy to conclude with neonatal fatality, after the initial stillbirth, seems almost too much to bear. Doubt concerning reproductive capacity has to be aggravated by such an experience.

A year after the death of the second baby the couple adopted a normal, healthy infant girl whom they named Debra. At about the time the adoption was made final, Karen accidentally became pregnant once more. She did not feel that she was emotionally ready to try again, and had the pregnancy terminated.

The choice to adopt seems thoroughly understandable in view of the Greens' strong desire for children, and expectation that in choosing an already existing child, prospects would be more favorable.

That Mrs. Green's new pregnancy was unwelcome is not surprising. Becoming a mother by adoption is emotionally demanding, without the advantage of the preliminary nine-month relationship with the baby in utero. Apparently the mourning for the little boy who so promptly died was not yet completed when the adoption and new conception occurred, so that pregnancy became an unallowable added burden.

When Debra was 2 years old, she became ill with leukemia, and she died at the age of 3.

The loss of this child occasioned fresh mourning, which probably revived the mourning for the two infants who had died earlier. The death of the adopted child retrospectively must have altered the Greens' attitude toward the elective abortion. After all, the discarded fetus might have been a normal child.

When Karen and David Green were referred for genetic counseling, it was a year after Debra's death. Karen's obstetrician had called first to inquire about procedure. I informed him that this was a satellite clinic associated with a university teaching hospital, and that the family would see me on their first visit and the medical geneticist on their subsequent visit or visits. He, in turn, said merely that he was referring a new patient of his who had given birth to an achondroplastic dwarf. He sounded as though he was in a great hurry, and volunteered no other information. I asked him to send me whatever medical records he had.

The next day, Karen Green called for an appointment for herself and her husband, and I was able to arrange one within the week. I described our procedure to her, explaining that a minimum of two visits was necessary, and that on the first visit I would take their family history and begin asembling their medical records. The telephone conversation was short and unremarkable.

A few days later they were seated in my office, their two chairs drawn up alongside my desk. With the door closed, the room was quiet and private. Settled in the chair closest to my desk, Karen seemed reserved and a trifle strained. David appeared warmer, but was content to sit back and let his wife do the talking.

I began the interview by asking if their obstetrician had discussed with them his reasons for referring them for genetic counseling. Karen explained that actually it was the other way around. She had asked him to send them to a center for genetic counseling. She said that after the birth of her son, Charles, it seemed as though no one in the hospital had had much time to talk to her. The Greens had been living in another state when he was born. A few months after his death they had moved to their present home, and they no longer had any contact with her previous doctor.

However, she had read several articles about genetic counseling in various magazines, and this had prompted her to ask her present doctor about it. He seemed to think it was a good idea, and had referred them to our center.

I asked if he had discussed the risk of recurrence of achondroplasia with them. She answered that he had said no one knew what caused it but it wouldn't happen again. However, he knew that she was nervous about another pregnancy, and so he had encouraged counseling.

In response to my questions, she described the results of her first two pregnancies—the stillbirth and the death of the dwarfed infant—in a flat, unemotional voice. At this point this was all that I knew of their family history. When I asked if there had been any other pregnancies, she hesitated, and then answered that they had adopted a daughter who died. For the first time her voice shook as she described the little girl's illness; her husband put his arm around her. Neither of them told me that she had undergone a third pregnancy which had been terminated.

Her story about Debra's death and her distress was extremely painful to me. Telling myself that I would return to it later, I changed the subject and began taking the family pedigree. I started with Karen, who had a large family. Although she herself was in good health, there was a strong family history of diabetes and heart disease. It took about forty-five minutes to do a careful pedigree.

David Green's family, in contrast, was small, healthy, and long-lived; it took only ten minutes to complete his pedigree.

> The poor family health history for Mrs. Green can alert us to anticipate that despite her own good health, she is likely to believe she is genetically loaded the wrong way.

I then explained that even though Karen had brought along her own medical records, we would have to have the hospital records of the first two babies. Karen was sitting closest to the desk; I asked her to sign the release forms.

She became agitated and upset, looked at me angrily, and said, "Why are you laying all the guilt on me?"

"Guilt? What guilt?" I asked, completely taken aback.

She pointed to the routine intake forms on my desk. "You put my name above my husband's; you asked about my relatives first; you took much more time with *my* family tree; and now you ask *me* to sign these releases."

I realized then that I had made a mistake earlier in the interview by changing the subject when she became upset. She had been ready then to tell me about her feelings, to describe in her own way what had happened to her, and her reactions to these events. Because her story was so painful to me, I had shied away from an opportunity. Perhaps the fact that I had retreated from the subject tended to confirm her own feelings of guilt. But before I tried to correct my mistake, some explanations were in order.

I explained that I always began a pedigree with the wife because not only will she know all about her own family, but she will often know more about her husband's relatives than he does. This had indeed been the case with the Greens. I told her that I had taken a lot of time with her family in the interests of thoroughness, even though the information we got might turn out to have no bearing at all on the main problem. And I had asked her to sign the forms because of where she was sitting. I had not suspected that all these details would appear so significant to her.

> Mrs. Green's agitation and accusation that the counselor is making her feel guilty are a psychological defense—denial coupled with projection: "It's *not* that *I* reproach myself as biologically inadequate; *you* are making me feel this way." The counselor, surprised, seeks successfully to mollify Mrs. Green and restore rapport. At the same time the counselor has learned of the burden of guilt and self-reproach Mrs. Green is carrying. Whether the earlier change of subject by the counselor was a "mistake" is debatable. The issue of guilt was bound to emerge.

I then broached the heart of the matter: "Why do you talk about guilt, Mrs. Green?"

"Because it's more my fault than my husband's!" she answered in a low voice. He sighed, shook his head, and said wearily, "No, it isn't."

I asked her what it was that she felt was her fault. She answered that the stillborn baby was perfectly formed and yet had died, so there must have been something wrong with her womb or her placenta. This defect, then, might have caused the second baby to be a dwarf.

"Did anyone at the hospital suggest genetic counseling to you after Charles was born?" I asked.

"No," she replied. Shortly after Charles's birth her obstetrician had come into her room in the hospital, while David was there, and informed them that the baby was a dwarf and might not live. They had a vague recollection that he had told them they could have normal babies in the future, but they had been so distraught at the time that neither of them could remember the conversation clearly. After the baby's death they had seen very little of the doctor, and soon thereafter had moved away. The nagging feeling remained with Karen, after two disastrous pregnancies, that she had some defect which prevented her from having a healthy baby.

She lowered her voice. "That is why," she said almost inaudibly, "I couldn't go through with my third pregnancy."

I asked, "Was there a third pregnancy?"

"Yes," she said. "Right after our adoption of Debra became final, I found out that I was pregnant. I was frightened—I wasn't ready—I couldn't bear to lose another baby. We decided that an abortion was the best solution. But what does an abortion have to do with genetic counseling?"

I replied that it didn't have anything to do with genetics, but it did help us to understand her feelings; and that was *very* important. I added that I understood why she had felt she was not ready for another pregnancy at that time.

Mrs. Green takes the major onus upon herself. It is striking that mothers, by virtue of being the host to the fetus for nine months, tend to take major responsibility for mishaps upon themselves regardless of the actual genetics in a situation. This is a fact of psychological observation.

The counselor's interest in the aborted third pregnancy underscores her concern about the Greens' total situation. This is conveyed especially with the empathic comment that she can understand why Mrs. Green had felt unready for another pregnancy. The rapport between counselor and counselee improves markedly at this juncture.

For the first time, Karen seemed to relax and let her defenses down. When she relaxed, so did her husband, who had been watching her with great concern. I asked him how he had felt at this period of their lives.

He answered that they had both been in bad shape since Charles's death; the birth of an abnormal child and the loss of a son had been a double blow. They had felt that things were changing for them when they obtained their baby girl, and the new pregnancy had been a threat. His main concern had been with his wife's happiness—he had thought that having the abortion was for the best.

I plunged in again: "It must have been difficult to recover from Debra's death." Karen began to weep, and David's eyes filled. We sat quietly for a few minutes, and then Karen began to speak. She described the ordeal of diagnosis, treatment, temporary remission, and final hospitalization a year ago. Her husband was holding her hand tightly. They looked young and vulnerable—it was hard to believe that they had gone through so much in only six years of marriage. Recently, she said, she had gotten a job teaching typing and shorthand in a business school, and going back to work had been a great help.

But, she continued, a job was not the answer for her. They still wanted a family, but they had to make a decision: whether to start the difficult process of adoption again or to attempt another pregnancy. They had been told that their chances of having another baby like Charles were small, but they were afraid. They felt that this decision was too difficult for them to make without assistance. They needed more help.

I explained that before we could talk about the risks involved in future pregnancies, we would have to see the baby's hospital records and X-rays in order to confirm the diagnosis of achondroplasia. I added that whatever the diagnosis, it had nothing to do with defects of the placenta or uterus, but I felt that Karen Green was by no means convinced.

We made plans for a return visit with the medical geneticist and myself after the records were received. We had spent about two hours together.

Three weeks later, Karen and David Green returned to the Genetics Clinic to meet with me and Dr. W., the medical geneticist. We had received the hospital records of the stillbirth, and the X-rays as well as records of the boy diagnosed as achondroplastic. This time the couple were open and friendly; the coolness and reserve were gone. However, both Dr. W. and I could sense their apprehension.

We began by trying to reassure Karen about herself. Fortunately, the records concerning the stillbirth included an examination of the placenta and cord, which indicated no pathology. The doctor showed the report to Karen, who seemed very pleased; her husband, as before, seemed only concerned about her reactions.

The next part, we thought, would be more difficult. The male infant, Charles, had been identified as achondroplastic at birth, but after

X-rays and autopsy the diagnosis had been changed to asphyxiating thoracic dystrophy. We ourselves had had the X-rays checked again by a pediatric radiologist, who had agreed with this diagnosis.

Karen Green's new obstetrician had never seen these records, nor had the couple ever been informed of the changed diagnosis. Although Karen and David had not had genetic counseling before, and their information was vague, we knew that they had been told that the risk of recurrence for achondroplasia was very small. Now we would have to explain recessive inheritance to them. We felt that we were going to give them very bad news.

We told them that, as sometimes happens, the initial diagnosis had been wrong, and had later been changed on the basis of the autopsy report and the X-ray findings. We stressed the fact that we had checked and rechecked the X-rays. We described asphyxiating thoracic dystrophy and explained recessive inheritance. By the Greens' questions we felt that they understood what a one-in-four chance meant.

David brought up the fact that Karen's obstetrician had said they wouldn't have another dwarf. We explained the difference between the two types of dwarfism and the meaning of "sporadic" inheritance in achondroplasia. If the original diagnosis had been correct, the risk of recurrence would have been virtually nil, as Karen's doctor had said. I watched Karen; she did not seem as crushed by this information as I had feared. I wondered if she really had understood. David appeared saddened, but he, too, was watching his wife.

She seemed to be mulling something over. "The baby got a bad gene from me and a bad gene from my husband; that means that his trouble came from *both* of us—isn't that right?"

It was David who answered her. "Yes, that's right!"

She looked as if a burden had been lifted from her shoulders. When she was convinced that she understood what we had been telling her, she tried to describe her feelings. She explained that even though her doctor had told her that no one knew the cause and that she would not have another dwarf, she had kept wondering why it had happened to her. She felt that there had to be some defect in her body that had caused her first baby to be stillborn and her second to be a dwarf. She had not been able to rid herself of a feeling of guilt. Now, at least, she could share some of this burden with her husband.

We asked him how he felt about this; he said he understood and could accept it, "especially if it helps my wife." He actually appeared relieved when he looked at her.

We discussed the options. Artificial insemination by donor was rejected immediately by both with finality. The possibility of another pregnancy was explored. They asked about prenatal diagnosis. We explained that although asphyxiating thoracic dystrophy could probably be diagnosed by X-ray or ultrasound toward the end of gestation, it could not be done early enough to terminate the pregnancy.

We discussed the fact that the child, if affected, would be likely to die in the neonatal period. The risk of having to care for a handicapped child for a prolonged period of time would be small. David interrupted: "No, the risk is too great. We couldn't go through that experience again." Karen nodded her head. "I couldn't bear to lose another baby," she said. "It helps to know that it's not because there is something wrong with me, but I'm not ready to take that kind of chance now. Perhaps in the future. . . ."

I noted without comment the fact that she did not consider the possession of a lethal recessive gene as "something wrong"; sharing the responsibility with her husband seemed to make all the difference.

Her husband noticed her reaction, too. He said, "I'm glad it turned out this way. Maybe life will be a little easier for us—for both of us—now."

They told us about friends of theirs who had adopted a child from South America. This was the course they had been considering; it seemed even more advisable now. They would keep in touch with us and let us know their decision.

Following their visit we sent them our customary letter reviewing the counseling session. A few months later we contacted them by telephone. Karen told us that they had started the process of adopting a Colombian child, and hoped to bring it to completion within a year. She sounded at peace with herself.

Further Comment

It is certainly difficult to imagine a more depressing series of circumstances. At the same time, this report attests to the strength of the young couple's desire for their own family—naturally or through adoption.

There is an ironic twist in the discovery that the original diagnosis was wrong. Based on that earlier diagnosis, the prediction of recurrence risk was very low. Yet Karen's sense of her own special responsibility for the disaster was irrationally high.

The correction of the diagnosis led to explanation of autosomal recessive inheritance, making plain the shared responsibility for the malformation by both parents. Karen—and, therefore, her husband—seemed somewhat relieved on learning this, even though it meant that the risk of recurrence was greater. We should, however, not be surprised if some guilt and self-reproach were to persist, since the early stillbirth remained unexplained.

Confronting the question of attempting another pregnancy, the

Greens commented, understandably, that for them the *possibility* of another wasted pregnancy was unallowable. They had already lost four children, if one counts the elective abortion in the total. For *another* couple, three chances in four to have a normal infant might be good odds. For the Greens, the odds for success were not high enough. The counselor's role in conveying risk data was to facilitate the Greens' making properly informed use of the information as they saw fit.

References

FILLY, R.; GOLBUS, M.; CAREY, J.; and HALL, J. (1981). Short-limbed dwarfism: ultrasonographic diagnosis by mensuration of fetal femoral length. *Radiology* 138: 653–656.

OBERKLAID, F.; DANKS, D.; MAYNE, V.; and CAMPBELL, P. (1977). Asphyxiating thoracic dysplasia. *Arch. Diseases of Children* 52: 758–765.

TAHERNIA, A., and STAMPS, P. (1977). "Jeune syndrome" (asphyxiating thoracic dystrophy), report of a case, a review of the literature, and an editor's commentary. *Clinical Pediatrics* 16: 903–908.

14

Genetic Counseling Within the Framework of Individual Cultural Needs: Orofaciodigital Syndrome Type I

Like the narrative set in Israel dealing with Duchenne muscular dystrophy (Chapter 8), here is another situation in which the specifics of the counselees' beliefs are decisive in regard to the option of elective abortion. In the situation reported here, involving an uneducated Spanish-speaking family, an added complication is the necessity to work through an interpreter.

The counselor for the Colimas draws them into the counseling process as far as the family will permit, at which point the interviews are discontinued. The manner in which the interviews have been conducted, however, develops a rapport which can be built upon in case of future need.

Orofaciodigital syndrome, type I (OFD I), is very rare; prevalence is estimated to be one in 50,000 in the general population. OFD I is an X-linked dominant disorder, lethal in males. Affected male fetuses will be spontaneously aborted early in pregnancy.

Females who are heterozygous for the mutant gene run a 50 percent risk of transmitting the affected gene in each pregnancy. Female offspring have a 50 percent risk of being affected. Affected females will express varying degrees of the syndrome, as explained by the Mary Lyon principle (see the Glossary).

It is highly unlikely for a female who is carrying the mutant gene for an X-linked dominant disorder to be completely asymptomatic. Penetrance is unknown, but assumed to be high. If the mother is not affected, the disorder is considered to be sporadic, the result of a new mutation.

Prevention is possible through prenatal diagnosis for sex determination. When the fetus has been identified as female, couples may elect therapeutic abortion.

OFD I is characterized by severe oral anomalies including cleft tongue, cleft palate, hyperplastic frenula, multiple dental problems, a broad nasal root, involvement of facial bones, and evanescent facial milia. Skeletal malformations include anomalies of the hands and feet. A variety of central nervous system disorders have been described. A basic biochemical defect has not as yet been identified, and life span is normal. Early and continuous treatment, including surgery, is required for frequently severe oral-cavity problems and related complex speech and hearing dysfunctions. In some cases, mental retardation further limits functioning.

Following the birth of a child with OFD I, evaluation of the mother for symptoms of the disorder is essential, and should be mandatory. Unfortunately, the mother in the current instance, Mrs. Colima, had not been so evaluated, and no genetic counseling had been provided. The Colimas' reproductive history is replete with failures of professional staff to provide genetic information adequate for family planning. These failures were exacerbated by the language barrier: This couple spoke virtually no English, so that all contacts required an interpreter's assistance.

Bella Colima, their first child, was born when Mrs. Colima was 21 years old and her husband was 24. (The couple are unrelated, and both are of Mexican descent.) Shortly following Bella's birth in a university hospital, the diagnosis of OFD I was made after consultation with the staff dermatologist. The family was then referred to the university's Craniofacial Center, where a multidisciplinary team provides comprehensive outpatient services. (The Craniofacial Center supplies management for speech, hearing, developmental, psychological, dental, surgical, dermatological, pediatric, and nutritional problems. The team includes a consultant medical geneticist and genetic counselor.) Alerted by the hospital's neonatologist, the center tried energetically but fruitlessly to establish contact with this couple, and they were lost to follow-up for two years.

At that point the family again came to university attention following the birth of their second child, Maria, who was also affected with OFD I. While still an obstetrical patient, Mrs. Colima was examined by a staff dermatologist, and predictably found to be mildly affected with the syndrome. She was found to have two hyperplastic frenula and large great toes. The next professional to enter this clinical problem was a pediatrician, who unfortunately provided incorrect genetic information. Although chromosomal anomalies are not known to be part of OFD I, chromosome examinations were ordered for this couple, further compounding the confusion.

Two months later, the cumulative effects of giving birth to two affected daughters, of having attention focused on her own symptoms, and of strongly suspecting ''bad blood'' were sufficiently disturbing to bring Mrs. Colima (and her husband) to the Craniofacial Center at last. These parents wished to learn ''why their daughters were born with these problems.''

On this visit, 2-year-old Bella was found to be developing within normal limits, as was Maria, now 2 months old. Both girls were relatively mildly affected with OFD I. Bella had a lobulated tongue, multiple frenula, and absent lateral incisors. She showed brachydactyly of her hands and feet and double halluces of her left foot. Her skin revealed petechial hemorrhages, and she had brittle hair. Speech development was within normal limits. Maria had a deeply grooved palate, midline pseudo-cleft of the upper lip, and multiple frenula. Brachydactyly of the hands and large great toes were present. Maria, too, had brittle hair and milia on her face and ears.

I approached the first genetic counseling interview with awareness that erroneous genetic information had been given to the Colimas and that Mrs. Colima was unquestionably affected with OFD I. I speculated that she might well feel guilty about having transmitted this defect to her daughters, or fear that her husband blamed her for the children's abnormalities.

I began our conversation by attempting to learn what Mr. and Mrs. Colima had been told about their daughters' problems, what they believed, and what concerned them most. I chose each word with great care. A problem developed immediately: Despite my meager knowledge of Spanish, I was able to determine that the interpreter was not translating me verbatim, and was also interjecting her own comments and personality. Instead of acting as an extension of me, the interpreter was usurping my position as the authoritative source of genetic information. Throughout this counseling session requests for verbatim translation were frequently ignored. Through the use of short words and phrases, I sought greater control of the interview, with only partial success. (This was the only interpreter available.)

For counselees to arrive at a proper genetic counseling facility with a narrative of earlier professional contacts of misleading, if not alarming, nature is unhappily too common. The expanding discipline of genetic counseling is now so complex that mastery of available knowledge requires full-time professional commitment.

The counselor's speculations concerning the inner mental state of the mother are in keeping with frequently observed trends.

Even when counselees have *not* had earlier professional consultation, it is well to inquire what their understanding of their problem is. Many have encountered comments in the popular press or heard things from friends and family that they have uncritically accepted as the truth about their own situation. What one expects to be told is a mélange of truth, distorted truth, and outright misinformation, which in summary describe just where the counselees are "at." Occasionally one must do a substantial amount of "cleaning up" of earlier misinformation before proceeding with new information.

Working with an interpreter is difficult. It would be best for the counselor to be bilingual, but failing this, she needs to work with a known and trusted interpreter who has been schooled to restrict himself to his assigned function.

At the beginning of the interview, Mr. Colima, an alert, intelligent man, was the spokesman for the couple. They did not touch each other, and Mrs. Colima's face was expressionless. She looked to her husband to respond to me. In his presence she spoke in monosyllables, nodding "yes" or "no," a common behavior among traditional Hispanic women. The couple believed that their "bad blood" explained their daughters' problems, although Mr. Colima thought his wife's oral-cavity problems might be associated. Mrs. Colima disagreed. "It was God's will," she said.

Mrs. Colima's denial of her role in the girls' anomalies suggests that the counselor's hunch about her guilt was probably correct.

When Mr. Colima was called from my office to assist with Maria's examination, I took advantage of his absence to speak with Mrs. Colima privately. It was important to build upon her strong religious faith to help explain the genetic facts. A shy, softspoken woman, Mrs. Colima was less passive and more communicative in her husband's absence. She calmly accepted the implications of her carrier status. In response to a direct question, Mrs. Colima urged me to tell her husband "the truth." "He will not blame me. It is God's will."

On Mr. Colima's return I explained that every female conceived would have a 50 percent chance of being affected and that a male carried to term would be unaffected. The mechanism of X-linked dominant inheritance was not explained. The availability of prenatal diagnosis for sex determination, and abortion was explained. Mr. and Mrs. Colima seemed to understand that only girls would be affected. Mr. Colima said they would consider abortion to avoid a third affected daughter and his wife concurred. Additional appointments for counseling were offered whenever the couple wished. They chose a return appointment six months afterward.

During the interim the Craniofacial Center acquired a new Spanish interpreter who translated verbatim and was sensitive to cultural differences and counseling dynamics.

I was unable to be present for the Colimas' second visit to the center, which was delayed until nine months after their first. Mr. Colima told the medical geneticist that Mrs. Colima would seek a tubal ligation as soon as possible, and Mrs. Colima nodded "yes." Interim birth control measures were stressed, since the couple was not using *any* birth control method.

When the situation was subsequently reviewed with me, I telephoned Mrs. Colima in order to discuss prenatal diagnosis and alternative birth control measures. I was concerned that Mr. and Mrs. Colima might not have understood their options and the irreversibility of tubal ligation. I was also concerned that Mrs. Colima, following cultural patterns, might be going along with her husband despite her own wishes.

Telephone communication, when a language barrier exists, is successfully accomplished by putting the interpreter on another extension in my office. Concentration on tone, inflection, timing, and content can be very helpful in ascertaining the client's state of mind even without visual contact. The following is a small portion of the telephone dialogue that took place.

MRS. COLIMA: My family in Mexico told me the pill drives women out of their mind.

G.C.: Do you believe this?

MRS. COLIMA: Yes!

G.C.: There are many stories and fears about the pill. There is nothing to show that it drives women out of their mind. Do you go to a doctor here that you have confidence in?

MRS. COLIMA: Yes.

G.C.: Can you talk to him about the pill and other methods of birth control?

MRS. COLIMA: I am going to the doctor's tomorrow and will talk to him.

It was important not to endanger my newly developing relationship with Mrs. Colima by strongly disagreeing with her comment on the pill. Encouraging her to speak with another medical professional in whom she already had confidence would hopefully provide her with accurate and acceptable information.

Strictly speaking, use of oral contraceptives may in certain women — a very low percentage of the total user group — produce mood changes of significance, especially depression. It is surely wiser to focus, as the counselor does, on the wisdom of a continuing relationship with a prescribing, monitoring physician.

Several weeks later a crisis developed. Mrs. Colima called to tell me she was pregnant. Her last normal menstrual period had occurred prior to the Colimas' second visit to the center. An immediate genetic counseling appointment was offered, but the Colimas elected to come several weeks later. She said she and her husband were interested in prenatal diagnosis and would consider abortion. Her voice sounded tentative, and again I had the impression that Mrs. Colima was going along with her husband's wishes. We had several other telephone conversations prior to the counseling session for prenatal diagnosis, giving me an opportunity to explore Mrs. Colima's feelings and offering her a chance to express them in her husband's absence. The following is drawn from the counseling session:

G.C.: Are you familiar with the words "sperm" and "egg"?
MR. AND MRS. COLIMA: Yes.
G.C.: What about the word "cell"?
MR. COLIMA: No.

This response is another of those important cues from counselees that they have no schooling to speak of in the facts of biology. It is hard at times for health professionals to keep this possibility clearly in mind, and to ask the essential question the counselor has posed here. Without this response for guidance, she might run the risk that counseling based on the missing knowledge of what a cell is would be wasted.

G.C: Let me try to explain. It is very difficult, so please tell me if you do not understand the way I explain it, and I will try to find a better way. [By shifting the burden of understanding from Mr. and Mrs. Colima to the difficult material and my own explanation, I hoped to help the couple feel less ignorant and more comfortable in asking questions. Mr. Colima in fact asked many questions during this session.]

G.C.: A man's hereditary messages are in the sperm in his body. During sex many sperm leave his body and enter his wife's body. If one sperm joins with an egg in the woman's body—and remember, the egg contains the woman's hereditary messages—a new life begins. The new baby begins and grows from the joining of the hereditary messages of the sperm and egg. [I selected the word "sex" from a number of other words that flashed through my mind, as it seemed direct, understandable, and hopefully unembarrassing to Mr. and Mrs. Colima and the interpreter.]

The counselor's tactful approach was plainly effective. Sometimes we are not so fortunate: Many counselees react to the interview experience with strong inner needs to respond affirmatively to questioning—whether they understand or not. Such false affirmations stem partly from the desire to appear intelligent. They are also meant to reassure the counselor of *her* wisdom, so that *she* will feel satisfaction in her professional role. Counselees want the counselor to be pleased with the interaction so that she will like them and continue to help. For obvious reasons one must be on guard against such "false positive" responses.

Mr. and Mrs. Colima did not understand this or several other explanations. Hoping to aid their understanding, I explained some basic facts about cells, chromosomes, and genes, using drawings and a magnifying glass to demonstrate that cells were so small that even the magnifying glass would not help us to see them. A much more powerful instrument, the microscope, did make it possible to see these tiny cells.

A coin was tossed to demonstrate probability. I concentrated on Mr. Colima in the hope that if he understood, he could explain it to his wife. Mr. Colima did grasp the basic points. However, as important as this understanding was, it was critical not to divert too much energy from the specific purpose of this counseling session: a discussion of Mr. and Mrs. Colima's current pregnancy and their option of using prenatal diagnosis.

Like the meaning of "cell," the concept of "probability" is basic to an understanding of risk. But the counselor keeps in mind that (1) top priority must go to planning for the ongoing pregnancy, and (2) there is a limit to the "dose" of new information that can usefully be conveyed to counselees at any one session. The dose varies from one counselee to another, and is not the same for one counselee at different sessions. Many factors affect a counselee's receptivity *on a particular day,* and only the conversational interaction between counselor and counselee reveals what the situation is for the period of time that they are together.

G.C.: How would you feel about having another little girl with this problem?

[Mrs. Colima looked at her husband and wrung her hands.]

Mr. Colima: It would be very difficult.

[Mrs. Colima was agitated. She looked nervously at her hands.]

G.C.: I understand. What part of the problem is most difficult?

Mr. Colima: The biggest problem with the older girl is we have been receiving all kinds of mental letters regarding mental problems.

G.C.: From whom?

Mr. Colima: Financial forms and income tax returns to help with the girls. All letters refer to a mental problem. I tear them up.

[Again, cultural and language barriers had led to misunderstanding.]

G.C.: Why do the letters bother you?

Mr. Colima: Why do the letters talk about mental problems? My girls are normal, play normal, talk. The oldest girl remembers everything—asks questions—she is bright.

G.C.: You are concerned because you think someone you don't know thinks your daughters have a mental problem, and we aren't telling you? There is no mention of mental problems in the girls' medical records.

Mr. Colima: Do you think that later on the girls will have mental problems? [Mr. Colima was very upset. This was the first time he had expressed his fears about mental retardation. Mrs. Colima remained expressionless, her eyes downcast.]

G.C.: I understand your concern and will try to answer your questions. The letters are from the Division of Services to Crippled Children (DSCC). They are routine, sent to everyone, not just your family. When you fill out the forms the DSCC will pay for your daughters' medical bills.

[In fact, Mr. Colima had not completed the forms, and the DSCC was not paying their medical expenses.]

G.C.: Your most important concern is how your daughters will do mentally. It is not possible to tell with very young children, with or without a problem, precisely how well they will do mentally. It takes time. When your daughters are older, we can test them to see how well they are progressing.

You know this disorder can be more or less serious. In the more serious form the people can have some slow mental development. They can be slightly or more severely retarded. In the less serious form, which is what Mrs. Colima has and what we believe your daughters have, severe mental retardation is not seen. The problem does not get worse with time.

Bella seemed to be progressing normally when we last saw her. Maria is still too young to evaluate. [Pause.] It is difficult, but we need to talk about how you would feel if you had another child with the problem.

Mr. Colima [with tears in his eyes]: We would feel even worse. I cannot find the words to tell you . . . it is going to be very difficult. The part of my wife that is affected doesn't bother her. No one in our family on both sides has any problems. [Mr. Colima's emotions had overwhelmed his understanding. He was having difficulty in accepting his daughter's problems, much less potential problems in his unborn child.]

G.C.: I understand that you feel badly about this . . . it hurts you. You want to know why this happened to you and not to anyone else. [Mr. Colima was relieved that I understood.]

G.C. [I now wanted to return to Mr. Colima's comment about no other problems in his family. It was important to avoid the impression of blaming his wife]: The same accident that happened to the two of you and your children could happen to any of us. It is an accident of nature. It doesn't mean there is anything wrong with you or that you did anything wrong.

Now that you know you have this special problem, would you like to take *active* steps to prevent it from happening again, Mrs. Colima?

MRS. COLIMA: The only thing I can tell you is that if God wants us to have children like this it is up to God.

G.C.: That's right. Why do you think God wants this?

[Mrs. Colima shrugs.]

G.C.: Do you feel God is singling you out to punish you for something you did?

MRS. COLIMA: No.

G.C.: You are right to feel this way. You are right, it is God's will.

MRS. COLIMA: What else!

G.C.: God has also helped scientists to develop this special test during early pregnancy. You can choose to use it.

The counselor, strictly speaking, does not need to tell Mrs. Colima that the latter is "right" to consider that her daughters' and her own hereditary difficulties are God's will. This is a matter of religious belief, and Mrs. Colima is a believer.

But the counselor does gain something through her comment: She acknowledges to the counselee the importance of religious belief in the latter's world view, and her respect for the counselee's belief. In so doing, the counselor enhances rapport with Mrs. Colima. Accepting this religious belief as one of the given parameters shaping the counseling situation, the counselor proceeds to indicate that God's will also directs human beings to learn how to help themselves.

However, the effort to shape the counseling interaction to the emotional and religious "set" of the counselees reaches a standstill over the issue of elective abortion.

MR. COLIMA: Does it [amniocentesis] mean [you can have] abortion to stop from having another girl with a problem?

G.C.: Yes, if you choose this. But it can also reassure you if the unborn baby is a boy.

The counselor is seeking to indicate that the use of amniocentesis goes beyond discovery of a female fetus.

In some instances, even if preliminary objection to potential abortion has been stated on religious grounds, counselee response to the knowledge that the fetus is female may be a surprise: Some suitable rationalization may be fashioned to permit religious proscriptions to be set aside.

MR. COLIMA: We are not going through with the test. We could not abort the baby and would only worry if it is a girl.
[Mr. and Mrs. Colima had understood prenatal diagnosis well enough to resolve their feelings about abortion prior to this counseling session. If there was a difference of opinion between them, it seemed Mrs. Colima had made the decision not to undergo prenatal diagnosis and possible abortion. I felt that Mr. Colima had not imposed his will on his wife. They would rely on luck and religious faith. Mr. and Mrs. Colima also had a support system in nearby family and friends.]
G.C.: We don't care which choice—[The interpreter interrupted me at this point and advised me not to use the word ''care'' in this context. The couple would think I didn't care about them.] We don't want to pressure you to choose the test. We care very much about you and your daughters.

Since the last visit I have telephoned the Colimas every week or so to reassure them of our interest and to learn how things are going. Mrs. Colima seems to feel calm and well. In an early phone call they were referred to an appropriate service for obstetric and prenatal care.

It is worth mentioning that during the months of counseling Mrs. Colima had been alerted that her sisters, like herself, might be affected and face similar problems with children. We expressed a willingness to see any relatives living in the area who would want to come in. She agreed to inform her sisters in the area, and we provided Mrs. Colima with a letter written in Spanish giving all pertinent information. This letter was to be forwarded to the sisters living in Mexico. To date we have not heard from others in this family.

This case illustrates some of the difficulties encountered in counseling an uneducated, non-English-speaking couple. The counseling would have been ineffectual if not modified in consideration of this family's specific needs. An important component in my approach was the utilization of the Colimas' cultural and religious beliefs to reinforce the genetic information given and the understanding achieved. Any effort to change or devalue these beliefs would have risked losing their confidence and trust, which was won slowly over many months.

The fine quality and sensitivity of the Spanish interpreter was pivotal to the counseling dynamics.

While Mr. Colima assumed his cultural role of masculine domination during the joint sessions, my private discussion with Mrs. Colima at the first counseling session and our numerous telephone conversations provided opportunity for her to express herself during her husband's absence. During these conversations I avoided suggesting to Mrs. Colima that she might disagree with her husband. Rather, I encouraged her to express her own feelings, which she was sometimes reluctant to do. This technique enabled me to acquire a better understanding of the feelings of both spouses without provoking a direct confrontation between them. It would have been a grave mistake to risk disturbing an intact relationship at a time of severe family stress.

While these discussions were going on, the Colimas privately effected a resolution of the questions of prenatal diagnosis and abortion. Their ability to work out this resolution for themselves is an indication of strength in their marriage.

Along with others we have been dismayed at the attitude of some medical professionals and genetic counselors who consider that genetic counseling in not suitable for uneducated people because they are incapable of comprehending biological information. The broader lesson of this case study is that uneducated people of lower socioeconomic background most certainly can learn and benefit from genetic counseling provided the level of discourse is tailored for their needs.

Further Comment

In recent years there have been changes in the makeup of the professional staffs of medical centers, tending toward greater ethnic diversity. But for a long time staffs tended to be of a fairly homogeneous middle-class white origin. Clearly, professionals of all origin will find it easiest and most natural to work with patients of similar background. To be confronted with patients of a different cultural origin poses an immediate challenge.

Within living memory there have been many medical center personnel who took the attitude that medical centers were really suitable only for those who had taken the trouble to master English, and who knew how to interact with health professionals. We now consider that it is part of the professional's task to make his or her knowledge available to the largest number of patients; and if in some instances that requires working through language and cultural barriers, so be it.

Considering the counselor's behavior with this couple, we would probably agree that the preservation of rapport remained more important than other counseling goals. There may be future need for special additional assistance with either of the two daughters or with the next child, should it also be an affected girl. The problem of contraception—now in abeyance—will again need to be considered. Despite their religious background, the Colimas may be more accessible to birth control through contraception than through abortion.

References

DOEGE, T., et al. (1968). Mental retardation and dermatoglyphics in a family with the oral-facial-digital syndrome. *Am. J. Dis. Children* 116: 615–622.

GORLIN, R. (1968). The oral-facial-digital syndrome. *Cutis* 4: 1345–1349.

———; PINDBORG, J.; and COHEN, M., (1976). Oral-facial-digital syndrome I. In R. Gorlin and J. Pindborg, eds., *Syndromes of the head and neck*, 2nd ed., pp. 562–567. New York: McGraw-Hill.

SUE, D. (1981). *Counseling the culturally different.* New York: John Wiley & Sons.

15

A Young Married Woman Discovers That She Has XO and XY Cell Lines: 45,XO/46,XY Mosaicism

The presence of male chromosomes in a phenotypic female, (a person whose appearance is female), is plainly a counseling challenge demanding the utmost tact. In the situation to be detailed, the particular pathway followed in the counseling is indicated by the young woman who presents herself to ask simple, direct questions: Can she have a family? Can she be helped to have menstrual periods? Will she develop into a man?

How these questions are dealt with to satisfy the counselee's need for information, and how the recommendation for prophylactic surgery is conveyed, constitute the essence of this difficult interaction.

The clinical expression of 45,XO/46,XY mosaicism ranges over a wide spectrum. Individuals may manifest female or male phenotypes, typical Turner syndrome or some stigmata thereof, bilateral streak gonads, mixed gonadal dysgenesis, bilateral undescended testes, no gonads and hypospadias. Virtually all individuals have a uterus, and 80 percent have ambiguous external genitalia.

In XO/XY mosaicism, tumors composed of gonadal tissue occur with high frequency. To avoid the risk of malignancy prophylactic surgery is recommended. Masculinization *may* occur at puberty *or* in the presence of a gonadal tumor. Phenotypical females with XO/XY mosaicism may benefit from hormone therapy. XO/XY mosaicism is not familial.

Phenotypic females who have a 46,XY karyotype may have complete or incomplete androgen insensitivity syndrome, both of which are inherited as X-linked recessive disorders but thought to be separate genetic entities. No uterus is found in either syndrome. Surgery to remove potentially malignant testicular tissue is advised for both syndromes but the recommended timing for the surgeries differs. Because tumors rarely develop in the complete form of androgen insensitivity syndrome prior to age 20, *and* masculinization does *not* occur, surgery is postponed until after puberty to allow testicular hormones the additional time to promote development of female secondary sexual characteristics. In the incomplete form, masculinization at puberty is to be *expected,* making prepubertal surgery advisable. Hormone therapy follows.

Distinguishing between these three clinical entities is critical for genetic counseling.

The clinical situation to be described is that of a 27-year-old woman whose physical findings were typical of Turner syndrome: short stature, infantile uterus, and bilateral streak gonads. She had been referred to our clinic, however, not with the diagnosis of Turner syndrome (45,XO), but with the finding of a 46,XY karyotype in peripheral blood cells. A later chromosome analysis revealed XO/XY mosaicism.

The counselee, Ann Gray, was referred to our genetics clinic by her gynecologist, Dr. A. Although most of our patients are referred by their physicians, usually the patient telephones for an appointment. In Ann's case the appointment was obtained by Dr. A.'s secretary, who informed me that she was being referred because "She is a 46,XY and the doctor requests that we repeat the chromosome study and counsel Ann."

When patients arrive at our clinic, the secretary requests routine information, makes them comfortable, and then escorts them to one of our consulting rooms to await the counselor.

These rooms are purposely furnished to be nonclinical in appearance. There are sofas, comfortable chairs, coffee tables, pictures, and so on. No one on the clinic staff wears a white coat. Our objective is to provide a relaxed, comfortable setting.

When I first met Ann, she was already seated in a counseling room. I introduced myself, and we spoke briefly about the difficulty she had had locating our offices. My first impression of her was that she was a delightful young woman, short, overweight, looking somewhat younger than her actual age.

Our initial conversation included the following:

G.C.: What is your understanding of why Dr. A. referred you to us?
ANN: Because I asked him to.
G.C.: Oh?
ANN: I read about girls with boy chromosomes and I don't think that fits me.

This is a startling bit of dialogue. Contrary to our expectation that such a genetic difficulty must be experienced by the counselee as catastrophic, this counselee speaks about the problem in a matter-of-fact manner. She is, of course, by no means unconcerned, as the vigor of her disagreement with her prior source of information testifies. It is also rather plain that she regards herself—and has been regarded throughout her life—as unequivocally female.

G.C.: What have you read?

ANN: I am in nursing school, and the textbook says that girls with boy chromosomes are *not* short, and I *am* short.

G.C.: What else did the book say?

ANN: I don't remember exactly. I guess I didn't understand most of it. I just don't think it fits me. I asked Dr. A. to do the test again. Are you going to repeat it?

G.C.: Yes, of course.

ANN: Good.

G.C.: First I would like to ask you some questions about your family and past medical history; then we will draw some blood for the chromosome test. Is that okay?

ANN: Sure.

G.C.: Tell me something about why you went to Dr. A. and why he did a chromosome test.

ANN: Well, you see, not long ago I went to the doctor to get birth control pills so that I could have periods and become pregnant. We have been married for three years, and next month I will be finished with nursing school and we want to start a family.

G.C.: You wanted birth control pills so that you could become pregnant?

ANN: Yes. I don't have periods unless I take pills.

Ann went on to explain that when she was 14, her older sister took her to a pediatrician because she had not yet developed secondary sex characteristics, nor had she started having menstrual periods. The physician gave her some pills, which in retrospect she assumes were birth control pills. She was told that the pills would help her to develop and "make her grow." She continued taking the pills for about ten years, grew a few inches (she is presently fifty-seven inches tall), developed minimal secondary sexual characteristics, and had regular periods. Ann stopped taking the pills when she married, believing that this would stop her periods and thus prevent her from becoming pregnant.

Ann provided considerable additional information about her family and her early circumstances. Youngest of four children, Ann had been surrendered for adoption at birth by her mother. Her adoptive father was her maternal grandmother's brother—her granduncle. Ann's actual parents were both still living, but she did not know her father and had met her mother only once just two years previously. All these details Ann learned from her adoptive father.

Ann had two sisters and a brother whom she doesn't see. These siblings are of average height, as Ann's parents were also reported to be. Menarche for the two sisters occurred at ages 12 and 13, and both sisters have normal children.

. Ann's mother was described as an only child. The adoptive father was unaware of any infertile females, short stature, or instances of gonadal malignancy in their family.

G.C.: So one month ago when you went to your local doctor for birth control pills, he examined you and did a chromosome study?

ANN: Yes, and after he told me the result, that I had boy chromosomes, I asked him to send me to a specialist.

G.C.: I see. So then you went to Dr. A., who is a gynecologist. What did he do?

ANN: He did some other tests.

G.C.: What tests were those?

ANN: I don't know. He tried to explain them to me. He said they were too high. I don't really understand.

[I assumed at this point, and it was later confirmed by Dr. A.'s medical records, that he had tested Ann's levels of follicle-stimulating and luteinizing hormones. These levels were increased, indicating ovarian failure. The discussion with Ann regarding these tests—and more specifically, regarding her purpose in requesting birth control pills—indicated to me that her ability or desire to understand normal reproductive physiology was limited.]

G.C.: I know that you and Dr. A. want the chromosome test repeated, and we will do that. But what is it that *most* concerns you?

ANN [after a long pause]: I don't think that I can accept the fact that I can't have a family. [Silence; then, lowering her eyes, she spoke softly.] Am I going to become a man?

G.C.: Oh, no, Ann. [Pause.] I can understand that you have been awfully worried about that.

Ann's understanding of the physiology of reproduction may be patchy, but she does have some grasp of the relationship between chromosomal makeup and sex determination. Her description of a major worry evoked by the cataclysmic disclosure of her karyotype could hardly be more direct.

[Ann nodded her head and after a few moments looked up, her eyes brimming with tears.]

G.C.: What are you thinking about that is making you cry?

ANN: I have wanted so very much to ask that question ever since they told me I had boy chromosomes . . . and I have been so afraid to ask.

G.C.: Afraid to ask that question or afraid of the answer?

ANN: Both.

Confronted by a counselee who is weeping, many professionals will either assume they know what has occasioned the tearfulness or will be inhibited about inquiring for fear of prolonging and/or aggravating the weeping. These professionals anticipate feeling guilty because of such an imagined sequel to their question.

This counselor, however, suffers no such inhibition; in keeping with the ambiguous meaning of weeping, the counselor has inquired about the stimulus. The outcome is very useful, the reply placing the counselor in a much more advantageous position to be of help to Ann.

We talked at some length about Ann's fears of suddenly masculinizing. She had not noticed any changes to justify this concern, but the chromosome test results were reason enough for such alarm. I explained to Ann that sometimes people who have male chromosomes do not develop as boys because the Y chromosome either does not work properly or because it is not present in sufficient numbers.

During our discussion I indicated to her that girls who have Y chromosomes may have a higher chance for tumors to develop in their ovaries, and because of this, the ovarian tissue very often needs to be removed as a precautionary measure.

ANN: But what about having a family?

G.C.: Until we repeat the chromosome test, we just don't know what is going on. It may turn out that you will have your family by adoption.

ANN: I was adopted, too.

Until this point in the conversation Ann had not mentioned her husband. I asked her how he felt about what had happened so far. She thought that she was far more concerned than he was about having children. Ann didn't think that Frank would have serious objections to adoption.

I drew a blood sample from Ann's finger and talked about how difficult the next two weeks would be while she waited for the results of the test.

The cytogenetics laboratory reported that Ann, indeed, did have a

46,XY cell line and, in addition, a 45,XO cell line. I met with the clinic's medical director to review the facts of Ann's situation prior to the second counseling session, which he was slated to attend. I explained to Dr. M. that she was already aware of the XY cell line, although she was probably hoping that a mistake had been made. We discussed Ann's fears of becoming masculine, as well as her deep concern that she might not be capable of bearing children. I alerted Dr. M. to my impression that Ann's understanding of female reproductive physiology was limited.

At the second clinic visit I introduced Ann to Dr. M. She seemed to be more at ease than she had at our first meeting. Dr. M. told her that the chromosome report indicated there were *two* different cell groups in her body: one group, which she was already aware of, the XY cells; and the other, a group of cells that had only one X chromosome and *no* Y chromosome at all.

ANN: Does that mean that I can't have children?
DR. M.: It means that you can have your children by adoption.

To an outsider Dr. M.'s reply may register as "fancy footwork" with words. It is a statement of the truth, is framed from the vantage point of Ann's known concern for having her own family, and is doubtless knowingly stated this way to emphasize the positive side of the situation. As such, it is a very skillful response from a psychological point of view.

Dr. M. explained to Ann that she was clearly a woman despite the fact that she had some cells with Y chromosomes. He told her he suspected that her ovaries had not developed normally, and that additional studies would be advisable to exclude the possibility of malignant changes in her ovaries.

I asked Ann if she had read anything about Turner syndrome in her nursing texts. She said she had, and thought her situation fitted that description very closely. Dr. M. agreed with Ann's diagnosis, since she does have an XO cell line. He explained that Turner syndrome women or girls have three basic problems: short stature, ovarian underdevelopment, and, in some cases, heart disorders. Dr. M. reassured Ann that she was fortunate not to have a heart disorder, and once again he emphasized that she could plan to have her family by adoption. He added that girls who learn they have Y chromosomes in their cells would naturally be concerned about masculinizing. Looking directly at Ann, Dr. M. inquired if she were worried about this. Ann answered that she had been *very* worried before she had discussed her fears with me, but was somewhat relieved about it now.

Ann told us that her gynecologist was waiting for the results of the chromosome test before deciding what to do next. We assured her that we would convey the karyotype report to him immediately. Dr. M. mentioned the probability of Dr. A.'s wanting to perform a laparoscopy study and asked Ann if she understood what a laparoscopy was. She nodded affirmatively, and said that Dr. A. had already discussed laparoscopy with her. We told her that the laparoscopy would provide us with gonadal tissue which we would send to the cytogenetics laboratory for additional chromosome analysis. When these results were available, we would invite her for another counseling session.

Approximately one month later Ann's gynecologist performed a laparoscopy, and obtained a piece of gonadal tissue for biopsy and chromosome analysis. Dr. A.'s report to us following the laparoscopy indicated the presence of streak gonads and an infantile uterus. Two weeks later the karyotype report was ready, again with the finding of XO/XY mosaicism, the greater percentage of cells being XO.

Our third meeting with Ann took place seven weeks after the second. This time we had our first opportunity to meet Ann's husband, Frank. We explained the results of the ovarian chromosome analysis, pointing out the preponderance of XO cells. We added that the presence of even a very few Y chromosomes in ovarian tissue called for the removal of all gonadal tissue in order to prevent the development of a tumor. Dr. M. reassured Ann that she need have *no* further fears regarding masculinization since she was well past puberty, which was the developmental stage when these changes might possibly arise. He added that the gonadectomy, which would eliminate the possibility of a proliferation of Y-bearing cells in the gonads, was additional insurance against masculinization and malignancy.

For a young woman who has come for counseling concerning childbearing to learn through the consultations that not only will she be unable to have her own biological children, but she must undergo a laparotomy for removal of gonadal tissue, is more than a bit much. The important recommendation for removal of the gonadal tissue has now been made for the third time, with the buttressing of the laparoscopy findings. During this period of time Ann has had the opportunity to get used to the idea, and is therefore better prepared to accept the definitive recommendation.

I again reviewed the information about Turner syndrome, indicating that it really was not so uncommon and that a great deal was known about it. I suggested that Dr. A. could provide hormone replacement in the form of medication for Ann so that she could have a period and maintain adequate hormone levels. Again we stated that she and Frank could choose to have their family by adoption. I asked Ann how she felt about adoption. She answered by saying that she and Frank had already discussed this possibility. She went on to say that even before there was any suggestion of the possibility of adopting, she had sometimes thought that maybe her own adoption was meant to be a preparation of some kind for the adoption of her own children. I reminded her that she initially had said that she was not yet prepared to *not* be able to have a family. Ann replied, "But you never told me that I couldn't have a family; you said I *could* have my family by adoption."

Frank appeared to be very supportive of Ann and gave the impression that her well-being was paramount to him—more important than her ability to bear children.

We asked if either of them had questions about Turner syndrome or about any of the information they had been given. Ann responded by saying that she realized there was probably a very long, involved medical explanation which we would be able to share with her, but at the present time she was very content with the way things were. She didn't think that a medical explanation would improve matters. As long as the door was open for her to return to us for additional information, she was satisfied.

This exchange provides an excellent illustration of how a skilled counselor governs her behavior with the guidance of the counselee's level of curiosity at the moment. Knowing that Ann is a nursing school student, the counselor might have assumed that she desired a fully detailed medical explanation of her situation. Foremost, however, Ann is a counselee, and her student nurse's curiosity is clearly secondary. Ann has indicated that the dose of information she is contending with is quite sufficient for the time being. A less sophisticated professional with a private agenda of information to convey might have bombarded Ann with more than she could digest. In the latter instance any patient would be likely to listen politely, and either become confused or at some point "turn off" and simply not hear the rest.

Overall I was fairly comfortable with the progression and resolution of Ann's counseling. At first, however, I was a little uncomfortable about the fact that we never did give her what I would consider an "adequate" explanation of mosaicism. Had we been able to do so, we would have explained normal and abnormal cell division and chromosome distribution which takes place after fertilization. Ann's unqualified request that we limit our medical explanation deserved to be respected. Our obligation at this point was fulfilled. We had supplied her with a correct diagnosis, paved the way for therapy, allayed her fears regarding masculinization, and presented her with the option of adopting her family.

Further Comment

Ann has been confronted with the frustrating news that her family will need to be an adopted one. That Ann herself was adopted may turn out to be a most helpful fact, making adoption a legitimate and acceptable option—especially if her experience with her adoptive parents was particularly good. At the present time, however, it is unfortunately difficult to exercise this option because there are few babies available through regular channels.

Ann's husband may be less concerned about having children than she for several reasons. One obvious difference between the two on the issue of family planning is that the exclusion of natural parentage for *him* does not occur through a physical incapacity of his, but is imposed from without by hers. His emotional support for her is a huge plus, assisting her in digesting all the distressing news. His response in the face of this rigorous cha'`enge suggests strength in their marital bond.

It is the writer's impression that situations involving clients of ambiguous sex are experienced by many counselors as particularly trying. The counselee is often a young woman with abnormal development and/or problems related to reproduction. For some counselors the information that the patient's difficulties arise from being genetically male (or both male and female) is "dynamite."

The counselor may experience guilt in anticipation of expected dismay on the part of the counselee when she receives this information. Occasionally the counselor may experience the news as a dreadful "secret," feel guilt about possessing such a secret, and sense an urge to blurt out the news like a confession, before weighing the best style in which to proceed. Such urges need to be restrained in order to be able to offer the most useful perspective.

Yet, as this narrative illustrates, it doesn't need to be so difficult an interaction. Ann's gender identity was established—as is usual for all of us—early in life. The consistent nurturing of Ann by her parents and others as a girl has led her to unambiguously experience herself as feminine.

To inform her that she is a woman with some male chromosomes acknowledges her identity as a woman, which will persist no matter what. Some writers suggest (see, for example, Rimoin and Schimke, 1971), that it may be equally suitable to tell such a woman counselee that her ovaries did not develop properly.

References

MONEY, J., and EHRHARDT, A. (1972). *Man and woman, boy and girl.* Baltimore: Johns Hopkins University Press.

RIMOIN, D., and SCHIMKE, R. (1971). *Genetic disorders of the endocrine glands.* St. Louis: C. V. Mosby. Co.

YUNIS, J. (1977). *New chromosome syndromes.* New York: Academic Press.

16

Counseling with Unexpected Disclosure

The highlight of this counseling report is the unexpected disclosure of an important piece of information by the husband. The impact of this disclosure upon the wife and the counselor, and the subsequent course of the counseling, is detailed.

Fred and Maria Jamar came to the United States from Colombia, South America, for the explicit purpose of obtaining a genetic evaluation. They presented themselves without an appointment at the admitting office of our Medical Center, requesting genetic counseling services. I arranged to see them that very day in consideration of their need to return to Colombia within three days.

Four months prior to this visit the Jamars had electively terminated a pregnancy at six months' gestation as a consequence of ultrasonographic studies which had revealed fetal demise. Autopsy findings were a two-pound, eight-ounce achondroplastic dwarf. The Jamars' physician recommended that the parents undergo chromosome studies.

Both Fred, age 30, and Maria, age 27, are of normal stature. They are well dressed, and speak and understand English very well. Fred is a civil engineer, Maria a housewife. Both are well educated and belong to the upper socioeconomic stratum of Colombian society. Their first child, a daughter, is a healthy 2-year-old. The second pregnancy occurred fourteen months after she was born. Maria was not pregnant at the time of this consultation visit.

This case was selected for inclusion in this book because of special problems: (1) There is a need for immediate counseling, with minimal follow-up opportunity. (2) An incorrect diagnosis is possible. (3) Tests recommended by the referring personal physician are not applicable. (4) Important concealed information is revealed by one spouse to the other only during the counseling process.

The couple's anxiety became apparent early in the session. This is not surprising, as almost all genetic counseling is motivated by some anxiety-provoking situation. Maria and Fred expressed great concern about having conceived one child with achondroplasia and about possibly conceiving another. I explained that if the diagnosis was correct, the risk of recurrence was extremely low, since achondroplasia is inherited as an autosomal dominant disorder and neither parent was affected. Where inheritance is ruled out, the occurrence of achondroplasia is thought to be sporadic. The literature indicates that sporadic occurrence is often associated with achondroplasia.

Since the pathology report had not ruled out thanatophoric dwarfism, I felt obligated to mention that the autopsy diagnosis of the stillborn child might have been incorrect. While some investigators now believe that an accurately diagnosed case of thanatophoric dwarfism represents a sporadic occurrence, others maintain that this disorder is inherited in an autosomal recessive pattern. If sporadic, the recurrence risk is negligible; if autosomal recessive, the recurrence risk is 25 percent.

A detailed family history did not reveal any significant findings relating to the present problem, or indeed, any other genetic disorder which would suggest the necessity for chromosome evaluation. In deference to the specific recommendation by the Jamars' Colombian physician, I felt obliged to honor Fred and Maria's request for chromosome studies. I was very careful to indicate that the types of dwarfism with which they were concerned were disorders whose causes could not be revealed by a karyotype. The taking of peripheral blood for chromosome studies was arranged for the following day in a deliberate effort to have the Jamars return for a second visit. In addition, I explained that our medical geneticists would review the pathology reports before this visit in an attempt to formulate a definitive diagnosis.

After I had spent almost two hours with this couple, Maria asked me what the risks would be for having another child with other abnormalities. This kind of question is not unusual. Patients often refer to friends or acquaintances who have children with Down syndrome, clefts, mental retardation, or other defects. I asked Maria if she was especially concerned about any particular disorder. She then referred to a friend of hers who had given birth to an anencephalic child. I informed her that without any significant family history of such abnormality she and Fred would have no greater risk for this disorder than any couple in the general population. We concluded the session at this point.

Counselees vary in their capacity for instant assimilation of even the most adroitly framed explanations. In a first interview, factual material indicating potential family-planning difficulties must be respected as possibly evocative of strong, conflicting emotions, which may interfere with ability to grasp new information. The counselor can utilize a second visit for multiple purposes, including the clarification of any uncertainty in the counselees' grasp of the previous counseling interview.

Following this meeting I could not shake off the feeling that there was more to this couple's misfortunes than they had cared to admit. My impression stemmed from nothing that was specifically stated, but from things that were left unsaid. I was glad to have a second opportunity to explore further the Jamars' problem and to reexplain the two implicated hereditary patterns if the diagnosis was still regarded to be ambiguous.

I planned to speak with each member of this couple privately, and then together, in an effort to obtain additional information for fuller understanding of their problem.

There is often great value in having private conversation with each spouse, as disclosures may be made that are inhibited by the presence in the room of the other spouse.

The Jamars returned the following morning, one and a half hours late for their appointment, very apologetic and very agitated. I began this meeting by reviewing our discussion of the preceding day. I then asked if they had questions concerning any aspect of our earlier discussion, or any other consideration, that had not been discussed.

After a moment of silence Fred began to speak. (He had been particularly quiet the previous day.) He stated that for the sake of his wife and future children, he had made a confession to Maria early that morning which he knew was important to discuss in my office. He had had an extramarital affair with a woman who had become pregnant and given birth to an anencephalic, stillborn child six months before the birth of Fred and Maria's dwarf stillborn. Maria had apparently suspected that this anencephalic child was Fred's, precipitating her inquiry on the previous day about just such an abnormality.

It obviously had taken a great deal of courage for Fred to make this admission to Maria, partly because of his infidelity and especially because he had fathered two defective children with two different women. Maria, he believed, would now have a firm basis for justifiably placing the responsibility for their defective child squarely upon his shoulders.

It was then necessary for me to explain the genetics of a third disorder with a completely different pattern of inheritance and entirely different ramifications. The fact that the anencephalic child was Fred's but not Maria's placed the couple at greater risk of recurrence than couples with no history of a neural tube defect, but at less risk than parents of an anencephalic child. Prenatal diagnosis using ultrasonography and amniocentesis for alpha-fetoprotein assay was recommended for any future pregnancy of the Jamars in order to detect open neural tube defects.

At this point in our discussion, I decided to speak to Maria and Fred individually. I looked to the private interviews for better assessment of attitudes toward future pregnancies and the integrity of the marriage itself.

I spoke with each spouse individually for approximately twenty minutes. Maria was first. She admitted that she had suspected her husband of fathering the anencephalic child, and this suspicion had generated fear of having a similar baby from the very beginning of her own terminated pregnancy. She had been unable to confide this fear to her husband. The fact that she gave birth to an anomalous child compounded all the issues involved.

Fred indicated his deep feelings for Maria, and fought hard to control his emotions while speaking to me privately. He had not wanted to hurt and frighten his wife by admitting paternity of another woman's defective child. He appreciated, however, that it was necessary to make this disclosure for the purpose of obtaining an accurate genetic assessment. Neither Maria nor Fred were considering separation or divorce, and both very definitely wanted to have another child. Each stated this individually without any hesitation.

An additional issue to be underscored concerning this couple is their particular cultural background. In Latin America men do not generally confide in their wives, and wives do not question their husbands. (I have learned this from many couples of similar background.) A husband's extramarital affairs are fairly commonplace. Both of these facts played a definite role in all that transpired before and during the visits to my office. The fact that Fred was able to discuss very personal features of his life situation with Maria and me was a significant step for him to take. Maria was cognizant of this atypical behavior. She stated that she was brought up in a society where a strict code of behavior was adhered to from early childhood. The woman's role was to serve her husband and bear his children. Overtly to question her husband's actions was unthinkable.

Unfortunately, the pathology report that the Jamars brought did not enable our department to provide a definitive diagnosis for their stillborn child.

Maria and Fred would need much more time to integrate all the information they had been given, to heal the still-open wounds created by the birth of their defective baby and the recently admitted infidelity. I promised to send them a written summary of the genetic counseling given. This letter included a complete explanation of the inheritance and recurrence risks of achondroplastic and thanatophoric dwarfism and anencephaly; chromosome study results; and the use of ultrasonography and amniocentesis for alpha-fetoprotein assays.

Such a letter can be very valuable, and should be written by the specific person who conducted the counseling and who therefore is best attuned to the counseled couple's frame of mind. Having the facts on paper so that reference can be made to them as often as needed permits the couple to digest the information at their own pace. A written record greatly facilitates correction of distorted recall.

My intuitive reaction to this couple was based upon earlier counseling experience. Pursuing my intuitive response had often been fruitful in the past, and made me bolder in this regard. It is not unusual for a couple to talk for two hours and then make a statement, such as Maria's comment on anencephaly, which suggests that important information is perhaps being withheld. While every remark cannot be regarded as having deeper significance, it is worthwhile to be alert to subtle clues such as facial expression, posture, and tone of voice. Such additional information may be among the most important items conveyed to the counselor.

Further Comment

This case offers a remarkably succinct illustration of the stresses that may suddenly confront the genetic counselor and the entire genetic diagnostic team. First, the counselor is dealing with a couple from a quite different cultural setting, although fortunately, in this instance, they are able to speak and understand English very well. Second, the entire counseling interaction must be compressed into a very brief span of time, involving logistical problems in getting hold of relevant documents, and problems conveying new information in dosages that can be assimilated by the counselees. And third, in the middle of it all, an important piece of new information is introduced that requires some prompt "gear shifting" by the counselor to recast the substantive information she will convey.

It must also be apparent to the reader that the professional counselor has to remain undisturbed by any private value judgments concerning the new information, in this example a report of marital infidelity. The range of startling disclosures that experienced counselors encounter is very considerable, though this fact in itself ought not to be surprising, considering that genetic counseling deals with the most private of private matters.

Although initially the counseling focused upon recurrence risks for dwarfism, the unexpected disclosure led to consideration of neural tube defects and the possibility of prenatal diagnosis to detect such problems.

References

RIMOIN, D., ed. (1976). Skeletal dysplasias. *Clinical Orthopedics* 114: 2–179.

SILLENCE, D.; RIMOIN, D.; and LACHMANN, R. (1978). Neonatal dwarfism. In M. Kaback, ed., *Pediatric clinics of North America,* vol. 25, pp. 453–483. Philadelphia: W. B. Saunders.

SUE, D. (1981). *Counseling the culturally different.* New York: John Wiley & Sons.

17

A Face of Her Own: Down Syndrome Mosaicism

As indicated in the Introduction to this volume, more than one case report deals with the same diagnosis, but with differing emphases and outcomes. The following report of the Collinses' experience in grappling with the news of a Down syndrome infant contrasts sharply with the account offered of the Reids in Chapter 9, ''Hazardous Pathways to Nondirective Conseling.'' In the present report the counselees are specially concerned with their daughter's individuality rather than with her categorical diagnosis.

The setting for this counseling is a Regional Center within a state, a center serving more than 3,000 persons with special developmental needs, in an area of 2,400 square miles. The center provides a fixed point within a community where clients can obtain diagnostic evaluations, lifelong planning services, and program management for developmental disability. There is no financial means test for eligibility for services.

Nina was born in a small community hospital to David Collins, age 35, and Sally Collins, age 31. The Collinses are college graduates who moved west from Chicago. Mr. Collins is employed by the state in a blue-collar position, and the total family income is approximately $20,000 per year. The Collinses had been married for three and a half years when they decided that they wanted to start their family. Approximately eight months later they were delighted to have confirmation of a pregnancy. Gestation progressed uneventfully, and terminated at forty weeks with Nina's birth.

The pediatrician in attendance at Nina's delivery noticed that she had some of the facial stigmata of Down syndrome. The parents were informed of his suspicions and consented to have a blood sample drawn

from Nina for a chromosome analysis. The sample was sent to a cytogenetics laboratory at a distant metropolitan hospital. While Mrs. Collins and Nina were still in the local hospital, the Collinses were introduced to a parent who had a child with Down syndrome. This parent
suggested that they call their local Regional Center.

When a mother is only 31 years old (or younger), one is not likely to be
much concerned with the possibility of a Down syndrome baby. It remains the case that most Down babies are born to younger mothers
simply because most babies are born to younger mothers.

Ten days after Nina's birth Mrs. Collins contacted our center and
asked for services to be provided for her daughter, who was thought to
be developmentally disabled. At this time the chromosome analysis was
still in progress, and Mrs. Collins was referred by Nina's case manager
(a social worker) for genetic counseling. I arranged for the family to
come in for the next monthly genetics clinic.

Well before this appointment I telephoned Mrs. Collins to give the
family an idea of what to expect during their visit with us. She was told
that she and her husband would meet in conference with the medical
geneticist, genetic counselor (myself), staff psychologist, and Nina's
case manager. We planned to discuss the chromosome finding, answer
the parents' questions, and offer options if indicated. Mrs. Collins said
that she understood our procedures, and that she and her husband were
looking forward to Nina's evaluation. Despite her calm, it was obvious
from Mrs. Collins' tone of voice that the "looking forward" was mixed
with anxiety, reluctance, and possibly suspicion. I told her to expect
consent forms in the mail, which would need the parents' signatures
before being forwarded to various medical facilities that would provide
us with their daughter's medical history.

This effort to prepare a family as to what to expect at a subsequent
evaluation seems very prudent. It is virtually invariable that families approach important medical consultations—in any specialty field—with
much anxiety and associated frightening anticipations. It is not possible
to prepare anyone for *everything* that will occur, as that cannot be known
till the actual occasion of the consultation itself. If one can prepare
counselees for the broad procedural outlines of the consultation,
however, at least that portion of the unknown becomes known, and its
share in the generation of anxiety is subtracted from the total. The
counselees should, in consequence, be that much more accessible when
subsequently seen for interview.

All pertinent records were reviewed by the medical geneticist and myself prior to the clinic appointment. The genetic diagnosis was determined to be Down syndrome mosaicism with a 2:1 ratio of abnormal to normal cells.

Our first counseling session took place when Nina was 7 weeks old. In some respects it turned out to be a surprise for all of the clinic team present: Although the Collinses had been forewarned of Down syndrome by their pediatrician at Nina's birth, had accepted referral to the Regional Center by a member of a Down syndrome parent group, and had "read up on Down syndrome," they were not expecting to be told Nina actually had the disorder.

The Collinses were asked to join the medical geneticist, myself, the staff psychologist, and the case manager around a conference table in a comfortable, informal room. We were seven, including Nina. She, sucking contentedly on her bottle, was being cradled in her mother's arms. Occasionally Mr. Collins, seated next to his wife, would glance at her comfortingly and stroke his little daughter. The Collinses impressed me as being a tense, concerned couple somewhat uncomfortable in this setting. I attempted to make them more at ease by introducing the staff and explaining that we were all there to help them better understand Nina's special problem.

The medical geneticist, Dr. V., began by explaining that the special laboratory test called chromosome analysis had been completed and that the results were now available. It was explained that Nina had a condition called Down syndrome mosaicism. The word "mongolism" was used as a synonym at this point, but not repeated.

In careful detail, Dr. V. next explained the chromosome arrangements in Down syndrome. (As this has been presented in previous case reports, it is not being repeated here.) Dr. V. went on to point out that in a small number of Down syndrome babies (about one percent) not *every* cell has the extra chromosome of trisomy 21. When a child has two kinds of cells, those which have 47 chromosomes (trisomic), and those which have 46 chromosomes (normal), he added, we say that the child has Down syndrome mosaicism.

We do not know whether the Collinses, both college graduates, have a background knowledge of biology. This explanation strikes the knowledgeable reader as simple and direct. To some counselees for whom "chromosome" and "gene" are new concepts, it would be a large dose of new information to grasp.

When the Collinses were shown Nina's two different karyotypes, which were used to illustrate and reinforce Dr. V.'s explanation, their concern turned to grief. What followed was a tearful admission that their pediatrician had expressed his opinion to them soon after Nina's birth, but they had not believed him because Nina did not "look as bad" as the pictures they had seen.

> The self-protective psychological mechanism of denial takes advantage of anything usable for buttressing itself, including such observations as these.

I asked the parents to partially unclothe Nina so that they could be shown some of the physical characteristics of Down syndrome. Nina's face in her large-brimmed bonnet was barely discernible. Her various layers of clothing seemed excessive in the midsummer heat wave we were experiencing. I pointed out some typical characteristics of Down syndrome: the round face, flat profile, oblique eye openings, epicanthal folds, protruding tongue, and small, low-set ears. Nina's hands and fingers were noted to be short and broad, and the palms of both hands had simian creases. At this time Mrs. Collins became overwhelmed with tears. I told her it was perfectly all right to cry, and asked her to try to put her feelings into words. She looked at her husband, then at me, and said over and over, "I feel so sorry for Nina." Then she added, "And I'm very mad!" I asked her to explain and she retorted angrily, "It isn't fair, it just isn't fair that Nina looks like other mongoloids—I want her to be a person, too! How can she be a person if she doesn't have her own face?"

> This exclamation of Mrs. Collins and the exchange of remarks that followed were very important components of the total interaction being reported. Mrs. Collins was indicating her response to the naming of the baby's diagnosis. After all, what to the clinic staff is one afflicted child in a large population of handicapped is for Mrs. Collins *her baby*, constituting 100 percent of her series of one infant. She therefore does not think "What do I do with this Down syndrome infant?" but "How do I help *my baby daughter*, Nina, to grow up when she is so handicapped?"

I had never heard anyone verbalize the situation in that way, and was startled and touched by Mrs. Collins' remarks. I suggested that although Down syndrome infants do resemble one another more than other babies, in time, with love and attention, Nina, like all babies, would develop her very own special personality, with a complete repertoire of likes, dislikes, and other emotions. Nina, like every other infant, had inherited half of her traits from each of *her* parents and would be a completely unique person with her own physical traits. I pointed out Nina's dark hair and brown eyes, which were like her mother's.

Then we looked at many photos of Down children and adults, noticing that they really weren't copies of one another.

Mrs. Collins had been attentive to what was said, and had calmed down. It was then explained that Nina's chromosome abnormality had been an accident of cell division taking place shortly after her conception. This accident could neither have been caused nor prevented by the Collinses. I told them that there was nothing physically wrong with either of them and said they could expect to have normal children in the future. Their risk of chromosome abnormality in future pregnancies was one percent. We then talked about the availability of prenatal diagnosis by amniocentesis, now advised in view of this history.

Until this time Mr. Collins had been very quiet. He had sometimes been tearful and always responded to his wife and daughter with affection and support. He continued to clutch his wife's hand as he asked, "What can we expect of Nina?" Dr. V. replied that Down children frequently have an increased susceptibility to upper respiratory and ear infections as well as heart defects. Then Mr. Collins amended his question. "Not physically. . . . Mentally, what can we expect?"

In the era of antibiotics, Down syndrome children survive as never before. Therefore, their potential for development becomes a critical factor, with obvious bearing on the prospects for ever achieving independence from their families.

Since Nina had been diagnosed as having Down syndrome *mosaicism,* I explained that some of these children attain a higher level of functioning than those who have Down syndrome (all cells have the extra #21 chromosome), but that Nina would probably be retarded. The parents seemed happy and at the same time sad to hear this prognosis. Mrs. Collins asked, "Does Nina's higher proportion of abnormal cells mean she will be more retarded?" We stressed that the chromosome analysis could not tell us the abnormal-to-normal ratio of cells in *all* tissues in Nina's body, and even if it could, we would be unable to predict her potential.

This statement accurately reflects our uncertain ability to predict the limit of functional achievement. By virtue of its honest ambiguity it leaves the door ajar for some hopefulness.

After one and a half hours the counseling session drew to a close with a plan to monitor Nina's developmental progress as well as her program needs. Between 9 and 12 months of age Nina would be tested by a staff psychologist, and between ages 12 and 18 months she would have a full hearing evaluation. The psychologist mentioned the possibilities of temporary respite care and placement options. Respite care is a form of temporary "sitter service" arranged by Regional Centers for parents of infants with special developmental needs. In-home (the parents' home) and out-of-home respite care is provided through community facilities.

Following the clinic appointment, a letter was sent to the Collinses and Nina's pediatrician. The letter mirrored the counseling in content and scope. Mr. and Mrs. Collins were requested to read the letter carefully and contact me if they had questions or wanted to share their feelings abut the counseling they had received.

Ten days later Mr. Collins telephoned to say how much he and his wife appreciated the opportunity to discuss their fears and concerns about Nina, and how much they had learned. He said, "I feel relieved that Nina has a disorder about which so much is known and so much can be done." He thanked me for the letter and the genuine concern shown for their family.

The second counseling session was held three weeks after the initial session and lasted for one hour. At this meeting, I briefly reviewed the events leading to mosaicism, the recurrence risk, and the availability of amniocentesis. The discussion then turned to the availability of temporary respite care. The Collinses responded quickly, almost angrily to my offer. They said, "We love Nina and want her to stay with us." Then Mr. Collins calmly said that he and his wife had discussed placement and they both had come to the decision that it was not for them. I supported their decision and reiterated that at any time they could reconsider or take advantage of short-term respite care. They seemed to appreciate my concern and apologized for "jumping down your throat." The session ended with a few more words about amniocentesis and the pending psychological assessment.

Three months after the first clinic session I telephoned the Collinses to inquire how they were getting along. Mr. Collins was not at home, but Mrs. Collins was happy to report that they were adjusting to Nina's disability. With the help of Nina's case manager and with Regional Center funds Nina had been enrolled in a special infant development program for Down children. The Collinses had joined the evening parent group and were being given an opportunity to share the fears, concerns, and joys of having a child with Down syndrome. Mrs. Collins told me that she and her husband were definitely planning to have more children. She said she would call "as soon as I know I am pregnant so that I can have the special test."

The psychological testing and evaluation follow-ups are planned as well as ongoing management of Nina's educational needs. Medical care will continue to be provided by Nina's pediatrician, who was and will be contacted throughout this process.

Further Comment

This narrative illustrates expectable difficulties for the counselees, beginning with their shock and denial of the distressing news concerning Nina. When the question of possible placement arises, we have to keep in mind that it is not a viable option for every set of parents. Some cannot tolerate bringing their Down syndrome infant home from the hospital, while for others placement is unthinkable, at least at the outset. As in this instance, counselors should avoid the pitfall of assuming that all parents react the same way, and that all will therefore opt for placement. Temporary respite may be more acceptable as a solution to the endless challenge of life modified by the special demands of an unusual child.

Parents' groups are very valuable, but some parents need help in joining. Inhibited parents speak of their indisposition to having the social disability of their children underscored by membership in such a group. Yet *their* need for the group's help is very considerable.

The parents' difficulties encountered in a situation of this kind are reflected in the challenge presented to the professionals: As the parents reminded the counselor with their reference to "a face of her own" — a reminder that this counselor so ably acknowledged — we should not think in terms of categorical statements about diseases. The affected baby is not just a Down syndrome infant; she is Nina, their particular baby, and invested with feelings by her parents who eagerly awaited her birth.

References

De Grouchy, J., and Turleau, C. (1977). *Clinical atlas of human chromosomes*, pp. 187–209. New York: John Wiley & Sons.

Koch, R., and De la Cruz, F. (1975). *Down syndrome: diagnosis and management*. New York: Brunner Mazel.

Smith, D., and Wilson, A. (1973). *The child with Down's syndrome*. Philadelphia: W. B. Saunders.

18

Uninterrupted Pregnancy with Prenatal Diagnosis of Open Neural Tube Defect: Cultural Influences on Access to Self-Help

The story of Gloria Robia's counseling experience has been selected for a number of reasons. It concerns a 44-year-old expectant mother who already has children (including one born with a congenital defect that was repaired), who has been referred for prenatal diagnosis because of her age. The case illustrates some of the problems encountered in cross-cultural counseling, and some of the problems associated with open neural tube defects.

Cultural differences between counselor and patient introduce complications to the genetic counseling process. Motivation to seek genetic counseling, acceptance of amniocentesis and carrier screening tests, and decisions regarding reproductive alternatives are known to be influenced by one's ethnic, religious, and economic background. Unfamiliarity of genetic counselors with the culturally based health care beliefs and reproductive attitudes of a client can lead to misunderstanding, inadequate counseling, and/or improper interpretation of the client's responses. The existence of a language barrier between counselor and patient further magnifies the difficulties of the counseling process.

Neural tube defects include a group of congenital anomalies, among them anencephaly and spina bifida. These defects are thought to arise when the neural plate (the embryonic precursor of the spinal cord and central nervous system) fails to close at some point along its length. In anencephaly, the most severe form of neural tube defect, many of the structures of the skull and brain fail to develop, a condition incompatible with life. Spina bifida cystica involves a midline defect of the vertebrae. If part of the spinal cord protrudes, the defect is called a meningomyelocele; if only a membranous sac is present, it is called a meningocele. The nerves in the exposed part of the spinal cord are stretched and damaged, producing varying degrees of neurologic impairment.

In the United States the incidence of neural tube defects is estimated to be 1 to 2 per 1,000 births. Ninety percent of cases occur in families with no previous history of a neural tube defect. Family and twin studies indicate that multifactorial inheritance is the cause of neural tube defects when anencephaly, spina bifida, or encephalocele (brain tissue protrusion) are the only defects present.

Neural tube defects also occur in a variety of disorders with other modes of inheritance. Aminopterin, a medication with recognized teratogenic potential, may produce neural tube defects in exposed fetuses and infants.

Therefore, when offering genetic counseling to a family with a previous history of a neural tube defect, it is essential to obtain a careful history and any available laboratory or postmortem reports in order to assure the accuracy of counseling and recurrence risk figures.

Gloria Robia, age 44, first sought prenatal care during the twentieth week of pregnancy, and was immediately referred by the hospital's Obstetrical Prenatal Clinic to the Genetics Division for pre-amniocentesis counseling because of advanced maternal age. This appointment was arranged by the clinic nurse. At the first counseling session Gloria was accompanied by her 18-year-old daughter, Rita.

At our Genetic Counseling Center all pre-amniocentesis patients receive by mail or just prior to counseling a detailed letter written by the genetic counseling team. This letter, written in either English or Spanish, discusses the indications for amniocentesis and describes the procedure, the diagnostic tests, and the reporting of results and fees. Each patient is asked to read the letter prior to her counseling appointment in order to familiarize herself with amniocentesis. In addition, the letter is meant to stimulate questions and concerns that can be discussed during the counseling session. It also serves as an informational record of much of the ensuing session, which the patient can review at home and share with family or friends.

All women referred by private obstetricians are contacted by telephone prior to their pre-amniocentesis appointment so that information about their pregnancy history, personal history, and family medical history can be obtained.

The timing for presenting the pre-amniocentesis letter and obtaining the intake information differs if the patient is referred by the Prenatal Clinic. Experience has taught that a language barrier, the patient's lack of a home telephone, and/or her lack of knowledge about amniocentesis make it advantageous to offer the clinic patient this letter to read just before the pre-amniocentesis session. We begin the counseling session by obtaining the intake information.

Gloria was given the Spanish letter to read upon her arrival at the Genetics Center. When she had finished reading it, I came out to meet her, along with an interpreter. She was invited to bring her daughter to the counseling session if she desired, and she did.

Interpretation for Spanish-speaking patients is provided by the secretary of the Genetic Counseling Center, who grew up in a bilingual home. Because she is employed in our unit, she is also extremely familiar with the genetic counseling issues being discussed.

Gloria was an attractive, plainly-dressed woman. During the counseling session she was shy and reserved, although gradually she became more open and descriptive. She was cooperative in that she willingly answered my questions, but she seemed to be somewhat ill at ease. She understood a little English, but said she was much more comfortable with Spanish.

First I explained to Gloria that she had been referred to the Genetics Division to discuss amniocentesis, a special test that her obstetrician was recommending because of her age. She was told that this meeting was an opportunity to answer any questions or discuss any concerns that she had about the test or its results, and that the decision about whether or not to undergo the test was up to her. I showed Gloria the intake history form and told her that the information she provided about her pregnancy, and the histories of herself and family, would be helpful to us. They would enable us to give her accurate information about which tests were appropriate for her.

While much of the information obtained through the intake is extremely personal in nature, we find that taking this history helps to establish rapport with the patient. Since the process involves filling in a set questionnaire, we reduce the likelihood that the patient may feel she is being singled out or scrutinized.

The intake revealed that this was Gloria's ninth pregnancy. She had four living children (ages 12 to 23) and had undergone three illegal elective abortions and one ectopic pregnancy. Her current pregnancy had been unplanned. Her family history revealed that one of her children had been born with a cleft lip and palate, which had been successfully repaired surgically. There was no other known incidence of birth defects or mental retardation in her or her husband's family. She had been married for twenty-four years to José Robia, age 45, who was a barber, and who had thirteen children in other relationships. Both Gloria and José came from Puerto Rico and were non-consanguineous.

Gloria did not appear embarrassed to share this information with strangers, or her daughter. Gloria's daughter was silent throughout the entire counseling session, but she did not appear embarrassed either, nor did she seem bored. I interpreted her presence as being supportive of her mother. Since José was not present at the initial counseling session or any subsequent session, it was not possible to assess their marital relationship or to get any impression of José as an individual.

G.C.: Gloria, do you have any questions or concerns about the amniocentesis test?

GLORIA: Will the needle hurt?

G.C.: Most women describe the pain as similar to the pain felt in a blood test. You feel the pinch of the needle during insertion and then a feeling of pressure while the amniotic fluid is being withdrawn. How do you feel about blood tests?

GLORIA: I don't like needles. They frighten me.

G.C.: Many people feel the way you do. The reason we are talking to you about amniocentesis is so that you can weigh the benefits and risks for yourself and decide whether you wish to have the test.

GLORIA: Will the test hurt the baby in any way?

G.C.: Most babies and pregnancies are not affected by amniocentesis. However, a small number of women—about one in every two hundred women who have amniocentesis—may experience a miscarriage that is apparently related to the procedure. There have been a few reports of babies that may have been injured by the needle, but these are very rare cases. Do you have any other questions or concerns?

GLORIA: No.

G.C.: Are you worried at all that this baby might be born with a cleft lip and palate?

GLORIA: No; the doctors were able to repair my son's lip completely, and he's fine now.

G.C.: How did you feel after your son was born?

GLORIA: I was very sad and worried, but his doctors reassured me that following surgery he'd be okay, and they were right.

These were Gloria's two main concerns. The rest of the session, which lasted about an hour, was taken up with discussing chromosome abnormalities and the reason prenatal testing was being recommended to her; reviewing the procedure and laboratory limitations; and briefly describing neural tube defects and how they were diagnosed by measurement of alpha-fetoprotein levels in the amniotic fluid. Gloria was familiar with Down syndrome because a neighbor had an affected child, but she had never heard of anencephaly or spina bifida. In addition, the two options open to her (termination or continuation of pregnancy) in the event of a positive test result were mentioned.

I had the feeling that Gloria was totally accepting of this pregnancy. Abortion was brought up at this time only in terms of an option for dealing with the pregnancy. Usually, unless the patient expresses her feelings about abortion, we do not ask, before the testing takes place, what she is likely to do if an abnormality is detected. At the conclusion of the session Gloria was asked if she needed time to decide whether to have amniocentesis. She said she wanted to have the test to reassure herself that "the baby would be healthy." I replied: "Amniocentesis can reassure you that the fetus does not have Down syndrome (mongolism) or a neural tube defect. Please remember that it cannot guarantee that there may not be some other type of birth defect, even though the chance of another problem is extremely unlikely." (Cleft lip and palate was used as an example of a nondetectable birth defect.) Gloria indicated that she understood.

Sonography and amniocentesis performed at the first available appointment, six days later, were uneventful. Gloria had come alone in spite of the fact that she was told a family member or friend would be welcome to accompany her. I saw her shortly after the procedure when she brought the amniotic fluid specimen to the laboratory. There are several advantages to having the patient act as messenger for the short distance between the Obstetrical Division and the cytogenetics lab; The specimens arrive promptly at the lab, one at a time about half an hour apart, thereby decreasing the likelihood of human error through specimen mixup, and the patient is reassured that the specimen has arrived at the lab safely.

Afterwards, I asked Gloria how she was feeling, and she expressed relief that the procedure was over. She added that it had been more painful than she had expected.

Results of the alpha-fetoprotein assay revealed extremely elevated levels of alpha-fetoprotein (above five standard deviations) in the amniotic fluid. Chromosome results showed a normal male 46,XY karyotype. Gloria was now almost twenty-three weeks pregnant. We immediately tried to contact her. She did not have a home telephone but had given us her cousin's phone number, where we could leave a message for her.

We reached the son of Gloria's cousin and asked him to have his mother call us as soon as possible. Gloria's cousin returned the phone call later that afternoon. Without revealing the nature of the problem we asked her to have Gloria call us as soon as possible or to come in to see us the next morning with her husband, if possible. Genetic disorders are family problems, and it is therefore preferable for couples to be counseled together. We have found that joint counseling increases the amount of information likely to be retained, and decision making is more likely to be shared.

In our Genetics Center couples with positive prenatal test results are counseled concurrently by both the genetic counselor and the medical geneticist. In spite of our concern that she wouldn't be given our message, Gloria arrived at our center the next morning. She was alone, however, explaining that her husband was unable to take time away from his job. Dr. I., the geneticist, was introduced to Gloria.

One of the major drawbacks of counselors not having the ability to speak and understand the counselees' language is that subtle, "in between the lines" feelings expressed by the patient are missed. The nuances of the language are likely to be lost even when the translation is as expertly done as possible. The counselor may therefore have to rely more heavily on the patient's nonverbal communication in order to understand more fully how she is feeling. This, too, is difficult to assess in a shy individual.

G.C.: I don't know if you suspect why we asked you to meet with us again. I'm afraid we don't have good news for you. One of your tests indicates that the baby has a problem.

GLORIA: Oh, no! That can't be. [Gloria's face became expressionless and she seemed very withdrawn, looking at her hands.]

[We sat for a few minutes in silence. When Gloria lifted her head and looked at us, we started talking again.]

G.C.: You may remember that we performed two tests on the amniotic fluid that we obtained. The chromosome test that can diagnose Down syndrome (mongolism) or other chromosome abnormalities was normal. So the baby does *not* have Down syndrome. However, the chemical test, where we measured the amount of the chemical called alpha-fetoprotein in the fluid, had abnormally high levels. This almost always indicates that the baby has an abnormality in the formation of its nervous system. Have you ever heard of "open spine" or "spina bifida" before?

GLORIA: No, I have never known anyone with this problem. Will the baby be retarded? [Gloria looked extremely sad.]

G.C.: The baby will probably not be mentally retarded. Retardation may occur only if other medical complications arise. However, because the nerves of the spine are usually damaged, children with spina bifida are usually paralyzed from the waist down. Most children need to use braces and crutches or wheelchairs to get around. Because of nerve damage some children may never have control of their bladder or bowels. The baby will most likely need a skin-grafting operation shortly after it is born, and it may need other surgical treatment during its life. [A drawing of a baby with a meningomyelocele was shown to Gloria to help her visualize what the defect might look like.]

It is probably a mistake to imagine that showing a picture of a meningomyelocele to a counselee under these circumstances is a measure taken only because there is a language barrier. Even when counselees may have some acquaintance with a technical term and no language barrier, the term may not register with appropriate impact. In Gloria's situation, it is probably quite important to give human meaning—by use of a picture—to a meningomyelocele to help her differentiate it from cleft lip and palate, a lesion she has had experience with and regards as therapeutically altogether correctable.

To readers this measure may seem rather aggressive and disturbing, but the counselor is balancing any such possible impact against the need for Gloria to be able to make the best-informed decision as to what she wishes to do, and to make it promptly.

G.C.: Very often though, children with spina bifida can participate fully in school, and can grow up to be independent, working members of society despite their disabilities. One limitation of the alphafetoprotein test is that we can't predict how severe or how mild the child's disabilities will be.

[During the conversation Gloria began to cry softly. We gave her some tissues and sat silently for a few minutes. From this point on there was little eye contact between Gloria and the counselors. Gloria had no questions at all, which made us worry about whether she really understood what we were telling her. Was the translation adequate? Was she able to visualize the problems we were describing?]

G.C.: I realize that what we have told you is extremely upsetting to you. Are there any questions that you have about what we have said?

GLORIA: No. I understand.

Two important dialogues are proceeding simultaneously here. The one is verbal, as noted in the narrative. The other is nonverbal, referred to by the counselor in her description of Gloria's ceasing eye contact and not responding with any questions. The reader may object that quite possibly the counselor has presented the facts with such consummately crystalline clarity that no one, with or without a language barrier, would have anything to ask. The counselor knows better than that. She observes the counselee's reaction to this large dose of bad news against a "backdrop" of many similar interactions with other counselees. She knows that the usual human response, provided no inhibition has quietly slipped into the interview, is at least some questioning by the patient, even if only to clarify what has been stated. Gloria had no questions, a negative observation by the counselor which she interpreted as meaningful and probably derived from the emotional onslaught of the bad news.

G.C.: There are a few other things about the testing and your pregnancy that we wish to discuss with you. Would you like to talk about them now?

[Gloria nodded affirmatively.]

G.C.: We want to recommend that you have another ultrasound test as soon as possible. We can schedule this test for you. Even though an abnormality of the spine is the most likely problem that the fetus is affected with, there are a few other birth defects that can also cause high levels of alpha-fetoprotein in the amniotic fluid. Some of these other problems are not as severe as spina bifida. The doctor performing the ultrasound can take a very careful look at the fetal spine to see if he can observe the abnormal opening. The information that you get from the ultrasound test may help you to decide whether you wish to continue the pregnancy or terminate it. You also may find it helpful to talk with a mother who has a child with spina bifida. She can tell you about her experiences in raising a handicapped child. There are also doctors who specialize in treating children with spina bifida, and they can give you more information about the medical needs of a child with this disorder.

[Gloria did not volunteer any comments or feelings.]

DR. I.: It's not necessary for you to make a decision about any of these things today. However, due to the fact that you are late in your pregnancy you have only a week at most to decide whether you wish to terminate the pregnancy. We would also be happy to meet with you again and speak with your husband if you feel it will be helpful to you.

GLORIA: I don't think I can terminate the pregnancy because I have been feeling the baby move for many weeks already. [Gloria had indicated during the first counseling session that although this had been an unplanned pregnancy, she was greatly looking forward to having this baby.]

G.C.: The baby seems more real to you because you can feel it move?

GLORIA: Yes it does. Even if the baby is paralyzed, I feel that I will have to accept it.

G.C.: Do you think it would be helpful to talk with other parents and doctors about raising a child with spina bifida?

GLORIA: I don't know.

Gloria did not have any further questions and did not appear to want to discuss her feelings or the difficult decision any further. Both the medical geneticist and myself felt that she understood the information we had given her. We offered to meet with her as often as she needed to work through her decision. She promised to call us within a few days to let us know what she planned to do.

A week later we still had not heard from Gloria. We called her cousin and left a message for Gloria to call us. We called again the following day. The cousin said during this conversation that Gloria understood what we had told her about the test results and spina bifida and that she had decided to continue the pregnancy and not to undergo any further testing.

Gloria had clearly stated during the previous counseling session that this was a wanted pregnancy, and that because she felt fetal movement, abortion was unacceptable for her. Now that she had had a week to consider her options, we accepted Gloria's decision as final and sent her a letter in Spanish reviewing the counseling sessions. We also telephoned Gloria's nurse in the Prenatal Clinic.

The nurse became very upset, and felt that because Gloria had decided *not* to terminate the pregnancy, she had not understood the counseling. The nurse was appalled at Gloria's decision, and found it impossible not to assume that her own feelings about the situation were identical with those of her patient. We tried to explain the philosophy behind nondirective counseling to the nurse, and finally had to insist that she not call the police to bring Gloria in for another consultation. Gloria had acted within her rights to refuse further counseling. The nurse indicated she would try to reach Gloria by phone.

We later discovered that Gloria missed several prenatal appointments and reportedly resumed her prenatal care well after the time a termination was medically possible.

We were informed by a resident in the Neonatal Intensive Care Unit shortly after baby Robia was born that the infant had spina bifida, and genetic evaluation was requested.

Genetic evaluation consultations for newborns suspected of having or known to have congenital anomalies are usually requested by the chief physician of the Neonatology Division or the patient's attending pediatrician. The medical geneticist will examine the infant, request specimens for indicated diagnostic tests, and together with the genetic counselor visit the infant's mother (and father, if possible) during her hospital stay.

The story was relayed by the Intensive Care Unit staff that José, the baby's father, had become extremely upset after its birth. When he came to visit, he acted as if he had not expected the congenital problems. Since we had never met with him, we had no way of knowing whether Gloria had shared with him the results of the test.

With the editor's advantage of hindsight, one gathers that whatever did or did not take place at home between Gloria and José, he did not comprehend the risk as she did. While there is no way to be certain, the suggestion is implicit that Jose's presence might have helped matters. Perhaps he might have assisted her in deliberating about the decision that had to be made so promptly. At the very least, his being prepared for the birth of the defective infant would have enabled him to be emotionally supportive of her both in the immediate postnatal period and in the later period when contact with helping organizations can make a considerable difference.

The counseling team tried to visit Gloria while she was hospitalized, but she told the attending physician that she was unwilling to see us. We left our names and telephone numbers saying that we would be happy to speak with her at any time. She never called.

Seven months later we received a call from the Pediatric Clinic referring baby Dennis Robia for a genetic reevaluation. An appointment was made, and we were surprised that Gloria actually kept it in view of her refusal to meet with us earlier.

Gloria brought the infant and her 12-year-old daughter. The counseling team consisted of Dr. I., myself, and the translator. The baby was a handsome child who appeared alert and amiable. He was well cared for and beautifully dressed. Gloria appeared shy and reserved, as she had during our previous meetings with her, but not reluctant to meet with us.

The baby seemed to be doing well in spite of severe paralysis of the lower extremities. He had no signs or symptoms of hydrocephalus. While the medical geneticist was making arrangements for the baby to be reevaluated by the Pediatric Neurology Division, I took the opportunity to talk with Gloria.

G.C.: Gloria, would you mind telling me about the medical treatment Dennis received after he was born?

GLORIA: Dennis was born with part of his backbone open, as you said. He couldn't lie on this back, and the doctors were afraid it would get infected. So when Dennis was three days old they operated on him to close his back.

G.C.: What did the surgeons do?

GLORIA: They had to take some skin from Dennis' thigh and backside in order to cover the opening. But they couldn't do it all at one time. About three or four weeks later he had a second operation to finish closing the sac. He had to stay in the hospital for about two months.

G.C.: Will Dennis need any other operations?

GLORIA: I asked his doctor and he said he can't tell yet. He has to see how Dennis grows and to watch him carefully to see that he doesn't develop water on the brain.

G.C.: Are there any special things you have to do in taking care of Dennis?

GLORIA: When I first took him home from the hospital I was very scared

I would hurt his back. But the doctor told me I could hold him and play with him like any other baby. He said, though, that because he can't feel pain in his legs and feet like we can, I have to be careful that his clothes aren't too tight and that he doesn't hurt himself and not know it.

The counselor is taking a detailed history of what has gone on since she last saw Gloria for several reasons, one of which is to reestablish rapport with her client after a considerable intermission. The details of the history will cue the counselor concerning possible suggestions for helpful services. She is about to inquire more directly concerning Gloria's mood and health, important ingredients in shaping her recommendations.

G.C.: What were you expecting would happen at today's appointment?

GLORIA: I don't know—I thought you would examine Dennis and tell me how he's doing.

G.C.: How have *you* been feeling since the baby was born?

GLORIA: I've been okay. [This was not at all convincing, since she looked sad and strained.]

GLORIA [tears welling in her eyes]: I had no idea how hard it would be for me. I wish you had told me what to do. I love the baby, but he's going to suffer so much.

Gloria expresses the emotional meaning of electing to have this infant. We recall, during the brief period of possible election to abort, that the counselor had suggested Gloria speak with physicians or mothers with spina bifida experience to make its human impact more vivid. But she could not do it. Her bond with the moving fetus was primary.

Was the amniocentesis therefore a waste of time? Knowing that she was to expect a defective baby, Gloria's "inner self" quietly, without any deliberate attention from her, "hardened" itself in anticipation of the shock. It can hardly be doubted that this silent preparation helped her to be able to collaborate with medical staff in numerous, rapidly made postpartum management decisions.

G.C.: Making the decision about whether to terminate or to continue the pregnancy was a very difficult one for you?

GLORIA: I felt I couldn't get rid of the baby because I had felt life.

G.C.: Therefore, you felt that you didn't really have a choice at all?

[Gloria nodded yes.]

G.C.: Is there anyone at home who is helpful to you?

GLORIA: My other kids are good with the baby. And my cousin helps me out. But they don't understand what it's really like.

G.C.: You feel they don't understand how you're feeling?

[At this point Gloria reversed herself, retracting some of her earlier feelings.]

GLORIA: It's really not that bad. He's a good baby.

G.C.: It's natural to feel that other people don't really understand what it is like to live through a difficult experience. This is why some parents like yourself who have children with spina bifida have formed an organization and meet with one another. They share their ideas and experiences, and help one another to solve some of the problems that other people don't have any experience with. You might find it helpful to meet with these other parents. I would be happy to introduce you to them if you wish. [The Spina Bifida Association is a nationwide organization of families with children born with neural tube defects. In addition to this Association, personal contacts with families willing to talk with others living through a similar traumatic experience can often be arranged by our clinic. These are families who previously received genetic counseling.]

GLORIA: I can probably manage.

G.C.: You are doing a beautiful job caring for the baby. He's really growing well! Sometimes it just feels good to talk with someone who really knows and understands because they have similar problems.

GLORIA: Maybe I'll take the number in case I want it later.

G.C.: You had mentioned earlier that you are afraid the baby will suffer. Is there anything in particular that worries you?

GLORIA: He won't be able to do what other children can do, and they'll make fun of him.

G.C.: Sometimes other children can be insensitive and cruel to people who are different from them. But your son can grow up to be independent, and a full member of society. There are special therapy programs that can help him develop to his fullest potential. I would like to give you the names and phone numbers of these programs so that you can call them. They may be able to teach you special exercises that will help Dennis.

While Gloria accepted both referrals, the genetic counselor detected some reluctance actually to follow through on these recommendations. Gloria was not interested in talking further about spina bifida or her feelings. She had not expected to talk about her feelings at this appointment. Speaking through an interpreter was additionally difficult and tiring.

For counselors this reluctance is hard to understand. Middle-class families usually welcome such referrals in order to fulfill the need to do as much as possible for their child. Was her reluctance culturally based? It was impossible to evaluate, since she wouldn't talk about it. Gloria did not wish to make another appointment with the genetic counselor at that time, and did not return a follow-up call several months later.

From a genetic counseling standpoint there is additional information to be given to Gloria and her family, such as inheritance pattern and recurrence risks. If she were receptive, more of her feelings might be explored. In reviewing this case, it was our speculation that Gloria's reluctance to meet with us was at least in part based on her past experiences with the medical community (as a Medicaid patient). She was accustomed to having physicians and nurses tell her what to do and not ask about her feelings. While we have no doubt about her need and desire to do everything possible to aid her son's development, her concept of herself as mother and head of her household and perhaps some feelings against seeking outside help may be contributing to her reluctance. Dennis' special needs will necessitate Gloria's obtaining help outside of her home community in surroundings where the customs are less familiar and the language difficult to understand.

Further Comment

Counseling situations often involve information that has powerful emotional impact, as here. Under such conditions it is often better to convey the troubling information to a few people simultaneously rather than just the patient alone. It is commonplace to learn later, if the patient has been present by herself, of the most dramatic distortions and falsifications of memory as to what actually was said or with what emphasis it was presented. The addition of a trusted relative or friend provides opportunities following the counseling session for the counselee to explore conversationally what went on, and, with the assistance of the third party, to correct such distortions.

This account of a woman who was unable to make additional use of the information conveyed in order to exercise the abortion option emphasizes several factors. The drive toward childbearing, even—or possibly, especially—at age 44 is very powerful, doubtless for many private reasons. The change in Gloria's bond to her fetus once movement was felt was dramatic, and in this instance (by no means unique) conferred an entirely different emotional complexion on the idea of abortion. Gloria had, after all, already undergone a number of elective abortions.

The clinic staff could not help but be impressed with Gloria's meaningful interruption of invited contact. Perhaps she expected clinic initiative would press her to rethink her decision, which she did not wish to do or even found intolerable to do. So she avoided the genetics clinic. Such was the measure of her disinclination for possible additional pressure to revise her decision that she also avoided the prenatal clinic until, from her viewpoint, attendance there was once again "safe."

The clinic staff commendably maintained their helpful stance when reapproached by Gloria with baby Dennis. Now the staff was oriented to a new, differently complex situation, the care of a handicapped infant and its parents.

The counselor was impressed with the patient's evident hesitancy in accepting a new set of helpful recommendations, including the invitation to return to explore further the expectable troubling feelings stirred up by the task of caring for a defective child. Why was the counselee "resistant"? The counselor speculated that she had been turned off by earlier interactions with medical center staff, and was not accustomed to sharing private feelings, perhaps not with anyone. The staff attempted to explain the resistance as an example, in part, of some characteristic of an ethnic subculture. An understanding of various ethnic cultures may shed light on certain client behaviors. Yet the more one engages in the laborious work of counseling across cultural lines, the more one becomes impressed with the differences among families even within a given subculture.

In Gloria's case, we may hazard some suggestions which differ from those of the genetic counselor but are equally speculative: Gloria may feel guilty about having permitted Dennis to be born, and consider herself unworthy to receive relief from her suffering. She may harbor within herself wishful images of miraculous improvement, making special help unnecessary—a variety of denial of reality. In the face of the sudden increment of specially difficult child-rearing tasks, Gloria may well experience feelings of rage and resentment at the baby for his very existence, and such feelings may well enhance this mother's guilt.

To follow the helpful recommendations for Dennis and for herself makes the actuality more real, which is depressing and probably can only be done a bit at a time. If José's surprise betokens genuine ignorance of what was expected, rather than his own repression of bad news from Gloria, there may be components of marital tension exacerbating this counselee's resistance, too.

References

Brock, D. (1981). Neural tube defects and alpha fetoprotein: an international perspective. In M. Kaback, ed., *Genetic issues in pediatric and obstetric practice*, pp. 471–488. Chicago: Yearbook Medical Publishers.

Fibush, E. (1965). The white worker and the Negro client. *Social Casework* 46 (no. 4): 271–277.

Sue, D. (1981). *Counseling the culturally different.* New York: John Wiley & Sons.

Swinyard, C. (1975). *The child with spina bifida.* New York: Institute of Rehabilitation Medicine, New York University Medical Center.

19

The Prenatal Diagnosis 47,XXX: Two Cases, Two Decisions

The pair of reports to follow have been selected because of the contrast between the decisions made by two couples contending with the same prenatal diagnosis. This may remind readers of the contrasting decisions we have already encountered in different instances of Down syndrome.

The following cases have special interest in that the two families are faced with the prenatal finding of a fetus with a chromosome aneuploidy (abnormal number), but one which does not usually have severe consequences.

In the report on the Sawyers further note of much interest is that unlike the situation in the case reported from Israel (Chapter 8), when the counselees' rabbi recommended *continuing* a pregnancy, the Sawyers' priest supported their decision to *terminate* the pregnancy. Once again this demonstrates that it is not possible to predict counseling outcomes.

Most aneuploid chromosome conditions have severe clinical consequences, and most are referred to as "syndromes" (e.g., Down syndrome, Edwards syndrome, and Patau syndrome, for trisomies 21, 18, and 13, respectively). However, the 47,XXX karyotype is rarely referred to as a "syndrome"; this presumably reflects the relatively mild clinical features of the trisomy X condition.

The frequency of the 47,XXX karyotype is estimated from surveys of consecutive newborns to be about one per 1,000 female births (Jacobs, 1972; Hamerton et al., 1975). The mean maternal age is 32.8 years, and the mean paternal age is 36.5 years (De Grouchy and Turleau, 1977).

Most women with the 47,XXX karyotype are phenotypically normal and go undiagnosed. Some patients have menstrual disorders, such as delayed menarche, secondary amenorrhea, or early menopause. [Some have excessive fetal loss.] Two-thirds of those cases brought to medical attention are intellectually normal and well adjusted, whereas one-third have delayed early motor and speech development, mild intellectual deficits, and/or disturbed interpersonal relationships.

Prenatal diagnosis of the 47,XXX karyotype is, in my experience as a genetic counselor, more difficult for families to deal with than is the diagnosis of other trisomies, such as trisomy 21 or trisomy 18. In the latter situations, because of the serious physical and mental defects anticipated most families will elect termination of the affected pregnancy. The decision of whether or not to terminate a pregnancy involving a 47,XXX fetus seems to be particularly difficult because of the relatively high chance for a normal, or nearly normal, pregnancy outcome. I have participated in genetic counseling sessions with three families in which the 47,XXX karyotype was diagnosed prenatally. All three amniocenteses had been done because of maternal age greater than 35 years. Following genetic counseling by myself and a medical geneticist, two of the three families chose to terminate their pregnancies. I shall discuss below one of these two families, as well as the family that elected to maintain their pregnancy. These cases illustrate the unpredictability of the decisions made by parents of 47,XXX fetuses.

Case No. 1

An amniotic fluid specimen from a Mrs. Zaragoza, who would be 45 at delivery, was sent to the cytogenetics laboratory. She lived about two-hundred miles away, in a city in which amniocentesis was not available, and so was referred to our obstetricians at the medical center at sixteen weeks' gestation for the procedure. She was not referred to the genetics service prior to amniocentesis.

About two weeks later, when the diagnosis of a fetal 47,XXX karyotype was made, the referring obstetrician was informed of the diagnosis, and of the difficulty in predicting the outcome of the pregnancy. He said he would discuss this with the family, and recommend that they come to us for genetic counseling. Two days later, Mr. and Mrs. Zaragoza did so.

The counseling session took place in a large conference room, with myself, the director of the cytogenetics laboratory (a medical geneticist), and the obstetrician who had performed the amniocentesis present. The couple were Mexican-American. Mr. Zaragoza was a professor at a large university; Mrs. Zaragoza had a college degree. The current pregnancy was the fourth for this couple. The first, when Mrs. Zaragoza was 31 years old, had resulted in the birth of a son who was mildly to moderately retarded, and who had congenital heart disease and hypercalcemia. They did not know the cause of their son's retardation. From photographs they had with them, a presumptive diagnosis of the Williams (elfin facies) syndrome was made. (This was later confirmed by the child's pediatrician.) Apart from the retardation, the son was doing quite well, attending a special class in a public school. According to the Zaragozas, he had strong musical interests and could play several instruments. Mrs. Zaragoza's second and third pregnancies, at ages 35 and 38, had resulted in spontaneous abortions at six and eighteen weeks, respectively. The current pregnancy had been unplanned, but contraception had not been used because of religious beliefs.

Mrs. Zaragoza came from a family that had four girls. One of her sisters had undergone two tubal pregnancies and had no living children. Her two other sisters had five and seven children, respectively, although each had had at least one miscarriage. Apart from Mrs. Zaragoza's son, her family history was negative for mental retardation or other serious disorders. Professor Zaragoza (as he referred to himself each time) also came from a large family, in which a first cousin was mentally retarded, and an uncle had seizures.

Professor and Mrs. Zaragoza understood their reason for referral to have been the identification of a fetal chromosome abnormality. Mrs. Zaragoza was very quiet, and appeared quite upset. Professor Zaragoza did most of the speaking, and asked most of the questions during the session. He was obviously concerned about his wife, and it became clear during the session that the Zaragozas' relationship was a very close, loving one.

G.C.: Mrs. Zaragoza, what does the diagnosis of a chromosome abnormality in the fetus mean to you?

Mrs. Zaragoza: That I can't have a normal baby.

G.C.: Do you feel that this is your fault?

[Mrs. Zaragoza, who had her head down, nodded affirmatively.]

G.C.: Mrs. Zaragoza, what do you know about your son's problems?

Mrs. Zaragoza: He is slow, but he has a very keen musical sense, and he is a good child. We love him.

G.C.: Do you think that something you did, or didn't do, caused his problems?

Mrs. Zaragoza: Yes.

G.C.: What?

Mrs. Zaragoza: I don't know.

G.C.: And you think that your two miscarriages indicate you can't have a normal baby?

Mrs. Zaragoza, with tears in her eyes, nodded. The medical geneticist proceeded to explain to the couple the presumptive diagnosis of the Williams syndrome, and its sporadic nature. The fact that this was an "accident of nature" was stressed. Then he explained that the risk for spontaneous abortion in any pregnancy is 12 to 15 percent, making sure to mention the fact that two of Mrs. Zaragoza's sisters had had miscarriages as well. He emphasized that there was nothing she or her husband had done, or had neglected to do, which had caused her son's problems, the miscarriages, or the fetal chromosome abnormality. She did not respond verbally, but the tears vanished, and her facial expression lightened somewhat.

Once again we encounter the common readiness of a mother to take as hers alone the responsibility for a child's defect despite absence of evidence upon which to base such an assignment. The fact of gestation as an experience of the mother only may, irrationally, be a partial explanation for this bias concerning responsibility.

The counselor proceeded to describe the chromosome aberration that had been found in the amniotic fluid specimen. The karyotype was shown to the couple. They were counseled that unlike individuals with other chromosome abnormalities, those with 47,XXX are not considered to have a clinical "syndrome," although subnormal mental functioning, schizophrenia, and menstrual and reproductive problems are known to occur with slightly higher frequency in 47,XXX individuals than in the general female population. We discussed the fact that the difficulty was not being able to predict, for their fetus, the precise outcome of the pregnancy.

Although this medical information is all factually correct, it may not be important to this couple. Their thinking will expectably be more in broad categorical terms of "normal" versus "abnormal," and less in terms of a distinctive clinical syndrome.

Mrs. Zaragoza asked about the risk to her of an abortion procedure. The obstetrician explained the 12 to 15 percent risk in mid-trimester abortion of complications such as hemorrhage or infection. Specific complications intrinsic to the use of a saline solution and prostaglandin as abortifacients (e.g., fever, nausea, and vomiting) were described.

The remote possibility that the cells analyzed had been maternal cells was also discussed. Mrs. Zaragoza was counseled that a buccal smear could be done to rule out 47,XXX in herself. Unfortunately, this focus upon her probably reinforced her feelings of guilt. She wished to have the test.

What an irony that this remote possibility—which can be ruled out—happens to coincide with Mrs. Zaragoza's bias concerning responsibility.

Several times during the session, Professor Zaragoza touched his wife's arm or hand and they looked at each other lovingly. When we had presented all the information we wished the Zaragozas to have, and they said that all their questions had been answered, the medical geneticist commented, "You both seem to be coping very well with this difficult situation. I can see you have a lot of emotional strength, and a lot of love for each other." They both smiled, and said, "Thank you." I then added, "Even people who are coping quite well on their own sometimes find it helpful to receive some support from a clergyman, or from a mental health counselor. Do you know such a person who you think might be able to give you some support now?" (Making this kind of suggestion can be risky. If one or both of the couple being counseled feel insecure, a suggestion to see a mental health counselor could be very threatening.) Professor Zaragoza replied, "Yes, we have a priest. I think it would be helpful to talk with him. Perhaps we'll talk with him." (From the tone of his voice, we could tell that he had received my suggestion in a positive way.)

Perhaps the counselor has intuitively sensed that this sophisticated couple would probably receive this recommendation in the best spirit, and not be intimidated or threatened by it. Usually, one would probably need to know a couple longer, and have a more specific notion of what *about them* needed "support," before venturing a suitably worded and presented recommendation for professional or priestly assistance. "Support" is a word from common speech, yet its meaning is very ambiguous. Its meaning becomes specific for the particular person or persons involved, and such specification requires time to know the counselees.

We ended the genetic counseling session by agreeing that we would contact the Zaragozas as soon as the results of the buccal smear were available; and that they were to call us in a few days with their decision regarding continuation or termination of the pregnancy. The other two professionals and myself all felt that the Zaragozas would continue the pregnancy, primarily because, as we assessed the situation, they both needed to have a normal child to prove they could do so, and would be willing to take their chances in order to have that child.

Considering that Mrs. Zaragoza is approaching age 45, the professional staff's prediction is not surprising. We should not, however, overlook as one of the ingredients of the Zaragozas' decision the fact that their experience with their retarded son has *not* been terrible.

The next day, when the buccal smear results were available, I called to tell them the results had been within normal limits. Professor

Zaragoza, with whom I spoke, told me that they were leaning toward continuation of the pregnancy. I responded, "I can understand your wanting to do that." He also said they were going to meet with their priest, and would call me when their decision was finalized. A week later, not having heard from them, I called and was informed by Professor Zaragoza that they were going to continue the pregnancy. I wished him and his wife well during the remainder of the pregnancy and said, "We're concerned about your family, and we'd appreciate your letting us know when your wife delivers the baby."

We then wrote them a letter, indicating our support of their decision, and emphasizing the importance of postnatal confirmation of the prenatal diagnosis for laboratory control purposes.

About two weeks after the expected date of delivery, I called Mrs. Zaragoza to find out how she and the baby were doing. She sounded very happy, and said all was well with her. The baby was entirely normal. She indicated that, all in all, the experience had been a positive one, and that if she were to become pregnant again she would undergo amniocentesis. She agreed to allow us to confirm the prenatal diagnosis by analyzing a blood sample from the baby. Since she was to take the baby to the pediatrician soon afterward, we agreed that I would ask him to obtain the blood sample and send it to us. She gave me the pediatrician's name and I telephoned him. Although he had known and worked with the family for many years, and said that he was the one who had suggested they have amniocentesis, he had not been informed of the amniocentesis results. He was very angry. We wrote him a letter, explaining that we had not been informed of his role in the referral for amniocentesis, but that we had learned from this experience the necessity of our requesting permission from the family to apprise the pediatrician of the situation.

Probably this faux pas was unavoidable, in that the genetics staff understood the referral to have been from the obstetrician, who *had* been informed of the amniocentesis result. The sequel underscores for us the fact that communication with the referral source is more than professional etiquette. In the present instance the mishap appears to have undercut a legitimate clinical-scientific intention.

The baby is now more than a year old, and to date we have not been able to confirm the diagnosis. Looking back over the case, I have a few speculations about various aspects of it. I think that Mr. Zaragoza's exclusive reference to himself as "Professor" was significant. I believe he needed to demonstrate that he was intelligent, even though he had "defective" offspring. I consider that the couple's religious beliefs probably made termination of pregnancy a difficult alternative; but it could not by itself have been the critical factor. Had the Zaragozas been unalterably opposed to abortion, they probably would not have undertaken the amniocentesis.

Case No. 2

Mrs. Sawyer was referred for amniocentesis at eighteen and a half weeks' gestation, because she was 42 years old. Like Mrs. Zaragoza, she had not been seen by the genetics service prior to amniocentesis. When the abnormal results of her amniotic fluid chromosome analysis became known at approximately twenty weeks' gestation, her obstetrician was informed. He discussed the situation with her and her husband and referred them for genetic counseling. They gave the following family and medical history.

Mrs. Sawyer's first marriage produced five pregnancies. She had three living children, all in their teens, and had had two spontaneous abortions. That marriage had ended in divorce.

Mrs. Sawyer had recently had a serious illness. Only after lengthy inpatient hospital investigation was the diagnosis of a rare infectious disease assigned. The outlook for eventual recovery was considered good.

As regards the present marriage, Mr. Sawyer had formerly been a Catholic priest. He had left the Church because of disagreements with some of its tenets, and had later married Mrs. Sawyer. He seemed to be fond of his stepchildren and to have a good relationship with them. This was the first time that he was faced with fatherhood. The pregnancy was unplanned, though no contraception had been employed. Mrs. Sawyer had been having frequent nausea, intermittent bleeding, and uterine contractions.

Mr. and Mrs. Sawyer were a highly intelligent couple. Mr. Sawyer had studied medicine for a short time, and was currently working with retarded individuals. They readily understood the genetic information presented to them about the triplo-X condition of the fetus. When we began to discuss the possibility of maternal contamination of the amniotic fluid cells, and the possibility of ruling that out by taking a buccal smear from Mrs. Sawyer, she responded, "Maybe one of my daughters is triplo-X. Should they have a buccal smear?" (I suspected that she was privately hoping to find a normal daughter with triplo-X, so that this unborn child with triplo-X could, by analogy, be assumed to be as normal.) The medical geneticist and I explained the low likelihood that either of her daughters was triplo-X and gently tried to redirect the discussion to the current pregnancy. Mr. Sawyer said, "I like kids. I would like to have the child, and would love her no matter what her condition. I am most concerned about my wife's health and her ability physically to tolerate the pregnancy.''

The reader may wonder what the basis was for the statement to Mrs. Sawyer that the likelihood of either normal daughter's being triplo-X was low. As stated earlier, two studies report the incidence of triplo-X in a series of consecutive newborns to be one per 1,000 female births, making the probability low.

The conversation continued as follows:

G.C.: What did Dr. W [the obstetrician] say about your ability to undertake this pregnancy, Mrs. Sawyer?

MRS. SAWYER: He's concerned, but never suggested I do anything about the pregnancy just because of my current health problem. He did tell me that if I choose to terminate the pregnancy, he wants to perform a hysterectomy at the same time.

G.C.: How do you feel about that?

MRS. SAWYER: Well, I'm not sure I want to end my reproductive career.

G.C.: Did Dr. W. say you could terminate this pregnancy without having a hysterectomy?

MRS. SAWYER: No, he didn't.

G.C.: You should be aware that you have another choice. You can have a pregnancy termination without a hysterectomy, and then have the hysterectomy at a later date, if you decide you want to have it done.

Mrs. Sawyer nodded that she understood. (The words "termination of pregnancy," rather than "abortion," were used throughout the discussion with this couple. They were struggling to do what was best for their family, in spite of their religious background, and we felt we could help them by avoiding use of "abortion.")

The genetic counseling session ended with the plan that Mrs. Sawyer would have a buccal smear, and the couple would discuss the situation with a priest they felt close to. The buccal smear results were within normal limits, but after discussion with the priest, the couple elected to terminate the pregnancy. Mr. Sawyer told me that the priest had agreed with them that the entire family situation should be taken into account in making the decision, and that a termination of pregnancy would be reasonable in their situation. (It was clear to me that they had chosen to seek the advice of a priest who they knew interpreted the Church doctrines liberally.) The pregnancy termination was, in fact, accomplished by hysterectomy. The prenatal diagnosis was confirmed by chromosome analysis of fetal tissue. I offered Mr. Sawyer an opportunity to come in with his wife for follow-up counseling. He wished to defer this until they contacted us, and we never heard from them again.

This case was very different from the first in a number of ways. In the first, the focus of the couple was on their ability to produce a normal child. In the second case, the focus became the wife's own health. In spite of the fact that they were religious Catholics, the Sawyers were able to locate a priest who supported Mr. Sawyer's view that his wife's health was paramount. From this we learned not to prejudge what decisions a couple will make solely on the basis of their religious background. It is interesting that the couple elected to have Mrs. Sawyer end her pregnancy by a hysterectomy. The medical geneticist and I both thought the Sawyers were dealing with their situation very appropriately. One may speculate that the decision to undergo a medically recommended hysterectomy was a means for this couple to avoid having to deal with issues of contraception, abortion, or sterilization in the future.

Further Comment

The fact that both families in the two cases reported are observant Catholics makes the contrast especially instructive. (Recall that the second father had even been a priest.) Religious affiliation may in some instances bolster a decision. In others, the affiliation may be altogether disregarded. Decisions to proceed with pregnancy or to undergo abortion are very complicated. They result from many factors—some quite conscious, such as genetic information, family history, parity, and the like; others more deeply unconscious.

One may argue that for the counselor even to guess what a given couple will decide—a kind of private game which, like any game, one enjoys "winning"—may risk introduction of subtle biases into the counseling. In the editor's view it is probably safer to concentrate on the clarification of issues and permit oneself to be interestingly surprised by the various solutions of different couples to the same or similar dilemmas.

References

DE GROUCHY, J., and TURLEAU, C. (1977). The 47,XXX karyotype. In *Clinical atlas of human chromosomes*, pp. 235-236. New York: John Wiley & Sons.

HAMERTON, J.; CANNING, N.; RAY, M.; and SMITH, S. (1975). A cytogenetic survey of 14,069 newborn infants. Part 1: Incidence of chromosome abnormalities. *Clinical Genetics* 8: 223-243.

JACOBS, P. (1972). Human population cytogenetics. In J. De Grouchy; F. Ebling; and I. Henderson, eds., *Human genetics,* pp. 232–242. (Proceedings of the 4th International Congress of Human Genetics, Paris, 1971.) Amsterdam: Excerpta Medica.

ROBINSON, A.; LUBS, H.; and BERGSMA, D. eds. (1979). Sex chromosome aneuploidy: prospective studies on children. In *Birth defects:* original article series, vol. 5, no. 1. The National Foundation–March of Dimes. New York: Alan R. Liss.

SIMPSON, J. (1976). Polysomy X in females and polysomy Y in males. In *Disorders of sexual differentiation: etiology and clinical delineation,* pp. 361–364. New York: Academic Press.

STEWART, D. ed. (1982). Children with sex chromosome aneuploidy: follow-up studies. In *Birth defects: original article series,* vol. 18, no. 4. March of Dimes Birth Defects Foundation. New York: Alan R. Liss.

20

The Need for Time to Work Through an Agonizing Decision: Werdnig-Hoffmann Disease

The report of a couple's struggle with indecision concerning childbearing in the face of the risk of recurrence of a particular genetic disorder demonstrates how intensely invested with emotion the drive to have one's own children is. In this instance the struggle continued for more than two decades, required periods of psychotherapeutic assistance for both husband and wife, and could finally be resolved only with the skilled intervention of the genetic counselor.

The counseling took place in two segments, separated by an interval of five years. The counselor offers comments concerning the need for that five-year interval. We are also able to observe how a rapport established during just two interviews—which did not lead to the desired result just then—was eminently serviceable five years later when the counseling could proceed to a satisfactory resolution.

Mr. and Mrs. Brothers were self-referred for genetic counseling. They called because they had seen an article about the genetic counseling service at our hospital in a local newspaper. Their first contact was with the secretary, who obtained the basic information. As is our usual procedure, I telephoned the couple to verify the reason for the referral; ascertain what medical records would be needed to confirm the diagnosis which concerned them and arrange for transfer of these records to our office for review by the clinical geneticist and myself prior to the first appointment.

I learned that this couple's only child, Leslie, had died four years before at age 2, with a diagnosis of infantile spinal muscular atrophy type I (Werdnig-Hoffmann disease). The autopsy report, subsequently received, reliably confirmed this diagnosis, and an appointment was scheduled. Since there was a confirmed diagnosis and no patient for whom a physical examination was required, the clinical geneticist was not present during any of the counseling sessions. The counselees were seen in my private office.

They arrived for the interview carrying a large cardboard tube typical of those used to contain a rolled map or poster. Once they were settled into their chairs, I began the interview as follows:

G.C.: Parking at our hospital has become quite a problem. I hope you didn't have too much difficulty.

MR. BROTHERS: No, we were lucky and found a space right away.

G.C.: When we spoke on the phone, you mentioned that you were bringing some family history with you. Could that be what you have rolled in that tube?

MRS. BROTHERS: Yes, we have been working on it for quite some time.

G.C.: I am very interested to see it, but first *I* would like to obtain some information. Please tell me what information *you* want to obtain during our discussions.

MR. BROTHERS: We want the facts about Werdnig-Hoffmann disease.

G.C.: You have had many opportunities to discuss the disease with the doctor who took care of Leslie. What did he tell you?

MR. BROTHERS: Leslie's doctor told us that Werdnig-Hoffmann disease is very rare and he had never seen it before. He read us facts from a medical textbook. Quite frankly, this was not very helpful. We didn't understand most of it, and it wasn't the kind of information we needed.

G.C.: What specifically would you like to know about Werdnig-Hoffmann disease?

MR. BROTHERS: Well, you know Leslie died when she was two years old. Do all children with the disease die so young? If we have another child, what is the chance that this child will also have it? And, I guess most important, is there prenatal diagnosis for Werdnig-Hoffmann disease?

[I noted down all their questions so that they could see I was preparing an agenda for our meeting, and I told them that I would return to each one of the questions. Then I continued.]

G.C.: I will answer each of these questions, but first it would be helpful to obtain some background information.

[With a series of questions I obtained the following history: Mrs. Brothers was 38 years of age, of Irish descent, Catholic, and working as a secretary. Mr. Brothers was 37 years of age, of German descent, Lutheran, and working as a skilled toolmaker. They had been married seventeen years. When they had been married for ten years, Mrs. Brothers conceived for the first time.]

G.C.: Was it your choice to wait ten years to become pregnant?

MRS. BROTHERS: Not at all. Before we were even engaged, my gynecologist told me that I would never conceive. He said I had an "infantile womb."

G.C.: Mr. Brothers, did you know before you were married that you would probably never have children?

MR. BROTHERS: Yes, she told me when we were engaged, and I accepted it.

G.C.: With any regrets?

MR. BROTHERS: I could accept it.

G.C.: How did you take this prediction, Mrs. Brothers?

MRS. BROTHERS: I was never the same psychologically after being told that I couldn't have children.

In taking the history, the genetic counselor asks the husband if he accepted the news from his fiancee that she was likely to be unable to bear a child. Whatever he then told his fiancee — "I could accept it" — has to be heard with the mental footnote that "acceptance" of such news is more than a momentary mental act. "Acceptance" involves the loss of actual children, and of the dream or ideal image of having children. Owing to the complex meanings of such a loss and its impact over years, this renunciation triggers a psychological process of mourning, which extends over considerable time. Mr. Brothers states he could accept it, but Mrs. Brothers readily acknowledges that she was "never the same" after learning the news. The difficulty in accepting such a fate is reflected through the balance of this report.

During this discussion Mrs. Brothers seemed depressed but willing and able to take an active role in the counseling situation. Mr. Brothers was tense, angry, serious, and very sincere. I felt that they were beginning to respond to me with some confidence regarding my intention and ability to assist them with information and understanding.

We continued with the history. The first pregnancy had ended with a spontaneous abortion. Shortly afterward, Mrs. Brothers conceived again. This pregnancy resulted in the birth of Leslie.

I asked them to describe their memories of the first few months following Leslie's birth.

MRS. BROTHERS: Of course, we were overjoyed to have a child after many years of marriage without the hope that we would ever be parents. We didn't realize that Leslie was not as active as she should have been because we had never had a child before.

MR. BROTHERS [interrupting]: I was worried long before my wife, but I was just plain afraid to suggest that there was a problem.

MRS. BROTHERS: You never told me that! [She paused a moment while she thought about this, and then continued.] Anyway, when I took Leslie to the pediatrician for her three-month checkup, the pediatrician said, rather off-hand, that he felt Leslie's muscle tone was not as good as it should be at that age. He suggested that we admit Leslie to the hospital for a few days for evaluation. He didn't seem really worried, so we didn't think there was a serious problem.

MR. BROTHERS: We got worried pretty soon because the doctors were entirely too interested in Leslie. Everyone came in to see her! They were always huddled over her bed talking in whispers while we stood around waiting for someone to tell us something. It was hell! We were terrified. Finally, after four days, our pediatrician took us aside in the hall and told us that the consensus was that Leslie probably had Werdnig-Hoffmann disease. Of course, we didn't know what this meant, but we could tell from his grim expression and sympathetic manner that it was really bad. We asked him what Werdnig-Hoffmann disease is, and he said that she wouldn't recover, but would get progressively weaker. He said that a muscle biopsy would be done, and we would know definitely in two weeks.

MRS. BROTHERS: Those were the longest two weeks of our lives. Again, we got the news in the hall. Of course it was bad, and we knew the worst.

> Whenever professionals show special attention to a patient in the hospital, as here, both patient and family experience magnification of their anxiety. Their imagination fills in the blank of diagnostic uncertainty with the direst speculations. Under the circumstances described, these parents' terror is predictable.
>
> The corridor is not the best place to tell bitter news. Even if it does sink in—if the listeners are not too shocked and stupefied—it will be harder for them to ask whatever questions are stimulated by the news. Professionals may, in view of discomfort at being the bearers of bad news, prefer it this way, however.

Mr. and Mrs. Brothers looked pained, their faces were tense and sad, and their voices quavered while they relived these experiences. I was seated with my chair facing them, and I leaned forward toward them and put my hand on Mrs. Brothers' knee.

G.C.: I can understand how difficult it is to remember this time in your lives. How do you remember feeling?

MRS. BROTHERS: I was angry. It wasn't fair. It was a tease ever to have become pregnant. We had already gotten used to not being parents and never becoming parents. When I did become pregnant, naturally we thought we were going to raise a child. Then we found out our child was going to be taken from us. It wasn't fair!

G.C.: You had good reason to feel angry. You had learned to live and plan your life without expecting to be a mother. Your hopes were raised, only to be destroyed. [Mrs. Brothers nodded.]

G.C.: Mr. Brothers, did you ever feel angry?

Mr. Brothers: Sure, and I still do. It was the first time in my life I had faced a problem I couldn't solve myself.

G.C.: That is certainly frustrating.

Mr. Brothers: Damn right!

G.C.: During this period of time you did have some discussions with the doctor. What did you learn about Werdnig-Hoffmann disease?

They said they were told that the disease was inherited, but they couldn't understand how this could be true because both of them were healthy and Werdnig-Hoffmann disease had never occurred in either family. At this point they opened the tube that they had brought and produced the family history they had researched and drawn out. In order to unroll the pedigree we moved into an empty, adjacent reception room because the pedigree was longer than my office. They had done all this work to prove to themselves and to me, ultimately, that their families were unblemished. We walked up and down looking at the fifteen or eighteen feet of beautifully drawn out family history while they pointed out its various features. Finally Mr. Brothers asked how they could have passed on a genetic disease.

I agreed that they came from fine, healthy families; but one would not expect to find evidence of Werdnig-Hoffmann disease in the ancestors of children with this disease. I then went on to describe autosomal recessive inheritance, beginning with a brief description of chromosomes as visible units of inheritance in each cell of the body. I highlighted the fact that each parent contributes one gene of each gene pair that the fetus receives.

It is important, I continued, to understand all this because Werdnig-Hoffmann disease develops in a baby who has a pair of genes coding for this disease in every cell of its body. The baby has received one of these genes from the mother in the egg, and the other half of the gene pair from the father in the sperm. Individuals who have only one gene for Werdnig-Hoffmann disease (like the parents of a child with the disease) never have any symptoms because the other gene of that pair is functioning properly. One properly functioning gene is sufficient to provide for normal development. The gene for Werdnig-Hoffmann disease is silent as long as the corresponding gene of that pair is doing its job.

When a couple who both carry one gene for Werdnig-Hoffmann disease conceive, there is a 25 percent chance that they will both transmit a gene for it and so have an affected child; a 50 percent chance that the child will be a healthy, normal carrier of one Werdnig-Hoffmann gene; and a 25 percent chance that the child will be completely free of the disease-bearing gene. And, of course, the chances are the same for each pregnancy.

I explained that for them to have had a child with Werdnig-Hoffmann disease, they both had to carry a gene for it, and that it was therefore probable that there are individuals in both families who carry the gene. Very possibly, I added, there had never before been a marriage between two individuals who carried this gene, and therefore no child with the disease had been born in either family, at least not in recent generations recorded in the pedigree.

Studies done in England, I said, reported that approximately one in 80 individuals carry the gene for Werdnig-Hoffmann disease. I didn't go any further with calculations to demonstrate the likelihood for a couple to both be carrying this gene ($1/80 \times 1/80 = 1/6400$) or the statistical chance for two unsuspecting individuals to have an affected child ($1/80 \times 1/80 \times 1/4 = 1/25,600$). My experience is that couples receive such information not as interesting facts but rather as facts that emphasize their misfortune to be the "one" on the wrong side of the ratio.

At the time of this first interview (1975), prenatal diagnosis was not possible for Werdnig-Hoffmann disease, and this information was communicated to Mr. and Mrs. Brothers. I asked them how they felt about a 25 percent recurrence risk without prenatal diagnosis. They felt that this risk was too high to accept. Their primary concern was the suffering of the affected child. I did caution them, however, that if they decided on another pregnancy, prenatal diagnosis would be recommended for chromosomal disorders, particularly Down syndrome, because Mrs. Brothers was already over the age of 35.

We went on to discuss Werdnig-Hoffmann disease in some detail. I explained that it is a neuromuscular disease suspected in a "floppy," or hypotonic, infant who may have been without symptoms in the first month or two of life. Ninety-five percent of cases are diagnosed at 3 months of age. The underlying problem is degeneration of nerve cells (anterior horn cells) found in the spinal cord. These cells normally relay impulses to the muscles of the arms and legs. The muscles in the arms and legs of these patients become atrophied due to lack of innervation. Muscle biopsy confirms the diagnosis when it shows this type of muscle atrophy. Postmortem examination provides confirmation of the diagnosis when it shows decreased numbers of anterior horn cells in the spinal cord.

Eventually a more generalized muscle weakness develops, and the child is unable to move, speak, swallow, or breathe independently. Weakness of the muscles controlling swallowing leads to repeated episodes of aspiration pneumonia and other respiratory problems and is the usual cause of death. The disease is particularly tragic because the intellect remains normal throughout. The average age at death is 7 months.

I particularly stressed that some children with Werdnig-Hoffmann disease have survived to age 5 or 6, unlike Leslie, who died at age 2. In families where survival is longer, the burden of the disease is greater, and this must be considered when one thinks about the 25 percent recurrence risk. When I stated that the intellect remains normal until the end, they both responded sadly that this aspect of their child's disorder was for them the hardest part of the experience. They were both tearful when they recalled Leslie as having been extremely weak but with bright clear eyes, comprehending everything that was happening around her bedside.

Then they put the expected question:

MRS. BROTHERS: What would *you* do about another pregnancy?

G.C.: It really wouldn't be helpful for me to answer that question for you because I won't have to live with the consequences of the decision. I believe I *can* be of assistance by helping you to discuss your feelings, to consider all options, and to understand the facts upon which your decision should be based.

MRS. BROTHERS: What *are* our options?

G.C.: There are several. What options can you think of?

MR. BROTHERS: Well, I could have a vasectomy, or my wife could have a tubal ligation.

MRS. BROTHERS: I could have another pregnancy. We could go on practicing birth control as we have been doing. Also, we could adopt a baby, or we could have artificial insemination.

MR. BROTHERS: We have been thinking about all of these possibilities for a long time, but we're unable to make up our minds.

[They looked tense and distressed.]

G.C.: These are obviously tough choices. Probably no one option seems ideal. We will have to discuss them carefully.

It was apparent that they needed time to digest the information I had already provided for them. They also wished to think about their options in view of these added facts. I suggested that we schedule another appointment, and they agreed. I then asked what form of contraception they were practicing. Mr. Brothers was using condoms. This method had been satisfactory, and they planned to continue with it at least until we met again.

They were just about to leave when Mrs. Brothers turned to say, "You know I'm Catholic. We have to use contraceptives, but it makes me feel terrible.'' Since we had been together over an hour, I replied, ''We must discuss this problem the next time we meet. Perhaps you should talk to your parish priest in the meantime. Maybe you can obtain official sanction to use contraception. I also urge you to talk openly to each other while you consider these different issues.''

We shook hands all around; they thanked me and left the office.

On their return four weeks later, I began as follows:

G.C.: When you left here four weeks ago, you were planning to think about the possibility of another pregnancy and the alternatives available to you. How do you feel about these questions now?

Mrs. Brothers: We talked a lot about artificial insemination. For a while we thought this might work out for us because half a loaf is better than none. But then we decided we couldn't do it.

G.C.: What changed your minds?

Mr. Brothers: Thinking about artificial insemination made me feel as if I was going off the deep end!

G.C.: Why was it such an upsetting idea?

Mr. Brothers: I'm not sure that a child conceived that way would have a soul!

G.C.: Why not?

Mr. Brothers: Because the pregnancy is not God's will. Conceiving like that is taking things in your own hands. . . . Dammit, it's like rape! I'm not so worried about the child while it's here on this earth; but without a soul, it couldn't go on to the Hereafter!

He spoke with great intensity and emotion. It seemed to me that he was sharing with me thoughts that he had never verbalized before. He came very close to tears. His wife listened with deep interest. While he had apparently never expressed these particular sentiments to her, she did not seem surprised at what he had said. The common denominator was the extent to which they had suffered and still were suffering as the result of their daughter's illness and death, and the dilemmas with which they were now struggling. The individual way in which each expressed this suffering could not generate additional emotion on the part of either spouse.

I was startled by Mr. Brothers' reasons for refusing artificial insemination. It is not unusual for couples to find it unacceptable. Typically this is because one or both simply cannot accept parenthood on this basis. Most frequently it is the father who feels he may have difficulty with his role. I would not have been surprised if the couple had refused because the donor could not be screened to determine if he carried the gene for Werdnig-Hoffmann disease. In fact, I would have raised this issue if they had shown interest in the procedure. They were not at all interested in donor selection or other aspects of the procedure itself. Their objections were on an entirely different plane. I responded as follows:

G.C.: Many people have strong feelings about artificial insemination. It certainly is not for everybody. You have obviously thought about it seriously and rejected it for valid personal reasons. Mrs. Brothers, what are your reasons for deciding against artificial insemination?

Mrs. Brothers: My major reason is that the Catholic Church considers it grounds for excommunication.

G.C.: Suppose there were no religious reasons. How would you feel about it personally?

Mrs. Brothers: To tell you the truth, that's just an excuse. I just don't want to conceive that way.

G.C.: Okay, I think that settles that issue. Let's talk about adoption. Did you look into this?

Mrs. Brothers: Yes, we did. It was very discouraging. We were offered only mixed racial or handicapped children. We can't even consider the added problems of raising such a child. We also met with my parish priest, by the way. That's the really big story. We asked him for permission to use contraception. We told him all about Leslie, of course, and the chance to have another child like her. He said no. We just couldn't believe it, even though I think we expected to hear just that. We were so upset that he suggested we arrange for an appeal to a tribunal.

G.C.: What is a tribunal?

Mrs. Brothers: That's like final arbitration. You go to talk to a number of priests, and whatever they decide is final. We have an appointment in two weeks. We're going to continue to use contraception 'til then, but I feel very guilty about it.

G.C.: I am anxious to hear about the outcome of that conference. Have you come to a decision about the possibility of a tubal ligation or a vasectomy?

Mr. Brothers: We still haven't ruled out a pregnancy at some time in the future, particularly if our financial situation improves.

G.C.: Shall we make another appointment after your meeting with the tribunal?

Mr. Brothers: No, we'll call you.

G.C.: Do you have any questions about the information we have already discussed?

Mrs. Brothers: No, it is really very clear. Thank you.

G.C.: I will be sending you a letter summarizing our discussions.

Mrs. Brothers called about three weeks later to say that the tribunal had refused permission for contraception. They were very disappointed but planned to continue using contraception anyway. They didn't want another appointment. I called six months later. Mrs. Brothers said that the situation remained the same. Again, they didn't want another appointment. She thanked me for the letter I had sent summarizing the counseling.

Five years later, in 1980, Mrs. Brothers telephoned to say that she was considering a tubal ligation. She wanted to make another appointment so that she and her husband could review the situation with me prior to making the decision about this permanent form of birth control. She told me that her husband had been hospitalized for a nervous breakdown twice during the five years since we had met. He had sought another type of job with less pressure because of the tensions he continued to feel.

When they arrived at my office a week later, we chatted for a few minutes and then I brought the conversation around to their present concern.

G.C.: I have been wondering why you are considering a tubal ligation at this particular time—after so many years.

Mrs. Brothers: Well, you know I'm 43 now. I guess I'm beginning to go through my changes, and my cycle is becoming irregular. Twice my period has been late, which is very unusual for me, and I thought I was pregnant. Each time we got very upset, which made us very aware that we didn't want a pregnancy. I realized that I wouldn't want an abortion, and I began to think that I should have a tubal ligation so that there would be no chance that I could conceive.

G.C.: I can understand your feeling about preventing conception in the most reliable way, since you now realize you don't want a pregnancy. Let's go back a bit. How did you react to the decision of the tribunal five years ago?

Mr. Brothers: That decision really blew my mind! They were so absolutely rigid!

Mrs. Brothers: That's what caused his first nervous breakdown. He hated to see me feeling so guilty about using contraception, and we really couldn't consider having sex without it.

G.C.: Did you rule out a vasectomy?

Mr. Brothers: I thought about it, and in a way I really felt I should do it and take the burden off my wife. But just thinking about it almost caused me to have another nervous breakdown. Later on, thinking seriously about artificial insemination caused the second nervous breakdown. Even after all these years in therapy, I don't know why I couldn't take thinking about these things.

G.C.: You were really on the brink for a long time.

When a patient is participating in psychological therapy, I avoid being too "analytical." I decided not to say that they should have called me or that I was sorry they hadn't called me. Why should I imply that they should feel guilty about not turning to me and make them apologize? Mr. Brothers obviously had had professional help during this period of time. With the degree of difficulty described, he needed the attention of a psychiatrist. I did feel distressed that they had refused a third appointment five years before. I had either failed to estimate fully the stress they had been under when I last saw them or it had developed after the last conference—depriving me of the opportunity to refer them promptly to a psychiatrist.

As is true of every interaction between a helping professional and a counselee, patient, or client, *both* partners to the encounter have feelings about what goes on or does not occur as desired. (This observation is illustrated many times throughout this casebook, whether specifically commented upon or not.) Every professional hopes to accrue daily the satisfaction of "functional pleasure," that special sense that one knows one's "business" and conducts it well, with observable benefits for those targeted.

In the present instance the counselor acknowledges *to herself* her sense of frustration that five years earlier the course of the interaction had deprived her of opportunity to be more useful *then*. Alert to the futility of voicing her frustration to the counselees—after all, five years earlier she could in no way have forced them to come for an interview they didn't, for whatever reason, want—this counselor proceeds rapidly to frame a new approach to the dilemma based on all information available, including the interim history.

There can be numerous factors that tilt a counseling interaction off the path desired by either or both parties, some of them controllable and others not at all. (A full discussion of them will be found in textbooks on psychotherapy and counseling.) Speaking categorically, four large groups of factors are skewing influences: (1) lack of knowledge, experience, and emotional resilience on the part of the counselor; (2) comparable lacks in the counselee; (3) "turn-offs" related to a specific mismatch between counselor and counselee, which are alluded to by such remarks as "I don't like how I feel with this person, and it makes it hard to pay attention"; (4) random or situational features, like geographical distance, or accidental intrusion by super-influential personages outside the bailiwick of the counseling.

Viewing the broad categories just described, one can appreciate that the factors in group 1 are those most subject to counselor control; group 2 factors are much less so, and those in groups 3 and 4 are usually not controllable by the counselor at all.

Novice counselors are subject to experiencing "miscarriage" of counseling personally: that is, as attesting to some disparagement of their net worth as counselors-in-training, or even as human beings. Once beyond this early phase of experience, having acquired a measure of professional respect and self-esteem, the counselor responds primarily in a curious or "analytic" mode to a defeat of her efforts.

Mr. and Mrs. Brothers wanted to know, before they went ahead with a tubal ligation, if it was now possible to make a prenatal diagnosis of Werdnig-Hoffmann disease. I explained that there had been studies of pregnancies at risk for the disease in which fetal movements were monitored with ultrasound. At approximately eighteen weeks' gestation an ultrasound examination could be done to note fetal activity. The procedure was without risk to the pregnancy, as far as could be indicated by available information. Of course it would be necessary to wait until the fourth month of pregnancy before doing the study. If the result showed decreased fetal activity, this would suggest that the fetus was affected. The reliability of this type of evaluation is not well understood; and not enough pregnancies have been monitored in this way to determine whether the outcome of pregnancy corresponds with the interpretation of the fetal movements. Mr. and Mrs. Brothers were not enthusiastic about the possibility of evaluating the pregnancy with ultrasound. Both of them were shaking their heads and looking disappointed that this was all that was available in 1980.

Since they didn't seem to be making any progress toward a decision, I decided to try a different approach. I suggested that they try to project the relief or anxiety that would be associated with the various alternatives available to them. I took a pad of paper and together we listed the following options: (1) prenatal diagnosis with positive results, which would lead to a termination of pregnancy; (2) prenatal diagnosis with normal results, which would lead to a full-term pregnancy with an indeterminate outcome because ultrasound evaluation has an unknown degree of reliability; (3) chemical or mechanical forms of birth control; and (4) permanent forms of birth contol (tubal ligation or vasectomy). I asked them to try to choose the plan or outcome that would lead to the least anxiety for the shortest period of time. We then considered one option at a time.

G.C.: First, let's consider the possibility that you would have sonography with results suggestive of Werdnig-Hoffmann disease. Following this report you would decide to terminate the pregnancy. How do you imagine you would feel?

MRS. BROTHERS: We couldn't terminate; we realize that now.

G.C.: Why not?

MRS. BROTHERS: Because terminating a pregnancy when the fetus had

Werdnig-Hoffmann disease would be like doing to the sick fetus what happened to Leslie.

G.C.: Do you agree, Mr. Brothers?

MR. BROTHERS: Yes.

G.C.: Let's consider the second possibility. Suppose you have ultra-sound with normal results and the pregnancy goes full term?

MR. BROTHERS: I would still worry that if the baby didn't have Werdnig-Hoffmann disease, it would have something else.

G.C.: Having had a tragic outcome to the last pregnancy, you feel vulnerable, isn't that so? I can appreciate how you feel. Statistics aren't much comfort to you, I know; but I must emphasize that every pregnancy has a 2 to 3 percent risk for a major abnormality at the time of delivery. The bottom line is that aside from Werdnig-Hoffmann disease your chance for a normal child would be the same as for any couple in your age category. This feeling of vulnerability may leave you unwilling to take even that chance.

MRS. BROTHERS: We could accept prenatal diagnosis only if it gave us a 100 percent guarantee that the baby would not have Werdnig-Hoffmann disease.

MR. BROTHERS: I'd want to know it didn't have anything else also. I don't even want the anxiety of waiting for test results from an am-niocentesis for Down syndrome or anything else. I don't think I could take the strain.

G.C.: Okay, let's think about the third possibility. How would you feel about some form of reliable contraception such as an intrauterine device?

MRS. BROTHERS: My gynecologist suggested an IUD or birth control pills, but they're not foolproof and there can be complications. I would be nervous about a diaphragm too.

G.C.: Mr. Brothers, we talked about a vasectomy a long time ago. How do you feel now about having a vasectomy?

MR. BROTHERS: I still feel so agitated when I think about it that I'm afraid of a nervous breakdown. I'm guilty about not being strong enough to do it, but I just can't.

G.C: Well, that brings us to the last plan on our list—tubal ligation.

MRS. BROTHERS: This is probably our best bet; but thinking about it is very upsetting.

[The problem seemed to be that the tubal ligation was not perceived as a good solution because they both felt a high level of anxiety when they considered it. I decided to explore the source of this anxiety.]

G.C.: Why do you find it so difficult to decide to have a tubal ligation?

MRS. BROTHERS: Needing to make this decision now has opened up everything again, and I've started to see a psychiatrist again every week.

G.C.: What do you mean that you have started to see a psychiatrist *again?*

MRS. BROTHERS: Well, I had been seeing a psychiatrist for two years between 1975 and 1977.

[I was now even more aware that a great deal had happened to this couple since our two previous meetings five years earlier. I wondered whether I could have explored their feelings more thoroughly during those two meetings. Perhaps they had not been ready to discuss their feelings with me at that time. Possibly the years of psychotherapy had helped them to open up. Perhaps it was simply the passage of time. Finally, I considered the possibility that my own skills had improved over the years. I returned to Mrs. Brothers' earlier statement.]

G.C.: What did you mean when you said that "needing to make this decision has opened up everything again"?

MRS. BROTHERS: I have never given up the hope that we would have another baby. Thinking about cutting my tubes is like cutting Leslie off.

G.C.: Why would it be like cutting Leslie off?

MRS. BROTHERS [in tears]: My psychiatrist told me that I am still hoping to get Leslie back. I guess that's why cutting my tubes is like cutting her off.

MR. BROTHERS [putting his arm around his wife]: I've been afraid for her to go ahead with the tubal ligation because something new might develop in prenatal diagnosis, and then we would regret having done it.

MRS. BROTHERS: My psychiatrist told me that I have enough trouble just going through each day. Another pregnancy would be too much. I couldn't even handle the first pregnancy.

G.C.: Do you mean when you were pregnant with Leslie? [This was actually her second pregnancy.]

MRS. BROTHERS [nodding]: I was so fearful during that pregnancy that I boiled all of our laundry to prevent germs from reaching the fetus. I was always cleaning the house. My psychiatrist told me that I had an obsessive-compulsive neurosis.

The reported psychiatric advice not to chance another pregnancy is understandable, but leaves us with an unanswerable question: The therapist believes he can foresee the consequences of adding a pregnancy to Mrs. Brothers' situation, and bases his advice upon that calculation. Can anyone, however, foresee the consequences to this couple, for the balance of their lives, of *not* adding a pregnancy, presuming that prenatal diagnosis one day becomes possible? The genetic counselor has opted all along for a neutral stance, leaving the couple to choose as freely as possible.

At the end of this discussion I summed up all the couple's responses and asked them what they felt would be the best choice for them. Mrs. Brothers replied, "Probably the tubal ligation, because look what the need to make this decision is doing to me. At least after that decision there would be no more decisions." Mr. Brothers agreed. "That's how I feel, too."

We went on to talk about their feelings and experiences during the years since our last meeting. They had continued over the years to talk about their remorse, hopes, and options. They had remembered Leslie as she was when she was an infant and throughout her illness when they watched her become more and more inactive, weaker every day, until finally she couldn't move or talk. When they entered her room, her eyes would follow them, and they knew she understood everything around her. Mr. Brothers said that he was glad they had had Leslie. It was better to have had her than never to have experienced being parents. Suddenly, Mrs. Brothers interrupted.

MRS. BROTHERS: I've been thinking about your first question, which was "Why are you considering a tubal ligation at the present time?" I suddenly realize why I can think about a tubal ligation now. All along I have had the hope that someday I would have another baby, and that the baby would not only be healthy but would be Leslie returning as a healthy baby. Your question made me realize that I can think about a tubal ligation now because I finally know that this is never going to happen.
[She started to cry and her husband came close to crying also. They looked at each other and held hands.]
MRS. BROTHERS [very wistfully]: We talked and talked so much over the years with you, with our therapist, with our doctors, and with each other. We seemed to be saying the same thing over and over, and all of those conversations led nowhere.
G.C.: Perhaps you should consider that it may have taken all of those "repetitive" conversations, including the years of therapy, to bring you to the point where you could reach a decision and be at peace. [They both nodded.]
MR. BROTHERS [with tears in his eyes]: I believe that we will catch up with her in heaven—or at least my wife will, because she is a Catholic and I am only a bad Lutheran.

This was the time to conclude the session. I asked them if they felt that they had reached their decision, and they said "Yes." I asked them if there was anything else they wanted to discuss with me, and they said "No." As they were leaving, Mr. Brothers said that they would be glad to make themselves available if they could be helpful in research efforts concerning Werdnig-Hoffmann disease. He thanked me for my help, particularly in the beginning, when, as he said, I was "the only one who laid it on the line" for them.

I spoke with Mrs. Brothers by telephone after the tubal ligation had been performed. She was depressed but not sorry. She was continuing to see the psychiatrist and anxious to get her life back in order. She said her husband had taken it well.

The pivotal point in this last interview was the one well-placed, on-target question asking why they were considering a tubal ligation at this particular point in time. The counseling session also served to focus their thoughts regarding the alternatives available to them. After many years of considerable distress this couple was visibly more at peace with themselves and their problem.

Further Comment

After ten years of marriage Mrs. Brothers did conceive and later had a spontaneous abortion. We do not learn the impact of this miscarriage, but remind ourselves that it is an event consonant with the gloomy prediction of the gynecologist prior to the marriage. The new conception, "shortly afterward," is in keeping with a popular belief that a prompt new pregnancy will somehow cancel the painful impact of a prior miscarriage.

When the counselor learns of the impact of Leslie's diagnosis on Mr. and Mrs. Brothers, she can empathize with their helpless passivity in the face of something they cannot control. In the discussion that ensues, the counselor gives a careful explanation of autosomal recessive inheritance, and properly emphasizes that the probabilities are the same with every single pregnancy. She is careful to avoid adding information that could possibly heighten the couple's sense of their misfortune. The Brothers' remark, in keeping with their experience with their affected daughter, that for them the one-in-four chance of a recurrence is too big a chance for them to take. This observation by the counselees highlights the fact that the longer a child survives, the more intense is the emotional bond with the parents, so that the pain of the eventual loss is correspondingly greater. The child's intellectual normality enhances the attachment and aggravates the pain of the loss.

When the counselor is pressed to advise what she would do about having another child in these circumstances, she adopts a strictly hands-off attitude and gives a simple, polite, direct explanation for it.

Religious precept and belief enter this complicated situation in a number of different ways, introducing important variables, although probably not the weightiest. Contraception, for example, is practiced in the face of religious proscription, attesting to the major impact of the losses already sustained. Artificial insemination is rejected for reasons that appear more idiosyncratic than strictly religious. The sequel to the clerical tribunal's proscription of contraception is not surprising. The Brothers' suffering has been such that their need for birth control overwhelms other considerations.

The response to questioning about the option to adopt a child is also of interest, offering a caution to those advisers tempted to say "You can always adopt." The fact is that there may be many reasons why the option to adopt is unattractive. As we later learn, both counselees have received psychiatric care in connection with their family-planning experiences, and in certain settings a history of this degree of emotional unsettlement may be regarded as disqualifying prospective parents for adoption placement.

Five years after the initial counseling experience the couple return to discuss their plan for Mrs. Brothers to undergo tubal ligation. It is strongly suggested that the experiences in the intervening five years with psychological illness as well as the approach to menopause have produced a major change in attitude about chancing another pregnancy. Until now, less aggressive forms of contraception have sufficed, suggesting that some feeling about the possibility of trying again is still quietly present in the back of the couple's minds. Indeed, they ask the counselor if there have been any new developments in making a prenatal diagnosis of their daughter's disease — which also suggests a lingering wish to learn if there is any way that they might proceed with less anxiety about giving birth to another affected child before making a final decision not to have their own children.

The news that Mrs. Brothers was in psychotherapy after the initial counseling sequence suggests how difficult it must have been to digest the news of her genetic dilemma, compounding as it did (1) the original gynecological prediction, (2) the long wait until first conception, (3) the miscarriage, and (4) the loss of Leslie.

For the couple, the prospect of tubal ligation means a final loss of the dream of a healthy replacement infant at the same time that it precludes the possibility of a new pregnancy's further disruption of their already troubled life pattern. We should also bear in mind that the emotional impact of tubal ligation or vasectomy is akin to that of castration, a more than adequate stimulus for eliciting anxiety.

Mrs. Brothers, perhaps because of the psychotherapeutic experience she has undergone, is able to be quite articulate in describing the meaning for her of a wished-for new baby in terms of the lost Leslie. The persistence despite everything of this cherished wish emphasizes to us what a long and tormenting process may be involved in arriving at a decision to forego any possibility of having a family. The length of time between the original pronouncement prior to marriage by Mrs. Brothers' gynecologist and her final decision to have a tubal ligation was at least twenty-three years.

References

EMERY, A. (1971). The nosology of the spinal muscular atrophies. *J. Med. Genetics* 8: 481–495.

MUNSAT, T.; WOODS, R.; FOWLER, W.; and PEARSON, C. (1969). Neurogenic muscular atrophy of infancy with prolonged survival. *Brain* 92: 9–24.

PEARN, J. (1980). Classification of spinal muscular atrophies. *Lancet* 1: 919–922.

21

A Divided Family: Counseling for Huntington's Disease

This chapter and the following one focus on problems caused by neurological maladies of late onset, characterized by progressive deterioration in most patients, and inherited as autosomal dominant disorders. The diagnosis of such a disorder has great impact on the life of the afflicted person with regard to the quality of his indefinite survival. Of course such a diagnosis also affects the family members with whom he resides, the marriage he may make, and the progeny he may conceive.

For the counselor the strain of working with such a family is very great and long protracted. Bearer of dreaded news, the counselor faces probably the greater part of his or her work only from that point onward.

The reader will appreciate that in such long-term situations, the counselor must be prepared to "go the distance" with the patient in order to be truly helpful, and that frustrations of the counselor's intentions are numerous. Long-term availability for follow-up is not a necessity unique to late-onset neurological disorders, but it is strongly highlighted in dealing with the counselees described below.

Ours is a large department of medical genetics, comprising a number of physicians specializing in medical genetics, a dentist, a pediatric orthopedic surgeon, a clinical social worker (myself), and patient assistants. Our outpatient clinic meets weekly, seeing fourteen patients on the average. The social worker makes every effort to meet all new patients and their families before they are seen by the medical specialists. We orient counselees to the routine of the genetics clinic and seek to allay initial anxieties.

After examination, diagnosis, and counseling by the medical geneticist several selected patients are presented to the entire staff and visiting staff at the afternoon case review. The social worker makes certain that she sees all patients and their families after they have been counseled to provide them with an opportunity to react to the genetic diagnoses, and to ascertain their understanding of the counseling they have been given. It is made clear that further communication is welcomed whether by letter, telephone call, or visit. This procedure is essential, particularly for those people who travel great distances to attend the clinic.

The counselor's contact with the counselees *following* their interaction with the medical geneticists is probably valuable to *all* counselees—not only those residing at a distance. The experience of medical consultation about family-planning issues is naturally a strong generator of anxiety. In some medical centers counselees are seen in settings in which numerous white-coated staff members are present, which facilitates the pooling of professional intelligence on a given problem but which most counselees find intimidating, and which interferes with absorption of new information.

Not rarely, counselee anxiety may obliterate or severely distort the information conveyed so that immediate recall, or recall the following day, is insufficient. For these reasons multiple contacts with counselees are invaluable for correcting distortions and improving the effectiveness of the counseling.

The social worker is often included in the genetic counseling session at her own request or that of the medical geneticists. Patients and families who seem to be particularly troubled are specifically referred to the social worker by the medical staff. She arranges psychological evaluation, further counseling, or referral to community services when indicated.

The case to be reported concerns a family who was in consultation with us over a two-and-a-half-year period. It has been selected to illustrate the special needs of a family struggling with the devastating dilemmas of a late-onset dominant disorder. A family in which the father had already been diagnosed elsewhere as having Huntington's disease (HD) had requested a clinic appointment. Dr. R., the medical geneticist specializing in neurological disorders, believed that the psychosocial burdens of a family already having one HD victim and in further jeopardy for this disorder required special attention. Consequently, he scheduled the Bates family for a non-clinic day, allowing me ample time to speak with them.

Huntington's disease is an unusual genetic disorder in that its symptoms are generally not apparent until adult life, usually between 35 and 45, although the full range of age at onset is very great. By the time an individual has been identified as affected by this disease, he or she has probably already had children and unknowingly transmitted the mutant gene to some of them. The gene for HD is dominant, which means, of course, a transmission probability of 50 percent with each pregnancy. If the offspring of an affected person does not inherit the gene, he or she will be free of the disease and cannot possibly transmit it to future generations. There are an estimated 25,000 Americans who have the symptoms of HD, and approximately 100,000 who are at risk for developing it. Because of the deaths of persons who have the HD gene but who die for one reason or another before symptoms become evident, statistics for gene frequency cannot be accurate.

Huntington's disease involves notable symptoms in both psychiatric and neurological categories. There may be severe mood changes noted even prior to any neurological manifestations, such as irritability and obstinacy. As the malady gets worse, the affected individual may behave violently toward property, self, or others. Suicide is not a rarity. Finer affectionate and ethical sensibilities are lost; paranoid trends, delusions, and hallucinations may appear as prominent features of a florid psychosis. Intellectual functions suffer, progressing to dementia. Tendencies toward withdrawal from social interaction steadily worsen.

As to the neurological manifestations, choreiform movements—involuntary, clumsy, jerky, and irregular—steadily affect more muscle groups, including those that affect the functioning of the upper extremities, face and neck, swallowing, speech, and gait. In the most advanced stages, the sufferer may be bedridden and helpless. Death intervenes usually from five to twenty years after the time of onset.

There is neither effective treatment nor a reliable means of detecting the presence of the HD gene before symptoms become clinically evident. It is understandable that the toll taken on the affected person and his family is horrendous. The counselor cannot allow his own feelings of hopelessness to add to those of the patient and family. Affected and potentially affected persons must be treated as responsible and responsive human beings as long as it is possible to continue doing so.

Genetic counseling frequently deals with very depressing conditions, and HD is an example of one which represents the most frustrating possible experience for the professional: From the outset one knows that health cannot be maintained nor death deferred. Yet affected persons must live till they die, and we try to ease, if possible, their path of torment. For a counselor to become depressed is expectable, but the professional deals with such feelings privately or with peer support to be able to remain effective.

I had arranged an appointment with Mrs. Susan Bates (age 50) and her 24-year-old daughter, Ruth. Ruth was to be examined by Dr. R. for early symptoms of HD. Ruth's 53-year-old affected father, Philip Bates, formerly employed by a large corporation, was temporarily hospitalized at a large medical center, spending only weekends at home. The Bates' had two younger children, a 17-year-old daughter, Lois, and a 23-year-old son, Daniel. The family lived some distance from our facility, making appointments difficult to arrange.

All described interviews took place in my office and lasted from thirty minutes to an hour. The following interview was with Mrs. Bates.

S.W. [after explaining what my position was on the genetics team]: Dr. R. tells me that you are here today because of your concern that your daughter, Ruth, may have inherited Huntington's disease from your husband. Is that your understanding of why you are here?

MRS. BATES [chain-smoking nervously]: Yes. But I am so hoping that I am only imagining things. When your husband is so ill with HD, there is a tendency, I suppose, to look for the symptoms in your children.

S.W.: That is certainly understandable. But is there anything in particular that has happened which causes you to suspect HD in Ruth now?

MRS. BATES: Well, yes. She was doing pretty well training to be a rehab counselor when she began dropping some equipment. Of course, she's always been clumsy since she was a toddler, so maybe this is nothing new. But then they ousted her from their program, and she has gotten so depressed as a result.

S.W.: This must have been upsetting to you, particularly in light of your apprehensions about your children inheriting HD. What is Ruth doing how?

MRS. BATES: She isn't doing much of anything, eats all the time, watches TV, and fights with Daniel, her brother. And she sits holding her hands tightly together for fear they will start shaking like her father's. I think she is terrified. She sees her father steadily going downhill.

S.W.: And you are frightened, too?

MRS. BATES: Yes, I'm frightened to death! I couldn't take two in my family. . . . But I really don't believe Ruth has it. She is much too young. Her father didn't show symptoms until he was 49!

S.W.: She *is* young, although there have been others her age who have had symptoms of HD. That makes is more difficult for you to accept the possibility that she has the disease.

MRS. BATES: I really don't think she has it. It's just that she's clumsy, and she's so close to her father than she imitates him (a circumstance that sometimes occurs).

In instances in which motoric abnormalities are shown by a close relative who is *not* affected, the process is likely to be a spontaneous, unplanned similarity (that is, an unconscious process of identification with the sick person by way of symptoms) rather than a deliberate imitation. Plainly, the daughter has become depressed—and understandably so.

S.W.: Tell me more about Ruth, about her interests, her hobbies. Is she a sociable young woman?

MRS. BATES: She has always been more or less a loner, except for people in need. She identifies with causes. She loves to read and listen to records. She particularly enjoys playing the guitar in her room. Actually, she has always put walls around herself. I can't get close to her.

S.W.: That must be difficult for you.

MRS. BATES: It is. But I have always been closest to Dan. I'm close to Lois, my younger daughter, too, but she doesn't need me the way Dan does. It feels good that he still turns to me for help. Maybe that's because Ruth and her father were always so close that I felt shut out. They went to bluegrass concerts and book fairs together. They were on the same wavelength somehow.

S.W.: Can you tell me something about your feelings toward your husband, now that he is so ill?

MRS. BATES [beginning to sob]: He's been sick for three years now. He never told me that his mother had died of HD. At first I was so angry at him. But I loved him very much. He was a real man! Now he is a weakling, a baby. I have to take care of him now. He even wets the bed! He sits home on weekends, watching TV and getting angry at us all. And I have to be the breadwinner. I have to be the strong one. It isn't easy. We had something good going for us. And now it's all gone [more sobs]. I just couldn't take it if Ruth is that way, too.

S.W.: You are naturally very angry at what has happened to your marriage because it was so good. You have managed remarkably well, but you are having to face the possibility of Ruth having what your husband has. And that is not easy.

MRS. BATES: That's right. All I have left now is my children. They are my sanity.

S.W.: You feel that you have nothing left with your husband?

MRS. BATES: We were so compatible—in every way. Our sex life was beautiful. He was so intelligent and sensitive. Now we have no sex; we never go out; I'm embarrassed to have friends over.

S.W.: That does not sound as if you're getting much satisfaction for yourself.

MRS. BATES: There is a man at work, really interested in me. But how can I do that to Phil, who always loved me and was so good to me? I could never forgive myself.

Mrs. Bates has lost both the man her husband was and her dreams of the life they would lead together as parents and grandparents. Her requirement to tend an invalid with deteriorating health and capacity to gratify her in any adult way serves daily to remind her of her past and expected future losses. Further, the temptation to be unfaithful adds a serious conflict of conscience.

S.W.: What satisfactions do you have for yourself now?

Mrs. Bates: My work. Thank God for that.

S.W.: I think it is essential that you continue to get some satisfaction for yourself and that you get away from home from time to time. We both know that you cannot avoid your problems at home permanently, but you can look for satisfaction for yourself elsewhere. In that way, you can be more helpful at home.

Mrs. Bates: It is so good to have someone concentrate on my own troubles and not just on Phil or my daughter. Thank you for listening to me.

From certain viewpoints the task of helping this burdened wife permits more room for maneuvering than the project of treating her afflicted husband.

Following her examination by Dr. R. that day, Ruth Bates was interviewed. She was a pleasant, soft-spoken 24-year-old who rarely looked at me while I was speaking to her.

S.W.: Ruth, what is your understanding of why Dr. R. sent you to talk to me today?

Ruth: He knows I'm worried, and he told me you are a social worker who might be able to help me with some of my worries.

S.W.: Want to talk about what's worrying you?

Ruth: Well, I think Dr. R. thinks I have what my dad has.

S.W.: And what do you think, yourself?

Ruth: I honestly don't know. I have feared getting Huntington's disease. I'm so like my father. But I'm too young.

S.W.: You are young, and you have plans for your future. I understand that your college training prepared you for a rehabilitation counseling program, but they would not let you continue with it. What are your feelings about that?

Ruth: Well [holding her hands tightly together], I don't know why they let me go. I really was shocked. They only gave me five days' notice. And just because I dropped something.

S.W.: Had you thought about the possibility that you might inherit what your dad has?

RUTH: Sure, I've thought about it a lot because I've always been so much like my father. But I never thought I would get it this young. We all got genetic counseling, but somehow I thought it could not happen to me. I paid for the training program myself, and now it's all money down the drain.

S.W.: You sound very sad and angry.

RUTH [tearfully]: I am, I am. . . . And I'm sorry for Mom. Because it's going to be rough on her if I really have HD.

S.W.: What other ambitions have you had for yourself other than rehab counseling? Perhaps you can consider another channel.

RUTH: Once I thought of being a nursery school teacher. I've always loved children. Children are so affectionate; you can do so much for them.

S.W.: You can do a lot for older people, too. We can look into some of these fields together, if you'd like, after you get the results of Dr. R.'s tests.

RUTH: Let's do that. Maybe we can arrange another appointment for next week?

The expression "results of Dr. R.'s tests" may be misleading to some readers. There is as yet no test that can diagnose Huntington's disease in someone who carries the gene but as yet demonstrates no symptoms. The neurological examinations that are offered in the effort to arrive at an early diagnosis are nonspecific techniques aimed at detection of abnormal involuntary movements. If such testing elicits no positive findings, the subject is "in the clear" for that point of his life but without implications for the future. Only after living through a considerable span of life can confidence in a disease-free future truly grow. It is probably impossible for outsiders to such family situations truly to be able to empathize with living indefinitely under such a Damoclean sword.

After Ruth and Mrs. Bates left, Dr. R. met with me to report that Ruth had definite signs of HD. He had told Mrs. Bates but not Ruth. His hesitancy in telling Ruth was based on his experience of several suicides resulting from patients' being informed of this diagnosis. I strongly believed that Ruth had a right to this information in order to plan her life as she saw fit.

The management of this young woman's case will be very difficult. If she is not told the truth, she must be told a lie or given some noncommittal response that she may well interpret as confirming her worst fears. Progression of symptoms will make the truth inescapable in time. Not to be told the truth may undermine trust in the professional group indefinitely.

It is hard to convey depressing news, especially if it carries a definite risk of severe depression and suicide. The one who does the telling must be prepared to work steadily with the depressed counselee or transfer the counselee to the care of someone who will.

Opinions of equally experienced professionals differ as to the best way to proceed.

Mrs. Bates and Ruth returned for counseling the following week. Mrs. Bates was seen first.

S.W.: I understand Dr. R. has told you that Ruth does have Huntington's disease.

Mrs. Bates [calmly]: Yes. Ruth does know.

S.W.: Are you sure?

Mrs. Bates: Well, it's hard to know for sure. She is more cranky than usual. She eats more and fights more with Dan.

These described alterations of mood and behavior do suggest an increase in Ruth's inner turmoil as manifestations of, and reaction to, her illness. We may inquire why, if she believes Ruth knows, her mother doesn't broach the subject with her directly. It is one thing to "know" a fact privately; it feels quite different to share that fact with an important other person. Doing the latter makes the fact much more "real." The wish to ward off the full impact of the misery subsides only after a struggle:

S.W.: It is very difficult for you to tell her the truth, isn't it?

Mrs. Bates [crying]: I can't, I can't. She will blame me. She blames me for everything. She blamed me for her father getting sick, even though she knew better. [Silence for a moment.] And why should we depress her further?

S.W.: It is hard for you to accept this yourself.

Mrs. Bates: Maybe the doctor is wrong.

S.W.: You would like very much to believe that; you want Ruth to be fine, and it's difficult to face this alone?

Mrs. Bates: Why me? Why does everything bad happen to me?

After further interchange, Mrs. Bates expressed anger toward her husband for not having informed her of HD in his family before they were married. After expressing this anger, she was able to consider Ruth's right to know that she had HD.

It is not surprising that Mrs. Bates angrily resents not having been told of the family history prior to marriage. There is an implication that forewarned, she might not have married. Since her husband was not then affected, however, and she loved him, it is equally plausible that she'd have married him anyway, telling herself he was probably one of the lucky ones.

Next, I interviewed Ruth.

S.W.: What do you think about what is happening? You've been waiting a long time to know.

RUTH: I think I knew before I came. My mother does not know I know. Maybe that's better.

S.W.: Is it better to have to go around in your own family, each person pretending, putting on an act, and not really communicating with each other?

RUTH: Let me think about that for a while.

S.W.: You appear to be calm today.

RUTH: As much as it hurts, it is almost a relief to know the truth. It was so hard not knowing—dreading the hard cold facts, wondering if I was imagining things. Now I know why I got kicked out of the program. And I feel even closer to Dad than I did before.

Most people—but not all—feel more tormented by their fantasies during periods of uncertainty than by the harshest truth. It is easier to focus one's coping capacities on bitter truth than on speculations.

S.W.: I can understand that it would be a relief to know one way or the other. Also, that you feel closer to your dad. But you may have days when you feel angry at others or feel sorry for yourself. You may have more questions for us. Please know that we are here to help, that you can call on us anytime.

RUTH: Somehow that feels good—knowing I have someone to call here. It's not always easy to talk to my family about what's really bothering me.

Six weeks later Mrs. Bates called, requesting that I see the other children, Lois and Daniel, who now knew Ruth had HD. Mrs. Bates explained that she had to tell them, particularly Dan, who was feeling the brunt of Ruth's frustration. At first Ruth had spent much of her time alone in her room, but now she was lashing out at Dan.

Next to be interviewed was Lois, Ruth's younger sister, a pretty, 17-year-old high school senior who resembled her mother. Lois worked in a store after school, and had been quite independent. She was close to her brother.

LOIS: I am nervous being here, but I need to talk. I'm glad you asked me to come in. I was feeling kind of excluded from what was going on.

S.W.: That is not a good feeling, being left out of family discussions and decisions.

Lois: Well, I've been feeling that way for a long time, ever since Dad got sick three years ago. Dad always seemed so close, but now it's as if he's disassociated himself from us, even when he's home. And I never really was as close to Mother as I was to Dad.

S.W.: Sounds as though you've suffered a very real loss.

Lois [crying]: And now the whole family is topsy-turvy. Mother escapes to work. Ruth yells at Dan all the time. And Dan is drinking and about to lose another job. Mother just can't accept the fact that Ruth has HD. She wants Ruth to carry on with her life, and yet she babies her. And I can't be Ruth's mother.

S.W.: It sounds as though you're feeling a lot has been put on you to be the family peacemaker.

Lois: That's right. But what about me? What about my own needs? It just isn't fair! [She cries again.] I am so scared.

S.W.: Can you talk about what you are so scared of?

Lois [pausing]: I am so afraid that someday I'll be like Dad and Ruth.

S.W.: That must be a frightening thought for you. You realize, of course, that there is just as much chance that you will remain *free* of HD. [We discussed her understanding, which was correct, of her "at risk" position.] What are you planning for yourself?

Lois: I'm going to keep on living my life as I would have anyway and face things if I have to when they come up. I'll get married someday and probably chance having my own kids, unless, of course, I'm sick or something. But dammit, I'm not going to let what's happening at home change my future and what happens to me!

Actually, Lois "escaped" her home situation as soon as she was graduated from high school by marrying her high school boyfriend. She was unhappy that her father could not be at either her high school graduation or her wedding. She still keeps in touch with her family, but from a "safe" distance. I gave Lois a great deal of support in handling her feelings. She knew that she could come back at any time, and subsequently she did bring her husband in for joint genetic counseling. They decided to take the risk of having their own children. Lois still feared getting HD but did not want to base her life on that unknown factor.

Occasionally, in just such a situation as Lois's, the opposite decision is made: The family's experience with the disease has been so shattering that the young married person is unwilling to run *any* risk whatever, and chooses to adopt.

Daniel, the middle child between Ruth and Lois, came in casually and reluctantly. He was unshaven, somewhat overweight, lived at home, was enrolled at a community college, and held a part-time job with a construction company.

S.W.: Daniel, do you understand why you are here today?

DANIEL: No, but I hope you can help me get Ruth and Dad off my back [indicating an alliance of the "sick" against the "healthy," perhaps].

S.W. [after explaining my role in the genetics clinic]: It sounds as though things are not going well for you at home.

DANIEL: That's putting it mildly. When Dad was home last time, he found out I was on pot. He tried to push me down the steps. Ruth is always fighting with me, and she gets more and more strange all the time. Lois leaves me alone, because she is always with her boyfriend. Mom is okay, but she expects me to graduate, and I can't 'cause I'm still on probation for shoplifting last year.

S.W.: How do you handle all this?

DANIEL: I drink, I smoke, I pal around with my friends. I can't stay home. Ruth drives me up the wall; she is so irritating. And Dad has always found fault with me.
[I discussed with Daniel the difficulty of living at home under these circumstances, and helped him begin thinking about alternative plans. He admitted feeling overwhelmed, but, interestingly, he did not follow up on any suggestions for alternative housing.]

S.W.: Do you find Ruth's behavior very different from before?

DANIEL: Not really. She has always bugged me. Maybe she's bugging me a little more now than she did before.

S.W.: Could that be because of her illness?

DANIEL: I don't know. I only know that I'm not going to end up like Dad and Ruth. I'm going to live it up while I can.

I saw Daniel twice more during the next three months. He was never able to face the reality of Ruth's illness, although it was obvious that he himself was frightened. His behavior became more and more erratic during the next two years, with his mother constantly siding with him against his bosses when he lost jobs and making excuses for him when he broke his probation. All her efforts suggested that she desperately needed this favored child of hers to be the "normal" one.

During these early contacts Mr. Bates was being followed at the medical center, and was receiving medical, psychological, and social services there. Ruth and Mrs. Bates continued to see me periodically during the next two and a half years, and were helped, in addition, by attending group meetings sponsored by the Committee to Combat Huntington's Disease, a support program for HD patients and their families. Eventually, the family was seen by a psychiatrist in family therapy.

I helped Mrs. Bates consider and eventually accept the alternative of a nursing home for Mr. Bates once he had to leave the medical center program. Mrs. Bates needed help in dealing with her feelings of guilt in "deserting" her husband. She also needed encouragement in seeking a higher-salaried position which would enable her to better satisfy some of her personal needs.

Ruth at first welcomed my help in sorting out what plans to make in the vocational line, setting her goals somewhat more realistically as she became more poorly coordinated. She enjoyed being treated as a responsible adult, someone who could still give to others and make decisions for herself. Her mother was ambivalent about Ruth's working, even in a sheltered workshop, and as much as she complained about Ruth's spending all her time in front of the TV, eating, and not getting out enough, she encouraged Ruth's dependence on her. Only when I focused on Mrs. Bates's own needs was she more able to stand aside and let Ruth try some of my suggestions.

The following work placements were arranged for Ruth, each of which lasted only a month or two and was only temporarily satisfying: a sheltered workshop, a vocational evaluation and training program, a nursing home, a center for retarded children and adults, and a hospital volunteer program. Eventually, a local family agency became involved in coordinating services for this family, such as looking into possible Medicaid and a temporary housekeeper for Mrs. Bates.

This family unfortunately was divided rather than united when faced with the nature of this genetic disorder. Family roles were reversed and revised, and family members became angry and apprehensive at the same time. If the genetic professional can find any satisfaction in this hopeless kind of situation, it is in knowing that he or she has given each family member a chance to be heard—to be anxious, to be angry, to be sad, to be accepting and accepted, and, most of all, to be considered a person who is capable of making informed decisions about the future, no matter how unreasonable these decisions might seem to others.

Further Comment

The late-onset, inherited neurological disorders constitute a category of malady with enormous potential for disrupting family relationships in myriad respects. All by itself in this case, the impact of the father's illness upon the family is very great. His care would be difficult enough in terms of the physical nursing required, but the alteration in his mood during his home visits makes matters much worse.

The addition of the newly established diagnosis of HD in Ruth at a rather young age for this has, expectably, hit everyone rather hard—each in a different way. Mrs. Bates now looks ahead to caring for two, rather than one. Lois bolts from this turmoil into marriage, although the example of Ruth's early diagnosis serves notice that Lois's fate will not be clarified for quite a few years to come. Daniel's uncertain situation adds to his mother's burden.

The entire family requires assistance. As can be discerned in these interactions with various family members, the counselor has been trying to help maintain some sense of meaningful existence for every member—those afflicted, for however much time remains for them, and those traumatized by the impact of life with the afflicted.

For the counselor the challenge is very great, as it is for all the professionals involved in this and similar cases.

References

FOLSTEIN, S., and FOLSTEIN, M. (1981). Diagnosis and treatment of Huntington's disease. *Comprehensive Therapy* 7 (no. 4): 61–66.

GIELEN, A., and ROCHE, K. (1979–1980). Death anxiety and psychometric studies in Huntington's disease. *Omega* 10 (no. 2): 135–145.

GUTHRIE, M. (1979). A personal view of genetic counseling. In K. Hsia, et al., eds., *Counseling in genetics,* pp. 329–341. New York: Alan R. Liss.

HANS, M., and KOEPPEN, A. (1980). Huntington's chorea—its impact on the spouse. *J. Nervous and Mental Disease* 168 (no. 4): 209–214.

SHOULSON, I., and FAHN, S. (1979). Huntington's disease: clinical care and evaluation. *Neurology* 29 (no. 1): 1–3.

WEXLER, N. (1979). Genetic Russian roulette, the experience of being at risk for Huntington's disease. In S. Kessler, ed., *Genetic counseling—Psychological Dimensions,* pp. 199–220. New York: Academic Press.

22

Waiting for the Axe to Fall: A Rare Late-Onset Neurological Disorder

As noted in the previous chapter, one of the most devastating tragedies occurs in a family when there is an individual with a progressively deteriorating neurological disorder which is inherited in an autosomal dominant mode and which becomes symptomatic after childhood, probably after children have been borne. Being prepared for tragedy does not necessarily lighten its impact.

This case is noteworthy for two reasons: It demonstrates the need for effective follow-up, even after an interval of several years, for certain families in which the younger members require different approaches as they grow older. It illustrates the fact that not all counseling situations can have results which are satisfying to the counselor and/or the patient.

A family in which a parent was slowly losing touch with reality, and deteriorating physically from a late-onset neurological disorder, came to our attention as a result of the thoroughness and sensitivity of a charge nurse at our hospital center. A young woman, Edith Kane, age 24, had been admitted for minor surgery. The hospital records referred to a progressive neurological disorder and indicated that other family members were afflicted with the same disorder.

Medical records complemented an extensive family pedigree: The mother, Mrs. Kane, and possibly three of her four children suffered from the same neurological disorder, which is progressive and inherited in an autosomal dominant mode. It appeared that the disorder began as a new mutation with Mrs. Kane.

When Mrs. Kane was 30 years old, she became severely depressed and was referred for psychiatric care. Other symptoms appeared over the next few years: impaired balance and coordination, blurred vision, incontinence, and failing memory. When we first became involved with the family, Mrs. Kane was 50 years old, confined to a wheelchair, and unable to do the simplest household chores.

The two oldest daughters—Edith, 24, and Rita, 25—appeared normal at birth. Rita developed problems with equilibrium at an early age, and by the fifth grade had difficulty learning. Over the years she became progessively confused and disoriented; exhibited a stiff, awkward gait; became affected with blurred vision; was occasionally incontinent; and became increasingly forgetful. Rita had become unable to walk and was bedridden.

When we first saw Edith, she exhibited a markedly decreased level of functioning. Neurologic examination revealed no obvious muscle wasting nor hypertrophy. There were signs of upper motor neurologic involvement, increased deep tendon reflexes, diminished motor power, and dementia. Edith had been well until age 13, at which time her IQ was 88. Problems were noted with increasing frequency at school, including a peculiar stiff gait, lack of concentration, blurred vision, and a tendency to fall. Her IQ at age 15 had decreased to 75.

The cause of this disorder is unknown, and it appears to be unique to this family: The combination of optic nerve atrophy, progressive dementia, and spastic paraparesis had not been previously reported.

Dominant hereditary disorders tend to be more variable in age of onset and severity than recessive disorders. Knowledge of what to look for can, however, call attention to specific symptoms and often makes definitive diagnosis possible earlier for succeeding generations. It is probable that Mrs. Kane's symptoms went unnoticed for years, or were even misdiagnosed, whereas her affected daughters followed a pattern made recognizable by their mother's condition.

We could not be of further help to the obviously affected family members, who were already being adequately aided by a variety of social services. Our principal concern was for Mr. Kane and the two undiagnosed younger children. When the age of onset of a disorder occurs well after infancy and possibly as late as the thirties, diagnosis cannot be made until symptoms become clearly definable. Children growing up in a family such as this can sense their risk and torture themselves with self-scrutinization. The fear of discovering symptoms is compounded by the fear of their confirmation.

This is one developmental vicissitude in children of such a family, but not the only possibility. In other families with similar disorders one may encounter children whose psychological self-protective mechanism of "denial" works very effectively—for a while. Such children may for long periods experience no focused anxiety about their own fate until confronting marriage or family planning. (Mrs. Kane did not become obviously symptomatic till age 30, but her daughters were not so fortunate.)

The burden on Mr. Kane, both financial and emotional, was enormous. He was married to a 50-year-old woman who was now incapable of caring for herself or her family, and he was watching two of his daughters slowly being destroyed by this monstrous disease. It was not surprising to learn, after many hours of investigation, that the family had undergone a genetic evaluation six years earlier, complete with pedigree analysis, neurologic testing of each of the children, and genetic counseling. He desperately wanted answers that he could handle. Since none were available, he was still searching.

One may speculate that Mr. Kane is expressing his own shock and his need to deny the prognostic gloom previously encountered by attempting to dismiss the grim information as possibly idiosyncratic to the earlier evaluating facility. Perhaps the new genetic disease center will "know more" and be less discouraging. This is an altogether understandable maneuver in these circumstances. As there is no specific treatment available, there has been no loss of important time.

After appropriate review and research, we counseled him regarding the inheritance of the disorder with which he was already familiar. Discussion of the genetics was clearly of less interest to him than his immediate concern of dealing with the day-to-day worsening problems of his deteriorating wife and two daughters.

We discussed his third daughter, Joan, who had been known to be unaffected since she had been examined at age 14, six years before. His son had shown possible minimal signs of the disorder at the time of the original investigation when he was 16 years old, but had not been informed of the findings. We offered to meet with both children individually, if they desired.

Joan, the unaffected daughter, contacted us and made an appointment to speak with us. She was now 20 years old, lived at home, and attended a local community college. She was familiar with the disorder and knew that she was unaffected. She was pleasant, nicely dressed, polite. Since she had requested the appointment, it was clear that she had some questions. The medical geneticist and I spoke with Joan.

G.C.: In summary, then, being unaffected means that you do not have the gene.

JOAN: I know.

G.C.: Therefore, since you don't have the gene, there is no way you can transmit the disorder to any of your children.

[Silence.]

JOAN: You mean—? [Silence. Tears appeared in her eyes.]

G.C.: You do not have an increased risk of having affected children. Since you are unaffected, you do not have the responsible gene. Didn't you understand that?

JOAN: No. I mean, I wasn't sure. And I guess I was afraid to ask. I didn't see how it was possible since it's all around me. Is it true?

The fact that Joan had evidently been previously assured she did not have any symptoms of the disorder, that the genetics had been reexplained to her in this interview but she *still wasn't sure,* is a piece of very meaningful and dramatic communication. We can presume that Joan, a college student, is intelligent. She has been told of the inheritance pattern, so that in the narrow, cognitive sense she *knows* she and her potential children have been spared. But she cannot quite *believe* it!

This indicates a complicated impingement of emotions upon cognition: Joan is in the emotional situation of someone who, for example, walks away unscathed from an automobile catastrophe in which the other passengers are seriously injured. She *knows* she has survived, but cannot *believe* her good fortune.

To a question as to how the genetics team could assume that Joan is free of the disease at age 20, given the fact that her mother is reported to have shown symptoms only at age 30, the counselor responded with the following additional information:

At the time of the first family evaluation six years earlier all four children were examined. Two of them, Edith and Rita, had manifested minor symptoms at a very early age, and their symptoms had worsened quickly. Joan had appeared well. The fourth child, Robert, demonstrated some positive signs. As a matter of clinical judgment, the staff inferred that if Joan had carried the gene, she would, like her siblings, have demonstrated some signs of the disorder by age 20. This was, the counselor emphasized, a clinical decision the truth of which the staff considered highly likely.

We went through the explanation again, slowly, step by step, with diagrams of the genetic mechanism. Joan's relief was evident, and she thanked us profusely.

The repetition of the genetics may have been necessary. Some inquiry about her astonishment, disbelief, and probably "survivor guilt" might have enhanced her emotional integration of the conveyed information and extended her sense of relief.

Joan is still undecided about whether to stay at home or move in order to create a more normal life for herself. The impact of her family tragedy and her possible guilt in being the only unaffected child may prevent her from doing the latter.

> For an adolescent or young adult to move away from the parental home is an important developmental thrust toward an independent life. This change of circumstances always entails overcoming difficulties, and even in our relatively enlightened era such a move is rather more difficult for women than for men. If to this gender difference is added the burden of Joan's guilt over leaving her family, we are impressed with the dimensions of the task. Such a challenge represents a quite sufficient basis for Joan to consider seeking specific professional psychological care.

Joan was eager for us to talk to her brother Robert, who had expressed no interest in speaking with us. Perhaps she was hoping we could give Robert similar good news. We encouraged Joan to speak to Robert about calling us.

As a routine follow-up, we sent Mr. Kane and Joan a letter soon after their visits, in which we summarized the highlights of the counseling sessions. The letter said that on the basis of the available information it was impossible to determine if Robert was affected, and we repeated our offer for him to have further consultation and evaluation.

A few days after the letter had been received Robert called to say he would come in, even though he "couldn't see any point in it," because his sister had urged him to do so. His hostility was evident during this brief telephone conversation.

Robert arrived on time for the appointment. He was an alert young man, 22 years of age, appearing to be in good health. He stated that he did not see himself as having the problems that the others in his family had. The previous year he had been graduated from college with a B.S. degree and a provisional teaching certificate. He had been home now for several months, and it made him very anxious and upset to be with his sick mother and sisters. He was currently unemployed but was looking for a teaching job "as far away as possible."

During the initial conversation, he related his experience of six years before when the family was first evaluated, and he spoke openly of his feelings of anger and disappointment with medical personnel. All of the family had undergone weeks of testing, some of it extremely uncomfortable, and were assured that the results would be discussed with them. This promise was never kept in his case. For six years he had suspected that the doctors felt he was affected, but no one would talk to him about it. Some early signs of the disorder had been noted and he had sensed this. Perhaps because he was young (16 years old at that time), no one gave him any information about himself.

This piece of spontaneously offered history is absolutely essential for the counselor to know. It explains immediately much of the reason for Robert's reluctance to meet with the evaluation team: He fears that the unfavorable experience will be repeated and that he will again be sent away to live in torment with his private speculations and imaginings.

This sequence illustrates clearly how past experience with professionals can color present expectations disadvantageously, intruding as obstacles to the counseling enterprise. The converse—the favorable carry-over of good experience with professionals—is also true.

At this point in the conversation, Robert said that he would not allow the same thing to happen again, that he wanted answers. "It's my body, my life, and I have a right to know anything you find out about me." He spoke loudly, firmly, and quickly. But the subtle undercurrent of "Help me" was perceptible. He had been living with his suspicions for six long years, but he had been functioning well and accomplishing things in spite of it. Now, he wanted to start his career and perhaps marry. (He casually mentioned a "fiancee," but would not elaborate on the details of their relationship.) He was afraid to make any long-range plans. His resentment at the lack of communication and understanding of his dilemma was repeated over and over, and he urged us to promise that we would tell him everything we found out. That promise was made without hesitation, and his attitude softened immediately.

Without this promise, no counseling could take place. Yet the counselor retains many options as to how to convey the truth—with what words and in what dosage, with what offers of assistance in coping with it. Who the patient *is* and how he or she copes with difficulties are of the greatest concern to us, rather than categorical imperatives about patients' rights to know all medical facts about themselves.

On the basis of his preliminary investigation the medical geneticist had the impression that Robert had some stigmata of the disorder. There was a suggestion of slurred speech, slight and intermittent drooping of the upper eyelids, and decreased muscle strength in the lower extremities. Confirmation could only be achieved with thorough neurological examination, and it would have been premature to share this information with Robert.

This is only fair and humane, considering the gravity of the situation.

After this preliminary evaluation, the geneticist explained several items to Robert: First, that it was impossible to state whether or not he was affected on the basis of the studies done previously or the physical examination just completed. He had to be seen by a neurologist. Second, that if he were found to be affected, the severity would not be predictable since the disorder had been expressed variably in his family. Whatever the severity, however, there would be a 50 percent (one-in-two) chance of his having affected children.

These remarks at this particular point pave the way for subsequent counseling through indication of the inherent uncertainties involved in this type of late-onset disorder. Other counselors might defer this added dose of information to a later meeting, hoping that such a resistant patient would meanwhile develop some added trust in the counselor. This is a matter of individual counselor judgment, since one might be fearful this counselee would break off contact after the one meeting and never be seen again.

Robert's hostility and disappointment were obvious. He became extremely agitated. "If, if, if! I don't need any more *ifs*. And more tests? I knew I shouldn't have come here. This is just the same thing all over again. I have to know what to do, how to plan!"

We assured him that only the neurological evaluation was necessary now, that we would have the results quickly, and that we would tell him exactly what they were. Without it, there could be no definitive answers. However, he had to realize that even after the examination, it was possible that there would still be nothing definite.

That this young man craves assistance with planning is dramatically underscored. "Planning" in such instances, owing to the uncertainties of prediction, requires considerable professional assistance beyond the reports of the consultants' examinations. One will certainly assure help with planning; the nature of which will depend upon reflective consideration of consultant opinion. Counselees make all manner of decisions on the basis of such information, from omission of marriage to adoption of children, to taking chances on conceiving their own. Counselees may, moreover, change over time their decisions as to what they want to do.

The counselor has to be prepared to be repetitively available over an extended period. Robert cannot know at the outset how complicated it will be "to know what to do." He will need assistance in accepting this irreducible complexity and persisting in grappling with it to some satisfactory resolution. Lacking that assistance, he will turn his back on the professionals, just as he did at age 16.

"Nothing definite" in this context means that he cannot be offered assurance that he is not at risk, and therefore able to forget about any such problem in himself or his progeny.

When I told Robert that an appointment for a neurological examination could be made for him, he slumped in his chair. "I'll think about it," he said. "You can make the appointment; I'll let you know if I'm coming." This became the pattern for every appointment we attempted to make for him. Perhaps this attitude gave him a sense of control over his life that he did not feel in most other areas.

Telephone conversations during this period alternated between complaints at having to wait for the evaluation; accusations that we were not treating him openly; anxiety about the actual tests; and threats that he was moving "far away" and might not be available for the evaluation or further counseling.

He eventually had the neurological evaluation, and he did come back for a follow-up consultation. This second consultation began poorly. Included in the genetics group on this occasion was a graduate student to whom Robert was introduced at the outset. Robert was noticeably angry and agitated. He told us that he had been terribly nervous and upset since the testing. He had the feeling that we had decided he had the disorder and were "just waiting for the symptoms to appear so that you can prove you're right." He challenged the student and wanted to know why she was there. We explained the nature of her involvement, and offered to exclude her from the conference if her presence upset him. Robert said that it was all right for her to stay, that he just wanted to know who she was.

He expressed his feeling that he is "a person," not simply an interesting case. He repeatedly expressed his resentment that "unfair" assumptions were being made about him. He was suspicious of everything and everyone, but could not express the primary suspicion that he had the dread disease.

We attempted to reassure him on each issue, but he was never told what he wanted to hear. The testing had revealed that he did have early signs of the disorder in a mild and subtle form. There were positive bilateral Babinski reflexes and pale optic discs but no progression over the past six years. Even so, there was no way to predict the rate of future progression. Periodic neurological examinations would be important in order to monitor these signs.

Another very important point had to be made. Since he was definitely affected, even if no further progression occurred in his entire lifetime he had a 50 percent chance of having affected children, and there was no way at this time of predicting how severely they might be affected.

Two bitter pills to swallow. Two impossible truths to accept. He was angry. He told us we had put him through so much and told him nothing new. He had come for answers and been let down again. What was he supposed to do now? How was he supposed to plan his life?

We agreed with him that the answers were understandably upsetting and frustrating, but repeated that there were no others at this time. We offered to speak with him again, with or without his fiancee. We suggested the possibility of referral to a psychiatrist who could help him to deal with his enormous problems. He refused it all and walked out angry, hurt, bewildered.

What Robert was told was exactly what is written in the report: that he demonstrated early signs of the family disorder in a mild and subtle form; and that by comparison with the report of his examination six years previously, the findings were the same. There had been no progression of the detected signs.

What he, of course, wished to hear, and what could obviously not be told to him, was that he showed no signs whatever of the affliction.

A telephone call to him the next day found him polite and distant. He had the possibility of a job in Puerto Rico, and he couldn't wait to leave his "messed up" home. He was not interested in further discussion.

The last contact came several months later when he called regarding his bill. He had succeeded in leaving home for a part-time teaching job in another state. The anger in his voice was familiar, but he was still not interested in further discussion of his problems.

We were unhappy and dissatisfied with the outcome of Robert's case and his reaction. In retrospect, we think that even if Robert had been treated more openly during the original evaluation (even if prematurely), his negative reactions would have still been expressed as a result of his untenable position and inability to face the uncertainty of his future. If he had been severely affected, he would have known there was no possibility of any future for him. As it was, there was no way of predicting whether his plans would have any chance of fulfillment. His basic good health only serves to tease him with the knowledge of what he may someday lose forever.

Robert needs psychiatric help to assist him in dealing with and accepting his burden. We will continue to contact him from time to time, to arrange for periodic neurological evaluations and to try to provide emotional support. We provided him with all the available facts, in a genetic sense, but we have not yet been able to help him as a human being. We have tried to help. We hope that we have done no harm.

Further Comment

In certain respects this family's situation is even more difficult than that of the family with HD in the preceding report. Each child in an afflicted family manifests a different response depending on a host of factors, of which the presence of early possible signs of the disorder is but one variable.

Robert enters counseling with his sister's encouragement, but his predisposition to trust interaction with the professional team has obviously been undermined in consequence of his counseling experience six years previously. His tentativeness in regard to appointment scheduling suggests the fragility of his rapport with clinic personnel.

Like most patients confronted with dreaded news about themselves, Robert is enraged and strikes out at anything or anyone handy to the purpose. "Unfair" statements *are* being made about him, but in this regard the professionals are only the conduit for the news. It is Fate that is unfair and generates his distress. How does one rage against Fate?

To work with a young man in such distress necessitates willingness to hear him out as he unburdens himself of some of the contents of his frightening private speculations and his rage. Such utterances are hard to listen to, but counselors must remind themselves not to take these harsh statements personally. The problem remains always the patient's. Our role is to *try* to be helpful. If we are able to sit still with such an angry young man without being distracted into defensiveness, if we can tactfully empathize with his distress, we will have a strengthened rapport.

If the patient can *not* be told that he demonstrates *absolutely nothing* suspicious, he is likely to infer that he does, indeed, have the feared malady. Although he may not say this in just so many words, he communicates his impression indirectly.

Robert wants "answers." The very word is quite ambiguous, and it is not rare for patient and professional to be employing it with different shadings. To some patients "answers" may be only the genetic verdict. For others — and Robert is among them — "answers" are plans for leading one's life, based upon the genetic diagnosis, plans that the counselor will try to help the patient to frame. The counselee must be assured that he will not be left to dangle in limbo with his bad news.

Robert has been offered additional counseling, and psychiatric referral has also been suggested. But the possibility of psychiatric referral was probably just too much to add to the one interview. Such referral requires most tactful presentation to be acceptable. One must know one's counselee fairly well to be able to help him deal with expectable reservations about accepting such a suggestion. The drama of this counseling session and the chance Robert would bolt probably forced the prompt mention of the option.

We hope we can get it across to the patient that the uncertainty of his future remains *whether or not* he continues with counseling. Furthermore, *whether or nor* he pauses to think about it, *he* will be shaping and carrying out plans, and we believe we can help him to frame the best plans possible.

The clinic's review of their conduct of the relationship with Robert is a commendable exercise for every professional. This clinical situation is one of the most taxing for anyone, with no certain guidelines that suit every counselee.

References

KELLY, P. (1977). *Dealing with dilemma.* New York: Springer-Verlag.

MURPHY, E., and CHASE, G. (1975). *Principles of genetic counseling.* Chicago: Yearbook Medical Publishers.

ROTHNER, A.; YAHR, F.; and YAHR, M. (1976). Familial spastic paraparesis, optic atrophy, and dementia; clinical observations of affected kindred. *New York State J. Med.* 76: 756–758.

23

The Undiagnosable Child: Special Counsel for the Parents

The high proportion of children who are undiagnosable at the time of initial evaluation—one out of three in this counselor's experience—pose very difficult, special problems.

The vicissitudes of family planning in the face of such uncertainty are illustrated by the three stories that follow. Given the persisting desire for all concerned to be able to assign a proper diagnosis, and thereby deal with more definite risk probabilities and treatment approaches, the counselor seeks to develop a relationship that will endure indefinitely.

It is impressive how much in the way of treatment and special assistance with development and education can still be done for a child despite the uncertainty.

Approximately *one out of three* patients seen for a diagnostic workup in our medical genetics unit can be placed in the undiagnosable category. The lack of diagnosis results in a unique vulnerability for both genetic counselor and parents, and may delay and/or disrupt the necessary process of parental adjustment. It is extremely difficult for parents to accept the fact that part of the impact of their child's disorder is the inability of the professionals even to supply a name for it. A genetic counselor can be of significant value to such a family by (1) maintaining an ongoing supportive and educative relationship; (2) anticipating problems which this group of parents commonly encounter; and (3) keeping the family informed of scientific progress which may, at some future date, result in a diagnosis.

This report will explore factors which are unique to, or more exaggerated among, parents of children with an undiagnosable condition. I shall identify these factors, explain their sources, and, with three families' histories, demonstrate how a genetic counselor can help families to grapple with their children's disorders.

The first job of the clinical medical geneticist is to provide a diagnosis of a child's medical problem. With a diagnosis, the medical team can explain to the family (1) the diagnosis (name) of the child's condition, including its etiology and ramifications; (2) the prognosis for the child; (3) the genetic aspects of the condition and recurrence risks for both parents and child; (4) the availability of carrier detection and prenatal diagnosis; (5) the management and treatment of existing and potential problems.

Having a handicapped child is troubling and bewildering to parents. When the medical problem eludes diagnosis, the parental burden is magnified and compounded. Special factors related to the absence of a definite diagnosis include vagueness of prognosis and recurrence risk prediction, conflicting medical opinions, inability to gain emotional support through identification with parents of similarly afflicted children, and prolonged retention of unrealistic hopes. Fear of the unknown and related feelings of helplessness delay adjustment to living with the problem.

Society conditions parents to expect physicians to make a diagnosis and "know all the answers." When a pediatrician in the community wants a family to consult a medical genetics team, he or she may idealize the capabilities of the team to ensure that the family does so. Such advertising reinforces societal conditioning to expect omniscience from medical personnel, and provides an added burden to the team when a diagnosis cannot be made.

The burden here is considerable: naturally, the team shares the preference of all professionals in any field to provide "all the answers." That is inherent in the notion of being a "professional" — one who has special, expert knowledge. In order to remain effective for the counselees, the professional team must be at ease with their own frustration and the accompanying dent in self-esteem.

For the counselors, the preliminary touting of the talents of the genetics team now has a devastating rebound: if *this* marvelously experienced team cannot come up with the diagnosis, then *nobody* can be expected to do so, and the situation is truly hopeless. Such an expectable reaction should receive professional attention from the team, because unaltered it can work mischief, preventing the parents from keeping the following in mind: (1) With further study, a diagnosis may become available at a later time. (2) It is not necessarily true that the quest will be equally unsuccessful elsewhere, as all clinics do not have identical experience. This is not to say that all frustrated parents should shop endlessly for additional opinons.

The genetics team needs to help the frustrated counselees express and reflect upon their disappointment and consider alternative courses of action. The problem, after all, continues with or without the diagnosis. At the least, the team can seek to establish an open, friendly channel of communication for use as needed.

When a clinical medical geneticist cannot arrive at a specific diagnosis, he or she can make predictions based only on general, rather than specific, experience. Parents are thereby left with a sense of shock and fear of what surprises may be ahead if additional problems come to light in their child. Having a diagnosis permits some separation of the known from the unknown, and makes it somewhat easier to begin to anticipate and be "braced" against the next crisis.

Without a diagnosis, it is common for parents to adapt by "taking one day at a time," not thinking about the future. This attitudinal change serves to protect the family against the pain of such uncertainty.

The "no diagnosis" diagnosis usually makes it difficult to establish a single recurrence risk for the couple's future children. Occasionally a family's pedigree will indicate a clear Mendelian inheritance pattern, but frequently the proband is the first child in the family to have "Disorder X." In many cases, families must be given an approximate recurrence risk, ranging from negligible to 25 percent. Invariably, no chance exists for prenatal diagnosis of the condition. Services a genetic counselor can provide for these particular families are: (1) to ensure that they understand why there is such uncertainty, and (2) to look for new information over the years that may apply to them. These considerations underscore one of the virtues of yearly follow-up appointments to the medical genetics unit, and establish a base for some realistic hopefulness.

Parents need hope, and hope is partly an outgrowth of what efforts they make to do something tangible to help their child. Despite the lack of diagnosis, affected children frequently benefit tremendously from correction and management, although parents are often presented with a full-time job in the provision of it. As an example, in Case 1 the patient has the following health professionals involved in her care: a pediatrician, the medical genetics team, a pediatric cardiologist, a pediatric ophthalmologist, a plastic surgeon, a pediatric neurosurgeon, a pediatric orthopedic surgeon, and a pedodontist. She spends a considerable amount of time in doctors' offices rather than in the classroom with her peers. It is left to the parents, the pediatrician, and usually the medical genetics team to integrate various medical opinions and establish the plan of action. "Experienced" parents often know that they are the best, and sometimes the only, advocate that their child will have, and they are willing to nudge the system to achieve worthwhile ends.

To help the parents of undiagnosed children deal with their chronic, monumental burdens, the medical genetics team can provide a tremendous service by bringing these particular families together and referring parents to community-based parent support groups.

Discussed below are three families who were thrust into this difficult situation. Each family has addressed to some degree the issues just presented, and I will attempt to point these out as they were encountered. Clinical information will be followed by a summary of the case history, including a representative dialogue. Please note that in each case, the history of the child prior to involvement with the genetic counselor is recounted by the family, and therefore may not be entirely accurate or complete.

Case 1

Melissa Paley is a five-and-a-half-year-old girl with a pattern of malformation which to date has not been described in the medical literature.

Melissa was born after an uneventful nine-month gestation to Mr. and Mrs. Paley, who were both 20 years old at the time. The Paleys had been high school sweethearts, and they married soon after graduation. At birth, Mrs. Paley noted that Melissa was "odd-looking," but this in no way impeded natural bonding and the love which she soon developed for her daughter. Melissa's pediatrician told the parents that she was "floppy" and that she had extra folds of skin around her neck. Since no other problems were mentioned, Mrs. Paley thought of her baby as completely normal until her regular nine-month checkup. At that time, a heart murmur was noted.

During the consultation with a pediatric cardiologist Mrs. Paley was told that Melissa had Williams syndrome and that she would be retarded. (A description of this syndrome may be found in D. Smith, 1977, pp. 54–55.) Mrs. Paley was crushed, and immediately went to see her general pediatrician. He told her that Melissa would never live to have children, and further, that Mr. and Mrs. Paley should not have any more children. Mrs. Paley relates that she doesn't remember how she managed to get her 9-month-old baby daughter home, but that she did somehow, and told her husband the news. To help them to cope, the family took a short vacation. On their return, Mrs. Paley found out that she was again pregnant. Following the advice of their pediatrician, and despite the fact that she and her husband desperately wanted more children, Mrs. Paley underwent a therapeutic abortion.

We are left to sense that if the general pediatrician suspected such a dire diagnosis, he had not let on. The Paleys, therefore, reached the pediatric cardiologist unprepared for the first thunderbolt. Reeling from that confrontation, Mrs. Paley sought out the general pediatrician, who supplied the second thunderbolt. Still no psychological assistance.

The gloomy prognosis for Melissa was quite a bitter pill to swallow, and the prompt prophylactic recommendation to forego further childbearing compounded its devastating impact.

The short vacation was a traditional, self-selected effort to gain some time in which to recover a semblance of emotional composure.

The prescribed therapeutic abortion added yet another to the rapid-fire series of losses with which the parents had to contend: first, the loss of the healthy infant, now recognized as defective; second, the loss of the dream of a healthy, natural family; and third, the loss of the new, desired pregnancy.

After the abortion, Mrs. Paley and her husband sought the advice of a genetic counselor at another hospital. Mrs. Paley thinks that she was given a 50 percent recurrence risk of having another child with the same disorder. She may have remembered this incorrectly, since there had been some discussion of Huntington's disease, a disorder present in her extended family. She was probably correctly told that Williams syndrome has to date been considered to be sporadic. In any event, Mrs. Paley became pregnant quite soon after this visit, continued the pregnancy, and gave birth to a healthy son.

Immediately before their appointment with us, Mr. and Mrs. Paley joined a prepaid health plan, which meant that they had a new pediatrician. In order to confirm the diagnosis of Williams syndrome, the pediatrician referred the family to Dr. E. of the Pediatric Genetics and Dysmorphology Clinic.

My first contact with Mrs. Paley occurred when I called the Paleys to reassure them about and prepare them for the appointment. Mrs. Paley and Melissa, who was then 3 years old, attended this first session. Mrs. Paley's purposes were to have Melissa's condition diagnosed, and to convince someone in the medical community that Melissa was not retarded. Her physical examination at that time revealed significant craniofacial abnormalities, which gave her a droopy-eyed, open-mouthed, dull expression. My initial impression of Melissa was of an obviously hyperteloric, unusual-looking child, unlike any I had ever seen before. Her specific abnormalities included: decreased facial expression, prominent nasal bridge, hypertelorism, down-slanting palpebral fissures, high arched palate, significant micrognathia, a notched mandible, fifth-finger clinodactyly, small hands, and mild pulmonic stenosis. We had obtained the results of developmental tests done on Melissa elsewhere and found them to be in the normal range, as were our own diagnostic genetic tests. These developmental evaluations measure intellectural growth.

During her appointment, three important events occurred: (1) We decided that Melissa's problem, although real, was not Williams syndrome. Dr. E. did not know what disorder she did have, but it was clear that it was possible to detach the label "retarded" from a child obviously functioning in the normal range. Mrs. Paley was elated that Dr. E. corroborated what she already knew, and it was at this point that she really began to trust our clinic personnel.

It is heartening to note that this mother, despite having received the dreariest news from professionals previously contacted, remained a staunch advocate for her daughter. She sought further expert opinion, since she was not to be dissuaded from her impression that the child was not retarded. In this instance her assessment was corroborated. (In other instances, it might not be, since parents may deny deficits obvious to outsiders.)

(2) Mrs. Paley was told that she and her husband faced a zero to 25 percent recurrence risk for any future pregnancies. (3) Although Dr. E. did not recognize her disorder, he felt that Melissa resembled a child he had evaluated during his fellowship. He promised to take Melissa's photograph and case history with him the next time he went to visit his fellowship instructor, Dr. H., in order to compare Melissa's history with that of the other child.

During the next four months Mrs. Paley called monthly to learn whether Dr. E. had visited with his fellowship instructor, and each time I had to tell her he had not yet been free to make the trip. I usually felt frustrated after these calls, because she so desperately wanted the waiting to be over. I sought to help her bear up with the long waiting period. I cautioned her that the consultation might possibly turn out to be unfruitful.

I learned something of the family dynamics in that Mr. Paley seemed indisposed to discuss Melissa's situation with his wife, claiming that to be "her area of responsibility."

Within a few months, Dr. E. did visit Dr. H., and discovered that on closer comparison Melissa did not resemble the other child. Dr. H.'s interest in Melissa's situation prompted him to ask to see her during his next visit to our hospital. Dr. E. asked me to call Mrs. Paley to determine if she wanted Dr. H. to examine her child.

Mrs. Paley was elated to learn of this possibility, and full of what I considered unrealistic hope. I knew that the setting of sessions like these was sometimes intimidating, since many students, resident physicians, and faculty would be present during her appointment.

I warned her, and I also wanted to prepare her for the possibility that even Dr. H. might not be able to assign a diagnosis to Melissa.

During the visit, 3-year-old Melissa and Mrs. Paley entered a room filled with people eager to see Dr. H. in action. Dr. E. and I presented Melissa's history to him, and Dr. H. examined her while simultaneously asking Mrs. Paley questions concerning the child's developmental achievements. At the end of the examination, he explained to Mrs. Paley that he felt Dr. E. had identified her major problems, and that he, too, had never seen or read about another child just like her. However, he did remark about the favorable results many children had achieved from surgery to correct hypertelorism: the Tessier procedure, which, depending upon the severity of the hypertelorism, moves the orbits of the eyes from their original position to one closer to or at the normal intercanthal distance. He explained that this surgery has had some mortality associated with it, and can take as long as fifteen hours to perform. Dr. H. also suggested a less dangerous but less productive alternative, which would involve surgically pinching in some of the extra skin from Melissa's wide nasal bridge. This alternative surgery would not correct the hypertelorism, but it would make it less noticeable. Dr. H. told Mrs. Paley that it was too early to perform either type of surgery, which is optimally done when a child is approximately 5 years of age. Mrs. Paley asked Dr. H. if he knew what her chances were of having another child with the same problem. He answered that he felt her risk was somewhere between zero and 25 percent.

She had heard from both Dr. E. and myself what the recurrence risk meant, and over the next few weeks Mrs. Paley would call and we would go over aspects of the consultation that were unclear to her. It took her a while to assimilate the new information, and she clearly had fixated on a word new to the medical vocabulary she associated with her daughter: surgery. When I felt that she had integrated the information, I told her that we wanted to see Melissa again in one year.

A few months later she called to say that she was pregnant. She was extremely happy. We discussed the fact that prenatal diagnosis was not appropriate, since we did not know what Melissa's diagnosis was. Further, I wanted to know how she and her husband felt about the risk that this unborn child would have the same problem as Melissa. She made it clear that they interpreted the zero to 25 percent risk as a low risk, and they were willing to take their chances. Having produced a normal child in between Melissa and the expected baby had made them realize that it was possible for them to have healthy children. I gave them my best wishes. When their second normal son was born about six and a half months later, Mrs. Paley called with obvious delight to tell me. She exuded tremendous relief at her son's apparent normalcy.

> This report emphasizes how individualized are the responses of different counselees to the specific numbers involved in a recurrence risk prediction. We may speculate that if Melissa had been mentally retarded, a 25 percent risk might well have been regarded by the Paleys as unallowable.

Melissa was approximately 4 years and 3 months old when she came in to see the medical genetics team for her annual checkup. She demonstrated that she was functioning very well from a developmental standpoint. Her growth was good, and her pulmonic stenosis was little trouble to her. The bulk of this appointment consisted of discussion about the possibility of the Tessier procedure for Melissa.

Over the next nine months we encountered serious problems with conflicting medical and surgical opinions. There were numerous telephone contacts with Mrs. Paley, and despite the fact that we were actively working toward the goal of surgery by our own craniofacial reconstructive surgical team, Mrs. Paley was not convinced that she would allow it to occur. This is a sample of dialogue that occurred before we knew our surgeons would want Melissa to have the Tessier procedure:

MRS. PALEY: Hello, Miss J., this is Darlene.
G.C.: Hi, Darlene, how are you? What has happened since we last talked?
MRS. PALEY: Well, I finally had my appointment with Dr. M., the surgeon at our health plan.
G.C.: What did he say?
MRS. PALEY: He said he didn't think Melissa needed any surgery at all.
G.C.: How did that make you feel?
MRS. PALEY: I was really upset. I asked him why he felt that way, and he said he thought that the Tessier procedure was too risky. He also said he didn't feel qualified to perform it.
G.C.: I can understand why he said he didn't feel qualified. It is very specialized surgery. Did you tell him about the reconstructive group at our hospital?
MRS. PALEY: Yes. He said that if we needed so much help from the outside we should change insurance plans.
G.C.: Good grief. How did you respond to that?
MRS. PALEY: I can't remember. I was pretty upset.
G.C.: It sounds like you still are, and I can understand why! Getting

back to when he mentioned that the surgery was too risky in his opinion—did you discuss that in depth?

MRS. PALEY: Yes. He tried to describe the surgery to me. He told me that other children had died from it. That scared me a lot!

Once more we encounter a highly idiosyncratic situation: In sharp contrast to situations in which a decision to forego surgery is likely to permit a serious defect to produce death, we have a decision focused on cosmetic appearance. One set of parents may well consider plastic reconstruction a worthwhile option only if virtually free of risk. To another couple, speculating on the potential quality of life for a girl with a notably different appearance, even risky cosmetic surgery may be regarded as essential.

G.C.: It is risky surgery. I think we all have to understand that fact. It also is the one type of surgery which can help Melissa the most if it works. If you had to talk about the one thing that bothers you the most, what would it be?

MRS. PALEY: That Melissa would die, and that I would be responsible. I would have been the cause of her death. I don't think I could handle that if it happened. But if she doesn't have surgery, I don't think I can handle the fact that it was my fear that kept her from looking more normal. It will be hard no matter which I choose.

G.C.: I understand that. You and Dave should make that decision together. First, we need to find out if the plastic surgeons feel Melissa should have the Tessier procedure, or the other surgery that Dr. H. suggested as an alternative. Let's get some more information, and then you and Dave can decide. I don't think it is helpful to worry about something that may not come to pass. What do you think is the next step?

MRS. PALEY: Well, if we want any surgery at all, we must get a second opinion from someone else. Then if they feel she should have the surgery, we can take that opinion to the health plan pediatrician.

G.C.: That sounds like a good plan. Do you have anyone in mind?

MRS. PALEY: No. Can you recommend someone?

G.C.: Well, I think we should have Melissa seen by someone familiar with both types of surgery. Dr. C., the head of the craniofacial reconstructive team, and the one who does the plastic surgery, would be my candidate, but he is gone for this month. Let's schedule an appointment with his associate, Dr. M. instead. He will be able to provide us with the information we need.

During this appointment Dr. M. decided that Melissa would benefit most from the Tessier procedure, and I decided that Mr. and Mrs.

Paley needed more input than I alone could give them. Fortuitously, Dr. C. was going to give a talk to a local parent support group on his return.

I telephoned the Paleys to tell them about the scheduled meeting. My motivations for wanting them to go were twofold: (1) I felt that if they understood Dr. C.'s concern for patients they would be more likely to put their daughter's life in his hands; and (2) I knew that Mrs. Lane, the mother of a little girl who had gone through the same surgery, would also be at the meeting. I felt that Mrs. Lane would be extremely helpful to the Paleys by sharing some of her experiences and fears with them.

Both Mr. and Mrs. Paley showed up at the parent group meeting, and I had the opportunity to meet Mr. Paley for the first time. He was, as Mrs. Paley had described him to me, incredibly shy. He appeared to be most uncomfortable talking. During the break in the meeting, we chatted for a short while and I introduced them to Dr. C. and Mrs. Lane. From the animation of their conversations, I knew that the family was benefiting from the experience.

The degree to which anxiety is reducible through identification with other parents who have successfully passed through a similar frightening challenge is very impressive.

The first thing next morning, I received a telephone call from Mrs. Paley.

MRS. PALEY: Hi, Miss J., how are you?

G.C.: Fine. How did you and Dave feel about the meeting last night?

MRS. PALEY: It was wonderful. Both of us learned so much. I feel like we will let Melissa have the surgery now. I feel much better knowing that Mrs. Lane's daughter get through it and did just fine. My husband said he liked Dr. C., that he trusted him.

We can well ask how it is possible for anyone to be able to repose trust in a total stranger, as Dr. C. is to the Paleys. In large part it comes about by a kind of "contagion," or spillover from the trust the Paleys have already developed in Miss J., Dr. E., and Dr. H. In part it is generated by Dr. C.'s willingness to permit himself to become somewhat known as a human being.

G.C.: I'm so glad. What do you want to do now?

MRS. PALEY: Well, I think I want to schedule an appointment for Melissa with the whole craniofacial team and get their opinion. That's what Dr. C. felt should be done next.

G.C.: Do you agree with him?

Mrs. Paley: Yes. I'm not as frightened as I used to be.

G.C.: Good. How does Dave feel about this? Is he worried?

Mrs. Paley: Yes, he's worried. I can tell.

G.C.: You mean he hasn't told you so? Have you tried getting his opinion on whether it should be done or not?

Mrs. Paley: Yes, but he says that it's my decision whether she has surgery or not.

G.C.: How does that make you feel? Do you think that's fair?

Mrs. Paley: Well, I wish he would let me know what he thinks. I don't want to make the decision alone.

G.C.: I agree. I think you should try and get his opinion. I think this is very important.

Looking back, I believe I should have asked both Mr. and Mrs. Paley to come into the office for a discussion about this issue of joint consent for the surgery. I had been feeling relatively content with the discussions that we had been having. I felt rather warm toward this family, and wanted to be helpful.

In such a situation as this, we can agree with the counselor that a joint conference with both Mr. and Mrs. Paley could possibly have facilitated the genuine sharing of responsibility for the important decision facing them. Husband and wife are sometimes able to say troubling things to each other with a professional in the room that they can not exchange while alone together. The presence of the professional reassures them that nothing will be permitted to get "out of hand."

During the consultation with the craniofacial team, which I attended, Melissa was assessed to be a good candidate for the Tessier procedure. Dr. C. said he would send a letter to the health plan's pediatrician requesting the health plan to allow the surgery to be performed at our hospital. Because of the considerable expense this would be for the plan, we knew that we might encounter some difficulty, but approval finally came after many weeks of waiting. Melissa was now 5 years old.

Due to the busy schedules of the plastic surgeon and neurosurgeon, the operation needed to be scheduled nine weeks from the approval date. This was an extremely difficult period for Mrs. Paley, because once she had decided that the surgery should take place she wanted it over with. She called me frequently to discuss her hopes and fears about the upcoming event. We also discussed how Mrs. Paley should prepare Melissa, the rest of her family, and Melissa's schoolmates for the anticipated abrupt change in her facial appearance. I remember feeling very impressed at her thoroughness in preparing Melissa. Using language that Melissa could understand, Mrs. Paley carefully explained what was going to happen.

A week before the operation, Mrs. Paley called to let me know that she had visited Melissa's class at school and told the children that Melissa would be going to the hospital, and what to expect when she returned. She asked me if it was possible to arrange a tour of the pediatrics ward so that she and Melissa could meet the ward personnel and become familiar with the surroundings. This was arranged with the head nurse; and the tour, five days prior to the surgery, included having Melissa role-play a patient, using a doll.

> The same principle of preparation that was discussed earlier for adults applies with even greater force to younger subjects for whatever expectably traumatic procedure lies ahead. A child has little prior experience to instill any sense of confident expectation concerning surgery and separation from parents in the hospital. That prior experience is, for Melissa, good, loving care at her parents' hands in her first five years of life. A child has limited cognitive capacity to understand strange new experiences without guidance. With such considerations in mind, the more specific details a child is told about in advance—naturally, in language and concept suitable for the child's age—the better the preparation will be.

After the tour, it was clear that the person who had benefited most from the experience was Mrs. Paley, whose anxiety level had been significantly reduced.

Melissa was admitted to the hospital two days before the day of the scheduled surgery, for preoperative tests and consultations. Because I did not feel that Mr. and Mrs. Paley had come to a joint decision about the surgery, I discussed the situation with the plastic surgery resident who would be most involved with Melissa's care. He suggested that he ask both parents to sign the consent form, and I heartily agreed that this might help the situation. This single event forced Mr. Paley to face the fact that he, too, by signing the consent form, was giving Melissa the chance to have a "new" facial appearance or die in the attempt. It helped bring Mr. Paley in touch with his feelings, especially his own tremendous fears for her safety. It also opened up a great deal of communication beween the Paleys.

Early on the morning of the surgery Melissa was taken to the operating room. I met with the Paleys for breakfast after Melissa had left the ward and discussed with them the signing of the consent form:

G.C.: How are you doing?
MRS. PALEY: I said good-bye to Melissa in the room. I couldn't let her see me crying, so I didn't go with her down the hallway.

G.C.: Dave, how did you feel?

Mr. Paley: I guess, after all this time, it really hit me last night. This has been a harrowing experience for both of us. I think it makes you realize how much your children mean to you. But we have to give her this chance.

G.C.: Did you both sign the consent form?

Mrs. Paley: Yes. Dr. J. felt it would be a good idea.

G.C.: So do I.

Mrs. Paley: I think we got to talk last night for the first time about what this really means.

Occasionally the concrete event of signing a consent form is needed to help a parent who has been dealing with a problem by self-protective distractions to confront his emotional conflict more directly.

G.C.: What does it mean?

Mrs. Paley: I guess . . . that Melissa might not make it, but that she probably will. Also, that we really have to stick together to help her. Dr. J. had to explain to Dave and me all the things that could happen to her. She might die, she might not die, she might need extra surgery if everything does not go as hoped, and it might go just fine.

G.C.: Dave, what does it mean to you?

Mr. Paley: More than anything, I guess it means that we have to worry, and hope that everything goes well. You know, it was easier when it was all up to Darlene. But Melissa is our child, and I know that I must help Darlene too. This has been very tough on her.

G.C.: It sounds like you two have really talked to each other.

Mrs. Paley: Yes. Last night we watched Melissa as she was sleeping. I felt I couldn't leave her. She was so helpless. I really needed to talk to Dave, and tell him how I felt.

G.C.: It's much easier sharing the responsibility.

Mrs. Paley: Much easier. I don't think I can worry about her and worry about Dave's reaction, too. It would be too stressful for me.

G.C.: I think it might be too stressful for anybody. I will stop in when I can with updates on how the operation is going. I will also stop by after work and wait with you.

Twice during the day I came up to the pediatrics floor and told the family that everything was going very smoothly. When I arrived after clinic hours, the operation had been going on for about nine hours, and everyone looked quite exhausted. I spent some time talking with Mr. and Mrs. Paley, and attempted to explain the surgery to the other family members there. They were appreciative that someone cared whether or not they also understood what was going on.

This thoughtful detail was of large importance: When people are left without information as to how matters are progressing—even when the news may not be the best—they have only their spontaneous imaginings to go by.

At 8:30 P.M., twelve hours after the operation started, the waiting was over. The operation had been a total success. Dr. C. askd Mr. and Mrs. Paley to come to the recovery room so that they could see Melissa's face before he put the protective gauze over her eyes to reduce the swelling. Melissa looked so different; she looked . . . normal. The operation was a success as far as Melissa was concerned—and also for her parents. They were now able to work together as a team in order to help their daughter.

I recently talked to Mrs. Paley about the inclusion of the case in this casebook. She was quite excited and said she wanted other families to benefit by her family's experience. She asked me to mention the following to other genetic counselors so that they might relay it to other families: (1) Doctors aren't always right; and (2) no one knows a child better than its parents.

The Paleys' adherence to these beliefs and a firm resolve to do what they considered best for their child helped them to achieve a monumental benefit for their daughter: a normal craniofacial appearance.

Case 2

Marie Morse was the carefully planned first child of Mr. and Mrs. Morse, two very responsible and intelligent parents in their late twenties. Since becoming aware of Marie's problems, they have actively pursued services available for her. Mr. and Mrs. Morse are college-educated, she a teacher and he an accountant.

Marie seemed normal at birth, but when she was 3 months old Mrs. Morse began to worry because she did not seem to be developing at an appropriate rate. Mrs. Morse took Marie to the pediatrician, who told her not to be concerned. Since Mrs. Morse was a new parent, she trusted the pediatrician, whose experience far outweighed her own. A month later, when Marie still failed to progress, Mrs. Morse's worries resumed. During the following appointment with the pediatrician Mrs. Morse was told that Marie was slow but still within the normal range for an infant her age. When Marie was 6 months old and was still making no improvement, Mrs. Morse actively sought the opinion of a specialist and was referred to our clinic.

Prior to their appointment, I telephoned the family. From Mrs. Morse I promptly gained an impression of dedicated and extremely concerned parents. She was incredibly eager to provide all the information necessary for the appointment, and asked myriad questions regarding what to expect.

After meeting Mr. and Mrs. Morse, I knew that these parents were going to need extra time for counseling. During Marie's examination Dr. E. noted that she was extremely slow from a developmental standpoint and had a few physical abnormalities including microcephaly, epicanthal folds, and metatarsus adductus. In order to date the onset of the microcephaly, I contacted the hospital where Marie was born, and learned from the medical record that her head circumference had been normal at birth. Mr. and Mrs. Morse were told that although Marie certainly had a problem, her physical examination and the history they had provided had not made it possible to assign a diagnosis for her condition. Diagnostic tests were recommended (chromosome analysis and amino acid screening), and with parental consent they were performed. I informed the Morses that usually the results of tests like these are normal, and that we would telephone them with the reports. An appointment was scheduled for discussion of the laboratory test findings and related questions.

The results of the amino acid screening were normal, and I called the parents. They were happy to hear the news but also depressed because we were back where we started. I told them that I would let them know when the results of the chromosome analysis were available.

A few days later, the results of the chromosome study showed that Marie had a possibly abnormal X chromosome. In order to discern whether it really was abnormal, the parents' chromosomes had to be tested. Arrangements were made to do this.

During their next appointment, Mr. and Mrs. Morse were informed that their X chromosomes were entirely normal. Dr. E. interpreted Marie's X as being a normal variant, unrelated to the child's medical condition. Because I believed the Morses were being offered much new information to assimilate, I resolved to call them and specifically review the X chromosome information. We discussed the recurrence risk they faced for future pregnancies (zero to 25 percent), spending a considerable amount of time detailing the reasoning behind it, and why we had to be so vague. After the visit, both Dr. E and I wrote letters to the family summarizing the results of the evaluation.

The twofold follow-up—initially by telephone, later by letter—responds to the expected "mind-blowing" tension of the actual interview. Although telephone contact can be more prompt, the careful summarizing letter has the advantage that it can be read many times over, in various moods of increasingly relaxed comprehension.

I would characterize their feelings after the appointment as shell shock. I think they had heard too much, despite their intelligence, and had had their hopes dashed twice in a very short period of time. I told them that despite the difficulty of not having a diagnosis, they were fortunate that something as serious as a problem with amino acid metabolism or chromosomes had *not* been discovered. I also tried to let them know that we wanted to see Marie as she got older.

In subsequent conversations Mrs. Morse raised questions about her comprehension of the recurrence risks, estimated in such situations as zero to 25 percent, the upper limit being that of autosomal recessive inheritance. Mrs. Morse observed that she really wanted to have more children, but couldn't face another like Marie.

In contrast to the Paleys of the first clinical vignette, the Morses reflect a negative response to the very same recurrence risk numbers. For the Morses, a repetition of the experience of having a retarded child is unallowable. (Melissa Paley was not retarded.)

The following dialogue is a portion of one of these telephone conversations.

G.C.: Have you thought about your plan of action at this point?

MRS. MORSE: Well, we are going to follow through with Dr. E.'s suggestion to see the orthopedic surgeon. We really want to help Marie in any way we can.

G.C.: Yes, I know you do. You have been among the most conscientious parents I have encountered. I think you are doing a tremendous service for Marie.

MRS. MORSE: Do you think so?

G.C.: Absolutely. In fact, I worry that you are neglecting yourself a little. In the long run, it will help Marie more if you have an opportunity to worry about yourself and keep yourself strong.

MRS. MORSE: It's hard not to want to do everything for her. She's so helpless.

Over the next six months, the Morses concentrated on finding ways to correct some of Marie's problems. She was seen by the pediatric orthopedic surgeon, who put casts on her to correct the metatarsus adductus. She was registered with the state agency which provides a number of services to developmentally disabled children, and enrolled in an infant-stimulation class. I also told Mr. and Mrs. Morse about the parent support group, and they faithfully attended each meeting. They even took notes when guest speakers discussed pertinent topics. They continued to be the ''perfect'' parents.

When Marie was reexamined six months later, she was just about one year old. During her appointment I spent a considerable amount of time with Mrs. Morse discussing how she had fared over the prior six months. Despite the fact that I had seen her at the parent support group meetings, I wanted her to give her own overall assessment of how the last six months had transpired. It was obvious that Mrs. Morse had spent little time on herself or her husband, and was emotionally exhausted. I again stressed the fact that she needed to get away, and that Marie would be better off in the long run if her parents did not "burn out" from too much giving and not enough support. After this appointment, Mrs. Morse called to tell me that she had taken this advice, and that she and her husband had benefited a great deal from their vacation together.

The counselor's caution is well intended. When parents' devotion to their child becomes utterly enervating—whether that child be normal or abnormal—they will eventually become joyless, irritable, angry, and depressed. Inevitably the child will become a target for some of that anger, as the agent causing the unhappy condition. This is unfair to all, and will exacerbate parental guilt and related self-reproaches.

At 13 months of age, Marie was seen by a staff pediatric neurologist, who felt that she should be hospitalized for detailed diagnostic evaluation. The Morses went along with this recommendation. A CAT scan (computerized axial tomography) demonstrated that Marie had cerebellar atrophy: a new potential diagnosis. At the end of this hospital stay the Morses were informed that the finding of cerebellar atrophy in combination with Marie's other abnormalities did not add up to any known diagnosis. During the evaluation, the pediatric neurologist asked Mrs. Morse about medications or illnesses she may have had during her pregnancy. These questions led her to worry that she had caused her daughter's problem. When she told me about the neurologist's questions and expressed her concern, I reassured her that we did not feel that these were the causes of Marie's problem. Mrs. Morse had frequently told us that she had been *extremely* cautious during the pregnancy, and had not experienced any symptoms of infection.

One offers such reassurance in the hope of reducing guilt. But some measure of parental guilt will persist inwardly, however irrational its basis.

After this episode, Mr. and Mrs. Morse began to realize that based on current knowlege, no one could give them definitive answers concerning Marie. This was quite an adjustment for them, and I feel that they now have a much more realistic attitude regarding Marie's condition. I meet the Morses at the parent support group meetings, and they are scheduled for their yearly clinic appointment soon. Mrs. Morse frequently uses our encounter to discuss Marie's progress, and sometimes asks that I refresh her memory about the genetics or other aspects of Marie's condition. At the present time, without more information, Mr. and Mrs. Morse are unwilling to risk having another child with Marie's condition. They are doing a good job of providing Marie with all the opportunities available to progress to the best of her potential.

Case 3

Jason Neustadt is now 7 years old, and burdened by an unknown dysmorphic syndrome. He carries, in addition, a reciprocal translocation between chromosomes #8 and #11. He is the first child of Mr. and Mrs. Neustadt, who had always wanted a medium-sized family. The Neustadts chose not to have additional children because no one could tell them their risk of having another child with the same condition as Jason. Mr. and Mrs. Neustadt are college-educated, intelligent, and precise people who are very cautious. Both dress meticulously, and despite the fact that they do interact in activities which help them or Jason, I have felt that they keep themselves somewhat at a distance from other people.

Jason was noted to be small and unusual-appearing at birth, following a totally uncomplicated pregnancy. At that time, no one could pinpoint the cause of his problems. He developed slowly, and was enrolled in a local center for developmentally disabled children when he was two and a half years of age. During the intake evaluation no diagnosis was made, and all tests including karyotyping were interpreted as normal. When Jason was three and a half, some of the doctors at the center told Mrs. Neustadt that they thought he might have Williams syndrome but weren't sure. When Jason was 5, his pediatric cardiologist felt very sure that he had Williams syndrome and referred the family to our clinic.

I was present during the initial appointment, and chatted briefly with Mrs. Neustadt. The bulk of this appointment consisted of a diagnostic assessment of Jason. The following problems were identified: prenatal and postnatal growth deficiency, maxillary hypoplasia, a long philtrum, a heart murmur, pectus carinatum, single upper palmar creases, and abnormal speech. He was clearly hyperactive when overloaded with auditory stimulation, and functioned in the educable mentally retarded range.

During the appointment, Williams syndrome was ruled out as a diagnosis, but no other diagnosis could be made for this pattern of malformation. Chromosome studies were repeated because of the presence of multiple dysmorphic abnormalities, and because it had been many years since the original study. The lack of diagnosis, the zero to 25 percent recurrence risk, and the reasons for both were explained to Mrs. Neustadt.

She was instructed to return with Jason after another year if the results of the chromosome study were normal. I told her that I would call her in a few days to see if she had any additional questions.

Mrs. Neustadt asked to review the reasons for saying Jason did *not* have Williams syndrome. I explained that the diagnosis of this syndrome is based on a pattern of problems in a child. Some children have a part, or a few parts, of the pattern, but only children with the Williams syndrome have the whole pattern.

If anything underscores the value of deferring diagnosis to a medical center, it is this variety of experience. No private solo practitioner can expect in an entire lifetime to see multiple examples of rare conditions. But the catchment of a medical center expectably pools the data of a much broader geographical region, providing a firmer base for certitude.

A representative conversation from this period of the counseling follows:

MRS. NEUSTADT: Almost half the children you see can't be diagnosed? I had no idea.

This piece of information has to reduce the client's depressing sense of being alone in misfortune. Not every center is equally relaxed in conveying the limits of current knowledge.

G.C.: It's true. There are so many things that can go wrong in a child, and given enough children, they will happen. We will want to see Jason in a year to see whether anything has developed that we can tell you about. If we can make a diagnosis then, we may be able to give you a more specific recurrence risk.

MRS. NEUSTADT: Really? We would love to have another child, but I just couldn't cope with another like Jason. I love him dearly, but I just couldn't handle two. I think I am still adjusting to Jason. He's going to school now, and is old enough for me to remind myself that I can't protect him all the time. It's very hard because I know how vulnerable he is, both physically and emotionally, and he can't understand why he's the way he is.

The task of adjustment probably goes on for a very long, perhaps indefinite, time period. After all, every new achievement of Jason's normal age-mates can only remind the Neustadts afresh of what Jason doesn't have or cannot achieve. This has to rekindle the Neustadts' mourning, even if only faintly.

An unusual finding in Jason's karyotype necessitated my phoning Mrs. Neustadt to come in and discuss the results with us. Dr. E. reported the presence of a reciprocal translocation between chromosomes #8 and #11 in Jason's cells. Dr. E. needed to test the Neustadts to determine whether either of them also carried this reciprocal translocation. The results for them were normal.

Dr. E. believed that the translocation in Jason may have resulted in the deletion of a small amount of chromosomal material, but he couldn't be certain. Because Jason's particular pattern of malformation has not been previously associated with the possible regions of deletion on chromosomes #8 or 11, Dr. E. could not feel absolutely certain his problems were due to the chromosomal rearrangement. The Neustadts were informed that many normal people carry small reciprocal translocations, and that this could be entirely coincidental to Jason's problems. If the Neustadts decided to have another child, there was no indication for amniocentesis, since the chance that the translocation would repeat itself in another child was felt to be insignificant. Later, summary letters concerning all this were sent by Dr. E. and myself.

Within a few months Mrs. Neustadt called me to say that she was pregnant, and that she and her husband felt confident that their interpretation of the recurrence risk (i.e., that it was low) was a reasonable one. They were prepared to take their chances that this child would have Jason's condition, although they now thought that it was a remote possibility. I tried to reinforce the positive feelings Mrs. Neustadt was expressing. We also discussed some of the problems Jason was experiencing at his school, and I gave her the names of some alternative schools.

The recurrence risk is still zero to 25 percent, as previously announced to the Neustadts. The risk that was formerly felt to be unallowable no longer is viewed that way. Why the change? In part, some of the discussions with counseling personnel have doubtless led the Neustadts—whether rationally or not—to suspect that *their* probability is nearer to the zero percent than to the 25 percent end of the stated range. We must not overlook, however, the impact on the Neustadts of their accumulating successful experience in raising Jason. Successful coping with a difficult reality silently accrues important increments of self-esteem and confident expectation.

During her pregnancy, Mrs. Neustadt attended meetings of the local parent support group, which I also attended. During these meetings I had short conversations with her, which allowed me an opportunity to reinforce what had transpired during the appointments. Mrs. Neustadt had an opportunity to share her feelings with other mothers who had undergone a pregnancy after having an affected child. They understood the reasons for her anxiety, and helped her a great deal.

The Neustadts' daughter, Marjorie, was born with a heart murmur but was otherwise completely normal. She is being followed by the same pediatric cardiologist who follows Jason, and is doing very well. The Neustadts are an example of a family who had to deal with changing medical opinions over time, and who additionally had the burden of trying to interpret ambiguous genetic information as it might affect their future children. Mrs. Neustadt has found the support of the parents' group very helpful through some of her stressful times during the pregnancy, and in coping with Jason. The Neustadts consider their life with Jason as a series of hurdles of different sizes. As they encounter and adjust to one problem, a new problem addresses them. They view life as a process of continual adaptation, especially when one has a "special" child.

Further Comment

In this casebook collection we have already encountered any number of instances in which uncertainty about diagnosis figures importantly in the counseling enterprise with a particular couple. The difficulties of having to endure periods of diagnostic uncertainty have been noted.

In the situations recounted in this subset of three, the need to live indefinitely with diagnostic uncertainty adds a special, but not unique, twist. What is particularly notable is how much assistance can be provided despite the diagnostic uncertainty; and some couples are even enabled to continue with their family planning. The counselor conveys all available information, maintains an optimistic attitude toward the possible assistance to be derived from further research, and cultivates (if possible) a lasting relationship with the counselees—one that will permit additional contacts over the months and years to come. The range of corrective measures available is presented to the counselees, and contact with the appropriate specialists is promoted.

It is instructive to note the different impacts on family planning of the uncertain range of recurrence risks for these three different couples. Melissa was not retarded, and a difficult cosmetic corrective was available to improve her appearance. Her parents had, moreover, given birth to a normal son after Melissa. These (and doubtless other personal factors) combined to facilitate the conception of a second normal son. Marie

exhibited some degree of retardation, and the many tasks involved in raising her, combined with personality factors not detailed in this report, led
to the decision not to attempt further childbearing. The situation with
Jason's parents began similarly, with appreciation of a degree of retardation. But it turned out that the tasks of rearing Jason were able to be accomplished without intolerable burden, leading to a revision of decision
about further children, and the birth of an essentially normal daughter.

Reference

SMITH, D. (1977). *Recognizable patterns of human malformation*, pp. 54–55. Philadelphia:
W. B. Saunders.

24

A Counselee Looks Back at Twelve Years of Counseling: G_{M1}-Gangliosidosis, Type II

In this account, the mother of a large family in which two children are affected with a heritable metabolic disorder recounts the assistance provided by genetic counseling over a twelve-year span of time.

This mother's capacity to articulate the character of her experience so impressed the editors that she is the only nonprofessional informant included in this collection.

This report concerns the Snow family, whose counseling began in 1968 and continues still. The strong bond of trust which has nourished this relationship was developed slowly and with great care. In addition to our medical knowledge and skills we were able to offer continuous availability, and we actively encouraged these counselees to be in touch with us as often as desired. Because the Snows live an hour and a half's drive from our Genetics Center, most contact after 1969 was by telephone or letter.

The opportunity to study the youngest child's rare genetic disorder and to counsel the parents and each of the three unaffected children through this long period has rewarded us professionally and personally.

Mrs. Snow (Fernanda) was very enthusiastic about the possibility of adding her family's story to this counseling casebook, so much so that she offered to help by writing a detailed summary of the family's experiences with two children affected with a neurologically degenerative disorder. Her backward look at twenty-three painful years provides us with material rarely available and therefore greatly appreciated.

Our initial contact with the Snows was through Mrs. Snow's letter to us in February 1968:

Dear Dr. T.,

I hope you may have time in your busy schedule to read my letter because I am hoping and praying that you may help us. Actually it is a long story, so I will try to make it as short as I can. We have a little girl almost 3 whose name is Marie. She cannot walk or talk. We took her to a children's hospital nine months ago, where she was evaluated for five days. Their diagnosis was that she was mentally retarded ("cerebral atrophy" was the name given), but that it was very probable that she would walk eventually.

The reason why I insisted on this evaluation at that time was that she had begun to regress at the age of twelve months, and I was in a very bad state myself because, you see, this is the *second* time this terrible thing has happened to us. We have had five children, and our third child was afflicted the same way. He gradually returned to an infantile stage and just wasted away, completely helpless. He died two years ago in an institution where he had been for six years. He was 10 when he died. Our fourth child is as active both mentally and physically as anyone could want, even more so. But Marie, now only creeping (she had begun to walk), is gradually going backwards. She cannot pull herself to a standing position anymore and her legs are getting stiffer gradually. Her fingers are curling a little, and about two months ago she started the same seizures that Joe used to have. We are trying to control them with Dilantin, as I believe the seizures weaken her considerably. Some mornings I think she might have had a slight stroke of some sort during the night, because she is sort of sagging on the whole left side of her body.

On the whole we feel perfectly helpless, and I feel I must exhaust every avenue before I give up hope completely. I just can't sit here and repeat this same horrible nightmare without one last try.

Could you tell us if there would possibly be anything at all to gain for her by our taking her to your hospital? You have been so highly recommended to us by Dr. D. But if needed, we could also get a referral from our family doctor.

Sincerely,
Mrs. Edward Snow

This very poignant account of a compounded family tragedy—one that has occurred more than once—highlights what from an emotional viewpoint is one of the worst features common to so many of these disasters: the feeling of *helplessness,* of being obliged to experience *passively* the impact of a deteriorating situation. This aspect of the situation breeds, in turn, a sense of *hopelessness* that enhances the family's depression. We can appreciate, therefore, that anything that professionals or family *can actively do,* regardless of eventual outcome, will lessen the sense of hopelessness and depression.

Dr. T. responded to this letter at once, inviting the Snows to bring Marie to the Medical Center for admission to be evaluated as an inpatient. He indicated plainly that although no effort would be spared, there was no guarantee that Marie's illness could be diagnosed. Mrs.

Snow's immediate telephone response to this offer resulted in an appointment that was to follow in three days.

When the Snows arrived, we arranged for them to stay with Marie until they were satisfied that she was settled into her new surroundings. Then we conducted them to our department for an interview. Fernanda (age 39) and Edward (age 40) appeared to be a deeply concerned couple, eager to give us as much information as possible. In seventeen years of marriage five children had been born to them: Marie, 33 months old, was the baby; Paul, 15 years old, was the oldest; Nicole, 14, next; Joseph, the third child, had died at age 10, about two years before; and Tom, the fourth child, was 5. Mr. Snow worked as a machinist for a large company. With the exception of one weekly trip to the supermarket, all of Mrs. Snow's time was spent at home.

This family is part of a very long-established ethnic group which has continually resided in the same geographical area. Although we were unable to pinpoint consanguinity, Mrs. Snow laughingly admits that if enough questions are asked, most people turn out to be "some kind of cousins."

The Snows told us much about Joseph's and Marie's similar illnesses. We explained during this first meeting that Marie would be examined, tested, and evaluated by the biochemical genetics, neurology, neurosurgery, and pathology departments and that her stay at the hospital might be as long as three to four weeks. We offered to make a room available to them in a home near the hospital to facilitate their expressed intention of trying to visit daily. The Snows politely declined this offer, explaining that they believed a prolonged absence from home at this time would be too difficult for their three other children, even though Fernanda's mother was able to stay with them. We encouraged them to visit Marie as often as possible and to make a point of stopping in to speak with us when they did. During the weeks that followed we had many informal conservations. They became comfortable with us and were not intimidated by their surroundings. Concerning this period Mrs. Snow writes, "We were very impressed with Dr. T. and Mrs. B.'s friendliness and genuine concern for us and for Marie. I felt that finally, we had found people who cared."

The following summary is drawn from Mrs. Snow's account of the course of Joseph's illness and the onset of Marie's illness:

> When we first became aware that there was something wrong with Joey, he was about 13 months old. We were a very young family then—I was 27, Ed was 28, Paul was 4, and Nicole was 3. Things had been going well for us up until then and we had been hoping to start building a house soon. Joseph had been fine and was beginning to take his first steps. He fell so often that I talked to our family doctor about him. An orthopedic clinic. . . .

We should bear in mind that having had the experience of developmental sequences with two normal children, Mrs. Snow was attuned, as parents become, to what is approximately expectable at different ages. A new, first-time mother may not react to developmental abnormalities with the same promptness.

An orthopedic clinic was recommended. There Joey was fitted with orthopedic shoes, and after a few visits he was recommended for evaluation to a medical center six hours away. We took Joe there and he stayed for seven weeks! By this time he had gone back to creeping and couldn't feed himself or even sit without help. My mother stayed with Paul and Nicole when we visited the hospital on weekends. At the end of his stay Joey was diagnosed as probably being retarded and having cerebral palsy. I heard of a clinic for cerebral palsy, and when Joey continued to get worse we took him there for two days of evaluation. This clinic was four hours from us. Their recommendation was for physical therapy and stimulation. After that, we acquired a walker for him and he was able to get around pretty well for a while. Then he began having seizures. Medication was prescribed, but the poor child got worse and worse. He was still on a bottle and in diapers, of course.

Our family doctor and others began to encourage us to institutionalize Joseph. I think we realized that almost all of our attention for the previous three years had been focused on him, and we were concerned about the effect this was having on Paul and Nicole. It was a very difficult decision, and it took us quite a while to agree to place Joey at a state institution for the retarded. Joseph was four and a half years old then. Having him there was something of a relief, but it was also a steady heartache.

The decision for institutional placement of a defective child is eagerly made by some families. For others, like the Snows, it is made reluctantly after heart-rending labor to resolve inner conflict.

We visited him as often as we could all through the years, and it created quite a hardship for us. It was expensive traveling the 600-mile round trip and nerve-wracking driving our old car on the dangerous roads during the uncertain weather conditions of our long winters. Leaving the children for the weekend, even though they were with their grandmother, added to the uneasiness and emotional exhaustion of the trip. Sometimes I would cry going and coming, but Ed was patient and always tried to calm me. I constantly wrote to the institution and inquired when I was there as to the extent of the physical therapy Joey was receiving. I guess I never really thought that he would *not* get better, and in itself that was quite exhausting. I always prayed for a miracle, that he would recover.

In the meantime, even though we had always wanted a large family, I was terribly afraid that I would become pregnant and have another child like Joseph. Our family doctor assured me that the odds were so great against it happening to another child that I had nothing to worry about. I was never able to fully believe him. When Joey was 7, I became pregnant. It was a *long,* fearful pregnancy. My prayers were answered, however, and our third son, Tommy, was fine in every way—a happy child, alert and proof positive that the doctor had been right. . . so I thought. Two years later, in May, our second daughter, Marie, was born. Four months later Joey died. We had not been able to visit him for months because Ed had been hospitalized for back surgery, I wasn't able to drive in the last months of pregnancy, and then Marie's birth kept us at home.

What a cruel irony that the birth of one and the death of the other affected child come so closely together! Some parents experience the concurrence of a birth and a death in terms of the new child becoming a replacement for the lost one. (Such a sequence has very complicated reverberations for the "replacement" child.) For the Snows this "replacement" involves a tragic twist of fate.

The lengthened intervals between visits to Joey—coupled with the expectable concentration on the current pregnancy, Marie's birth, and her early months—may have combined to attenuate the bond with the absent Joey. As a consequence, the wrench of his death may have been somewhat eased.

We were called to his bedside at the end, but it was too late, and the attending doctor advised us against seeing him. The doctor told us that Joey had returned to the way he was in the womb and had literally wasted away. Ed insisted that I take the doctor's advice.

Fernanda yearned for a final look at their unfortunate son, but Ed and the physician in charge overruled her. There is no assuredly "correct" pathway to select in this circumstance, which may be encountered soon after the birth of a defective infant, rather than ten years later as in this instance. For some parents it is "better" not to view their child. For others, *not* to view their child (or neonate) a final time leaves an uncomfortable sense of an aspect of their life that hasn't been "completed" or "resolved." Counselors in such circumstances may be useful in helping a couple to clarify what suits them best.

On the way home, I remember feeling relieved that I would never have to go back there again. After nine years we were free to return to normal living.

Our relief was very short-lived, however, because eight months later Marie, who had been active and healthy, who had started talking and walking, began falling backwards and dropping her spoon when feeding herself. I knew that the horrible nightmare was beginning again. The worst thing about it was that I couldn't convince anyone else. All I could think of was that I had to get help for her, and right away. I went to a different orthopedic clinic and after that a children's hospital. After a week of evaluation we were told that Marie was mildly retarded and nothing more. I remember thinking that we could take that, if only she could walk. Then the seizures and crying spells began. Nicole, now 14, slept in the same room as Marie, and I worried greatly about the effect all this was having on her. In desperation I wrote dozens of letters to hospitals and doctors and foundations, thinking that there must be someone who could help us. One of the letters was in response to a tiny ad in our local newspaper referring to the March of Dimes Birth Defects Foundation. This was one of the few letters that was answered. I was referred to a Dr. D., who in turn recommended Dr. T. as a person who was doing research in the field of neurological disorders.

At the Genetics Center, our initial impressions of Marie were of a well-nourished, irritable, retarded, spastic child with a shrill, piercing cry and little spontaneous movement. A general physical examination showed no abnormality. A variety of elaborate biochemical and other diagnostic studies were done in the next four weeks, including a brain biopsy. At the end of that time the diagnosis of G_{M1}-gangliosidosis, Type II, was made. This disorder is characterized by an excessive accumulation of G_{M1}-ganglioside in the nervous system and a profound deficiency of B (beta) galactosidase. This metabolic defect is inherited in an autosomal recessive pattern and is extremely rare. Marie was one of the very few living individuals in whom G_{M1}-gangliosidosis, Type II, had been identified, and at age 16 she was to be the oldest known survivor of this progressive, untreatable disease. Both parents showed significantly decreased B (beta) galactosidase activity in their leukocyctes, indicating their status as carriers.

Before Marie was released from the hospital, we had a lengthy meeting with the Snows. We felt that knowledge of the diagnosis, although very painful, would at the very least satisfy their need for an explanation of the disorder that had tragically befallen two of their children. We intended to offer them a program of medical supervision, our ongoing counseling and moral support, and testing for carrier status of their three unaffected children. Mrs. Snow writes of this meeting and what followed:

> When they finished their testing, we were told the name of Marie's illness and that she could not be cured. We were made to understand that research had only begun about three years before. Dr. T. took the time to draw pictures on the blackboard to help us understand how Marie had inherited this condition and the chances for any child that we conceived to become a victim of this disorder. We realized that our other children, too, might have had it. We, ourselves, proved to be carriers, and Paul, Nicole, and Tom would have to be tested to see if they were carriers. Dr. T. talked to us about death, how when a loved one dies suddenly, their family suffers for a long time afterward; but when a person suffers a long time before death, there is a sense of relief that their suffering is over.

The physician's easy acknowledgment that there can be a great sense of relief when an individual in agony succumbs is a valuable intervention. With the full force of professional authority, he "legitimizes" the experience of relief. Why is this of any value? Because many families experience guilt over their sense of relief, regarding the latter emotion as uncomfortably close to plain death wishes: "I wish this tormented child would die already!" Individuals with usual consciences recoil in distress at awareness of such wishes about loved ones.

> Of course, those are not his exact words, but his meaning has carried me for a long time and may have changed the course of my life. It was a shock, but at least now we knew. We were told that if we ever had any problems, night or day, we should call and ask for Mrs. B. This meant more to us than anyone could imagine, as there really wasn't anyone in our community who understood our problem. In fact, we noticed that people in general had avoided talking about Joseph and now Marie. I used to think that they were uncaring until one day I met my uncle, who said to me, "I've always meant to ask you about Marie, but I didn't want you to feel bad."

For many friends and family members it is difficult to broach what is expected to be a very sensitive topic. Commonly the fear in so doing is that the grieving family member will be moved to tears. The inquirer anticipates feeling guilty about having provoked the fresh show of grief, and so avoids the topic altogether.

The parent of an affected child may interpret the absence of inquiries as lack of interest—or may conclude that others cannot, themselves, tolerate speaking about such a distressing subject. And so a collusion may develop between parents and outsiders to maintain silence concerning the defective child.

This situation does not help the parents, who, as the Snows did, need opportunities to speak with interested people about their dilemma.

> Back home, armed with the information we had received, and determined not to become pregnant again, I went to my family doctor and told him I wanted a hysterectomy. He did not approve, but sent me to a surgeon who commented that I should have been sterilized years before. I knew that I could have had a tubal ligation, but it would not have reassured me as much as the hysterectomy. After it was done, I was tremendously relieved.

Our summary letter to the Snows included the diagnosis and an explanation of the genetics and risk of recurrence. It mentioned the parents' carrier status and the availability of carrier testing for the children. Recommendations for Marie's care and special equipment were also included.

The Snows let us know that as soon as Mrs. Snow had recuperated, they would be eager to return to the hospital in order for Paul, Nicole, and Tom to be tested for heterozygosity. They understood that these children would not become ill with Marie's disorder but felt it wise to obtain tangible proof of this information for them. After talking it over, Dr. T. and I agreed that if the family was willing, we would drive to their home and take the blood samples there. Mrs. Snow writes of this visit:

On Memorial Day 1968, Dr. T. and Mrs. B. came to our home and it was quite a day for all of us. To think that these busy people would actually care enough to drive all this way and sit down to have a meal with us! My husband often talks of it, and the children still remember that day. The children had blood samples taken, and about ten days later we received a call from Mrs. B. telling us the wonderful news that *none* of the children were carriers. We explained this to the children, and told them they need never worry about this disease again.

The Snows made every effort to cope with Marie's deteriorating condition. Her seizures became more frequent, and she cried for long periods of time. Both Ed and Fernanda were suffering back pain, which was exacerbated by having to carry Marie everywhere. Their family physician suggested that they begin to think about custodial care for Marie at a newly opened state facility only an hour from their home. Fernanda called us to talk about this possibility, reporting that Marie was now in need of twenty-four-hour care. We agreed that it would be only a matter of time before this step would be unavoidable. Fernanda commented, "This is a very hard thing for all of us. You know, I always came away from visiting Joey with a bad feeling. I never felt sure that he was being cared for properly. The thing that was especially troubling was that I had never been able to see where he actually slept." When we were finished talking, she said she thought the time had come to take the steps necessary to place Marie. Application was soon made, with some small relief felt as a result. Unfortunately, a letter to the Snows informed them that there was a year's wait for admittance. Mrs. Snow became so distraught that her doctor placed Marie in a local hospital, for temporary respite. Mrs. Snow telephoned me and exclaimed, "It's too much! After finally deciding, we have to wait a year!" I told her that we would do what we could to hasten placement. Dr. T. made some calls and was able to gain entrance for Marie in just one week. Mrs. Snow talks about this time:

Giving Marie up was hard on all of us. At first we visited her regularly, perhaps every other week. "Too often," everyone told me, but I needed to go and did. Ed always understood this. For him it was over once we were satisfied that Marie was getting good care—and we were very satisfied. We were never refused access to any building. The staff was made up of local people who prized their jobs. I insisted that the children visit Marie, feeling that it was good for them to see the less fortunate and learn compassion. That summer we took Marie to a local lakeshore for a picnic. It was a disaster; the children were miserable, and of course Marie didn't know the difference. I realized then that my stubbornness was having a bad effect on the children, especially on Paul and Tom. I couldn't make the trip alone for a long time; Ed and Nicole would come along. Marie is hardly ever awake now and always thinner than the time before. The worst times are when she is struggling and choking while being fed, and yet I always feel a little better after having seen her.

Dr. T. and Mrs. B. see Marie occasionally, as they are still investigating this disease. We are happy to give permission for them to take blood or skin from Marie. Perhaps in time something good will come of all this. After seeing Marie, Mrs. B. or Dr. T. call or write and let us know how they found her and what progress is being made in their research. I have kept all the letters and reread them from time to time. They seem to comfort me.

Over the many years that we have known Dr. T. and Mrs. B. there were many times that we would receive a friendly phone call from the Genetic Center asking how I was and what the children were doing. Usually I spill out everything, good and bad, and often there were problems. My husband had back surgery three times during our married life; how much of that was due to stress we will never know. Paul had migraine headaches and Nicole stayed away from school. They were both helped by their counseling. Tommy had his troubles, too. We had noticed that he always hated to see us go away in the car. When he was 8, he developed chronic stomach pain. This was about the time that Paul was getting ready to leave for college. After our family doctor could find nothing wrong and his pains continued, I called Mrs. B. She arranged for Tom to be admitted to their hospital for tests. When no physical cause for pain was found, Mrs. B. arranged for Tom to be seen by a staff psychologist. He was found to be an anxious child, worried about the death of his parents, brother, and sisters. He inquired of the psychologist whether college was like a hospital. He was afraid he would never see Paul again once Paul had left for college.

When Nicole, living across the country, became pregnant, she became very concerned about the child she was carrying. She must have forgotten her counseling. I wasn't able to convince her or her husband that they had no reason to worry that the child would have gangliosidosis. I called Mrs. B. and asked for help. In a few days Nicole received a lovely explanatory letter which reassured her about this worry. A copy was sent to us.

At one time, after Marie was placed, I went through a siege of unexplainable aches and pains and was certain I had cancer. A call to the center, and an appointment was arranged for me at a clinic at the hospital. As recently as this summer I called Mrs. B. and asked for medical advice about my sister, who is very ill with a rare blood condition. There has been no time when I called that I wasn't able to speak with Mrs. B. or Dr. T.—unless they were on vacation or at a meeting, and in that situation someone else was made available in their place.

Soon after Marie was placed, Fernanda was offered a part-time job at the local grade school teaching learning-disabled children to read. She felt that she wasn't at all ready to leave her home to work. Ed, however, persuaded her to accept the offer and she reluctantly agreed to try to do the job. After a little training and much encouragement Fernanda came to enjoy her work. This position became the first unplanned step toward continuing education and more responsible positions for Fernanda. Eleven years later she earned a bachelor's degree and has since completed studies for a master's. During this period she has functioned as liaison between the school and community, and is counseling evenings at a college in the area.

We have great admiration and respect for this remarkable family.

We have helped them, but mostly they have helped one another. They have made every effort to further our research by allowing us to continue to study Marie, and by searching their community for children who also seemed to be affected with disorders like Marie's. Mrs. Snow found some children and sent them to us. They did not have G_{M1}-gangliosidosis, Type II, but we were able to refer them for the special help they required. Mrs. Snow sums up this way:

> Dr. T. and Mrs. B., with their counseling and caring, helped me to realize that what happened to Joey and Marie was *not* my fault, that it was really out of our control. Since I could do nothing to prevent what happened, I was finally able to focus my energies where it can do the most good—on my family and on the children in the community. I have always felt that God had given our children a little something extra to make up for Joey and Marie, and I have always told that to them. We have been through a lot, but it has brought us all very close.

Fernanda Snow contacted the editor in December 1981 with news of the children's latest achievements, the growing number of grandchildren, and Marie's more frequent bouts of pneumonia. She ended her letter with the observation, "I have a very fulfilling job, and I still feel that I have received many graces from God along with the heartaches."

In February 1982, Marie died at the age of 16.

Further Comment

Although this report is based primarily on counselee recollection rather than counselor appraisal, we have included it for several reasons. First, it illustrates the fruitful integrative results of a lengthy interaction with the professional staff. Second, it demonstrates that a useful collaboration does not necessarily require personal visits and geographical proximity. Invaluable work can be done by telephone or letter.

In the latter portion of the narrative there are notations of physical difficulties experienced by Mr. Snow, Paul, and Tom, with the added question of the possible role of emotional stress in these problems. To know what each member of a family is experiencing specifically as "stress" in a genetic counseling situation requires knowing a good deal of the emotional "inside story" of each, perspectives that outsiders other than mental health professionals usually cannot gain access to. Everyone in a family has thoughts and feelings—some shared and others kept forever private—about the family member who is ill. How can it be otherwise? For the Snows, the continuing interest of the Genetics Center staff was invaluable, helping the family to further utilize the perspectives conveyed at the time of the original consultations.

When Nicole became pregnant, it appeared to her mother that she had "forgotten" her earlier counseling. Any woman may be anxious about the outcome of her pregnancy. For Nicole it is likely that her worries drew upon—and distorted—the family experience with counseling regarding the gangliosidosis. Timely intervention by the Genetics Center staff was important for Nicole and her husband.

Some readers may consider that Mrs. B. and Dr. T. involved themselves with the Snows in many contexts other than medical diagnosis and discussions of recurrence risk. A narrow definition of genetic counseling excludes other interventions. A broader view leads to assistance with all manner of reverberations of the original evaluation. Some of the assistance for the family took the form of direct counseling, but other help came as appropriate referrals to other medical specialists, or as intervention with the administration of the institution where Marie was placed.

In commenting upon her counseling experience, it is very impressive that Mrs. Snow singles out as one of the most useful features the reduction of her personal feelings of guilt about the defective children. She indicates how such feelings sap energy that can otherwise be put to very constructive uses.

References

O'Brien, J. (1978). The gangliosidoses. In J. Stanbury, J. Wyngaarden, and D. Fredrickson, eds., *The metabolic basis of inherited disease,* 4th ed., pp. 841–865. New York: McGraw-Hill.

Wolfie, L.; Callahan, J.; Fawcett, J.; Andermann, F.; and Scriver, C. (1970). G_{M1}-gangliosidosis without chondrodystrophy or visceromegaly. *Neurology* 20: 23–44.

Glossary

Abortus: a dead or nonviable fetus following miscarriage or abortion.

Acrocentric chromosome: one whose centromere is near one end.

Amenorrhea: absence or abnormal stoppage of the menstrual period (menses).

Amniocentesis: the withdrawal by transabdominal needle puncture of amniotic fluid for the purpose of prenatal diagnosis.

Anencephaly: congenital absence of the cranial vault, with the cerebral hemispheres completely missing or reduced to small masses.

Aneuploidy: abnormal chromosome number; in humans, when the chromosome number in somatic cells is other than 46.

Antimongoloid: having a feature opposite to one characteristic of Down syndrome, e.g., an antimongoloid slant of the palpebral fissures is a downward slant to the eyes.

Apgar score: a numerical expression of an infant's condition, usually determined at 1 and 5 minutes after birth, based on heart rate, respiratory effort, muscle tone, reflex irritability, and skin color.

Artificial insemination: the collection of seminal fluid followed by its introduction into the vagina or cervix by syringe.

Atrophy: a wasting away; a diminution in the size of a cell, tissue, organ, or part.

Autosome(n.): any non-sex-determining chromosome; in humans there are 22 pairs of autosomes. (Autosomal, adj.)

Banding techniques: staining methods eliciting specific landmark cross patterns characteristic of each chromosome.

Brachydactyly: abnormal shortness of fingers and toes.

Buccal smear: a scraping of cells taken from the cheek lining used to study sex chromosome complement.

Carrier: an individual who is heterozygous for a normal gene and an abnormal gene which is not expressed phenotypically, although it may be detected by laboratory examinations.

Centromere: the constricted portion of the chromosome separating it into a short arm and a long arm.

Chondrodystrophy: a disorder of cartilage formation.

Chromosome: a microscopically identifiable unit of genetic material.

Clinodactyly: permanent deviation or deflection of one or more fingers.

Coloboma: an apparent absence or defect of some ocular tissue; it may affect the eyelid, iris, lens, optic nerve, retina, choroid, or ciliary body.

Conceptus: the product of conception.

Consanguineous, Consanguinity: blood relationship; kinship because of common ancestry.

Cytogenetic: relating to the cellular constituents concerned in heredity, i.e., the chromosomes.

Dementia: organic loss of intellectual function.

De novo: anew, for the first time.

Diploid: the number of chromosomes normally present in the somatic cell nucleus (in humans, 46).

Diuretic (adj. and n.): acting to increase urine excretion or the amount of urine; an agent that promotes urine secretion.

Dominant gene: a gene which causes a visible effect when present in a single copy. A dominant disorder results from the presence of a single mutant gene.

Dysgenesis: defective development; malformation.

Dysmorphic: pertaining to defective form or structure.

Dysplasia: abnormality of development.

Ectopic pregnancy: extrauterine pregnancy; development of the fertilized ovum outside the cavity of the uterus.

Epicanthal: pertaining to a vertical fold of skin on either side of the nose, sometimes covering the inner canthus. (The inner canthus is the angle of the eye opening nearest the nose.)

Etiology: the cause (of disease or defect).

Exocrine glands: those that secrete externally via a duct.

Expressivity: the range of manifestation (type or severity) of a particular genetic condition.

Facies: the face; the expression or appearance of the face.

Fetoscopy: direct visualization of a fetus made possible by the introduction of a fiber-optic system through the abdomen into the uterus.

Frenulum (pl. frenula): a folded mucous membrane attaching the gum to the deep surface of the lip.

Galactosidase: an enzyme that catalyzes the conversion of galactoside to galactose.

Gene: the unit of genetic information responsible for the production of a specific physical or biochemical characteristic and transmission of this characteristic from one generation to another.

Germ cells: egg and sperm cells.

Gestation: the period of development of the embryo or fetus beginning with the fertilization of the egg by the sperm and ending with birth.

Gonadectomy: removal of a gonad (an ovary or testis).

Gravid: pregnant.

Halluces: the great toes.

Haploid: the number of chromosomes found in a normal germ cell (egg or sperm), which is half the number found in a somatic (diploid) cell, (in humans, 23).

Heterozygous: possessing two alternative genes for the same trait. In recessive disorders, refers to the carrier state with one normal and one mutant gene.

Homologous chromosomes: a matched pair, one from each parent, having the same gene loci in the same order.

Hydrocephaly: a condition characterized by abnormal accumulation of cerebrospinal fluid within the skull, usually resulting in enlargement of the head, atrophy of the brain, mental deterioration, and convulsions.

Hyperplasia: abnormal increase in the number of normal cells in a normal arrangement in an organ or tissue, which increases its volume.

Hypertelorism: abnormally increased distance between two organs or parts (here, referring to the eyes).

Hypertrophy: enlargement or overgrowth of an organ or part due to increase in size of its constituent cells.

Hypoplasia: incomplete development of an organ or tissue.

Hypospadias: a developmental anomaly in the male in which the urethra opens on the underside of the penis or on the perineum (pelvic floor).

Hysterectomy: removal of the uterus.

Karyotype: the ordered arrangement of a cell's chromosomes according to convention.

Laparoscopy: examination by means of a laparoscope, an optical instrument that is introduced within the abdominal cavity.

Laparotomy: incision through any part of the abdominal wall.

Lobulated: made up of small lobes.

Locus: the actual location of a gene on a chromosome.

Mary Lyon principle (also referred to as Mary Lyon hypothesis): describes the functional inactivation of all but one X chromosome in every cell. This inactivation occurs randomly early in fetal development and persists throughout life affecting the same X chromosome(s) in all the descendents of that cell. The inactivated X chromosome(s) stain darkly in interphase and are called Barr bodies.

Meiosis: the process of cell division leading to the formation of mature germ cells having the haploid number of chromosomes (in humans, 23).

Menarche: establishment or beginning of the menstrual function.

Mendelian: refers to genes and resultant traits or disorders being transmitted according to specific patterns as elucidated by Gregor Mendel; Mendelian disorders are also referred to as ''single-gene'' disorders.

Metacentric chromosome: one whose centromere is close to the middle.

Metatarsus adductus: a congenital deformity of the foot characterized by inward deviation of the forepart.

Microcephaly: abnormal smallness of the head.

Micrognathia: unusual smallness of the jaws, especially the lower jaw.

Milia: superficial inclusion cysts in the outer layer of the skin. They appear as pinpoint-size, slightly raised pearly spots, often on the face, and are transient.

Mitosis: the process of cell division involved in the duplication of somatic cells so that each new cell will have the diploid number of chromosomes (in humans, 46).

Multifactorial: refers to the responsibility of more than one factor for the development of a physical trait or clinical disorder; usually implies a combination of genetic and environmental factors.

Mutation: a permanent transmissible change in a gene's chemical makeup.

Neonate: a newborn infant.

Nondisjunction: the failure of sister chromatids to go separate ways during mitosis or meiosis; the failure of homologous chromosomes to disjoin during meiosis.

Obligate carrier: an individual whose carrier status can be inferred from family and personal histories without necessity for laboratory testing.

Occiput: the back part of the head.

Palpebral: pertaining to the palpebra, the eyelid. Palpebral fissures, are the eye openings.

Paraparesis: partial paralysis of the lower extremities.

Parity: the state of a woman as regards the fact of having borne children.

Pectus carinatum: pigeon breast.

Pedigree: the stylized, graphic way of portraying a family history; a family tree.

Penetrance: refers to whether or not a genetic trait is expressed at all. If the trait is expressed, no matter how slightly, the gene is penetrant, and if not expressed, it is nonpenetrant.

Petechial: refers to a minute red spot caused by escape of a small amount of blood; a pinpoint-size hemorrhage.

Phenotype: the observable or measurable characteristics of an organism.

Philtrum: the vertical groove in the median portion of the upper lip.

Polydactyly: the presence of extra digits on the hands and feet.

Polyploidy: an excess of chromosomes per cell resulting in a number which is a multiple of the haploid number (e.g., triploidy, 69 in humans; tetraploidy, 92 in humans).

Prenatal: preceding birth.

Proband: the affected individual whose disorder brings a family to genetic evaluation and counseling.

Propositus: See proband (q.v.).

Ptosis: paralytic drooping of the upper eyelid.

Pulmonic stenosis: narrowing of the opening between the pulmonary artery and the right ventricle of the heart.

Recessive gene: a gene which must be present in duplicate in order to produce a phenotypic effect. A recessive disorder results from two mutant genes at the same locus.

Reduction division: See Meiosis (q.v.).

Renal: pertaining to the kidney.

Sclera: the tough white outer coat of the eyeball.

Sex chromosomes: the X and Y chromosomes.

Sibling (sib): any of two or more offspring of the same parents; a brother or a sister.

Simian crease: a single transverse crease across the palm of the hand.

Sister chromatids: the complementary halves of a chromosome.

Somatic cells: all body cells except egg and sperm cells.

Sonography: ultrasonography (q.v.).

Sporadic: refers usually to the occurrence of a disorder in a family for the first time—a new mutation. This is possible when the condition is autosomal dominant or X-linked recessive.

Teratogenic: tending to cause developmental malformations.

Translocation: a chromosome rearrangement in which there has been a transfer of a piece of one chromosome to another.

    a. balanced translocation: when the chromosome rearrangement results in no more or less genetic material than is normal.

    b. unbalanced translocation: when the chromosome rearrangement results in more or less than the normal amount of genetic material.

    c. reciprocal translocation: a chromosome rearrangement in which there has been a mutual exchange of segments between two chromosomes.

    d. Robertsonian translocation (also known as centric fusion): a special class of unequal reciprocal translocation involving 2 acrocentric chromosomes, each of which has a break on opposite sides of its centrome. The long arms of these 2 chromosomes (one of which carries a centromere) fuse to form one metacentric chromosome. Usually there is loss of a minute centric fragment. The total chromosome number of the carrier of this translocation is reduced by 1 to 45.

Trimester: a period of three months during gestation.

Trisomy: the presence of three chromosomes instead of a pair, e.g., trisomy 21.

Tubal ligation: tying of the fallopian tubes so that they are constricted.

Ultrasonography: the visualization of the deep structures of the body by recording the reflection of ultrasonic waves directed into the tissues.

Vas deferens (also known as spermatic duct): the secretory duct of the testicle which carries sperm.

Vasectomy: surgical removal of a segment of the vas deferens.

Visceromegaly: enlargement of any large interior organ in any of the four great body cavities, especially in the abdomen.

X-linked: refers to a gene carried on the X chromosome.

Zygote: the cell resulting from union of a sperm and egg cell.

Index

Abortion
    elective, 18, 22, 25, 29, 62, 63, 65,
        75, 77–81, 113, 115–119, 122,
        129–133, 137, 140, 144, 146,
        148, 150, 153–156, 167, 182,
        184, 187, 188, 190, 192, 195,
        198–202, 249, 250
    spontaneous, 66, 105, 200, 206,
        219
Achondroplasia, 102, 135, 137, 138,
    141, 167, 168, 170
Adjustment
    to the diagnosis of a disorder, 17,
        19, 20, 23, 35
    when there is no diagnosis, 246,
        247, 262–266
Adoption, 27, 62, 64, 65, 131, 132,
    137, 141, 143, 161–165, 210,
    212, 220, 231
Advanced maternal age, 74, 113,
    181, 182, 192, 198, 209
Alpha-fetoprotein, 127, 170, 171,
    183–187
Amino acid screening, 260, 261
Amniocentesis: see Prenatal diagnosis
Androgen insensitivity syndrome,
    157, 158
Anencephaly, 168–171, 180, 184
Anger toward spouse, 226, 229
Artificial insemination by donor
    (AID), 23, 24, 25, 27, 50, 142,
    210–213, 220
Asphyxiating thoracic dystrophy,
    135, 136, 142

Autopsy: see Postmortem examina-
    tion
Autosomal dominant inheritance, 37,
    38, 43–45, 48, 49, 51, 53, 135,
    168, 222, 235
Autosomal recessive inheritance, 13,
    22–25, 44, 53, 60, 113, 114, 117,
    136, 142, 143, 168, 208, 209,
    219, 273

Balanced translocation, 67, 69, 70,
    71, 91
Banded chromosome analysis,
    107–109
Bayesian analysis, 74
Birth control (contraception), 18, 20,
    149, 156, 159, 160, 196, 200,
    210, 212, 213, 215, 216, 219,
    220
Buccal smear, 197, 198, 200, 201

Carrier, 16, 119, 121, 123, 148,
    273–275
    identification, 13, 180, 247, 274
Cesarean section, 27, 28, 136
Charcot-Marie-Tooth disease,
    44–49, 51
Child placement, 89–93, 95–100
Chondroectodermal dysplasia
    (Ellis-van Creveld syndrome),
    113–117
Chromosome abnormality (aneu-
    ploidy) or rearrangement, 32,
    67, 69, 70, 101, 108, 146, 177,
    183, 196, 197

Chromosome studies or analysis, 31,
    67, 85, 88, 95, 103, 104, 114,
    146, 157–163, 167, 168, 171,
    174, 175, 177, 200–202, 260,
    264
Clarifying counselee's meaning, 68,
    147, 148
Coercion, 96, 98, 100
Collusion of silence, 274
Committee to Combat Huntington's
    Disease, 232
Communication
  of bad news, 207, 228
  nonverbal, 171, 186
  telephone support, 19, 20, 153, 277
  telephone versus letter, 52
Concealing anxiety regarding preg-
    nancy outcome, 14
Concealing genetic illness, 20, 33, 42,
    90, 91, 97, 98
Consanguinity, 48, 270
Counselee
  anxiety, 67, 70, 71, 77, 128, 168,
    174, 223
  frustration and dissatisfaction, 96,
    98–100, 239, 240, 247, 248
  gratitude, 38, 95, 96, 178, 218,
    219, 238, 258
  guilt, 106, 110, 111, 193, 238, 239,
    262
  hostility, 15, 18, 239, 241, 244
  intimidation, 223, 252
  lost to follow-up, 41, 42, 51, 111,
    192
  private agenda, 71, 83
  preparation of, 85, 86, 125, 126,
    132, 163, 174, 252, 256, 257
  relief, 39, 40, 71, 129
  resistance, 94, 111
  unresponsiveness, 69, 71, 93, 95
  willingness to inform extended
    family of possible genetic
    defect, 39, 42, 154, 259
Counseling
  counselees' evaluation of, 96–100
  dose limitation, 16, 17, 81, 151,
    164, 171, 175, 186, 209, 240,
    241

interaction hindrance, 214
  pitfall, 179
Counselor
  assumptions or predictions, 28, 71,
    202
  discomfort, 99, 138, 139, 164, 165
  self-evaluation, 27, 28, 50, 117,
    164, 214, 215
  staff frustration or dissatisfaction,
    51, 71, 110, 111, 214, 224,
    243, 247
  value judgments (bias), 97, 171
Crisis intervention, 88
Cultural
  differences and beliefs, 13, 149,
    152, 154, 155, 180, 192, 193
  group pressures, 86, 90, 92, 94,
    95, 97, 100
Cystic fibrosis, 13–20, 68
Cytogenetic study, 30, 66, 69, 101,
    102, 163, 174, 195

Delayed development, 107, 109, 259
Denial, 14, 15, 29, 30, 35, 37, 44,
    45, 47, 51, 52, 139, 148, 176,
    179, 193, 236, 237
De novo translocation, 67
Desire for a son, 75, 76, 130
Disbelief reactions to tragedy, 84, 85,
    87, 176
Dissatisfaction with the medical pro-
    fession, 103, 104
Down syndrome, 30–35, 42, 74,
    83–90, 97, 103–111, 127, 168,
    173–179, 183–185, 194, 209, 216
Down syndrome mosaicism,
    175–179
Duchenne muscular dystrophy,
    73–81, 145

Ectopic pregnancy, 182, 196
Emotional response to the diagnosis
    of defect, 22, 23, 24, 26, 186
Environmental agents, 109, 110
Erroneous genetic information, 146,
    147, 167
Expressivity, 37, 38

Familial translocation, 62, 65, 91
Family
  acceptance of disorder due to fre-
    quent occurrence, 42
  and/or friend support in crisis, 20,
    68, 82, 154, 183, 192
Father's
  denial of child's defect, 27, 31
  helplessness expressed as anger, 15
  ignorance of prenatal diagnosis,
    188, 189, 193
Fetal alcohol syndrome, 101–111
Fetal sex determination, 74, 75, 119,
    126, 127, 145, 148, 154
Fetal X-ray, 24–28, 143
Fetoscopy, 113–117, 122, 123

G_{M1}-gangliosidosis, type II, 268–278
Gambler's fallacy (probability), 49
Gonadal malignancy, 157, 158,
    160–163

Hemophilia, 119–123, 126, 130, 133
Hope, realistic, 248
  and unrealistic, 247, 251
Hospitalization of child, 23, 28, 262,
    269–271, 273
Huntington's disease, 43, 57,
    222–233, 243
Husband's willingness for wife to
    assume responsibility, 14, 15,
    18, 251, 256
Hysterectomy, 201, 202, 274

Infant or child loss, 14, 24, 114,
    135–144, 204, 208, 210, 218–220
Infant-stimulation program, 34, 89,
    178, 261
Infertility, 74–76, 160, 206
Institutionalization or foster home
    care, 34, 92, 93, 271, 272

Joint consent for surgery, 256–258

Karyotype, 31, 32, 69, 121, 158, 163,
    168, 175, 181, 197, 263, 265

Language
  barrier, 146, 149, 152, 155, 185,
    192
  interpreter, 145, 147–149, 154,
    155, 182, 189, 191
Late-onset neurological disorder, 44,
    51, 222–245

Mandibulofacial dysostosis, 38–43
March of Dimes Birth Defects Foun-
    dation, 273
Marital harmony, 33, 105, 106, 132,
    155, 193
Marital infidelity, 169–171
Mary Lyon principle (hypothesis),
    145
Masculinization, 157, 158, 160–163,
    165
Medical-ethical dilemma, 76, 81
Meningomyelocele, 181, 185, 186
Mental retardation, 30, 33, 38, 42,
    88–90, 105, 106, 146, 151, 152,
    168, 177, 185, 195, 196, 198,
    250, 251, 253, 261, 263, 266,
    267, 269, 271
Metabolic screening, 107
Misdiagnosis, 53, 57, 101, 135,
    141–143, 167, 269, 271
Mother assumes major responsibility
    for defect, 15, 16, 20, 32, 69,
    139, 140, 142, 143, 147, 196,
    197
Mourning, 18, 137, 206, 265
Multifactorial inheritance, 181
Mutation, 74, 75

Neonatal death
  as affecting spouse relationships, 62

Omniscience expected from the gene-
    tics team, 247
Open neural tube defect, 170, 171,
    180–193
Orofaciodigital syndrome type I,
    145–156
Osteogenesis, 22–29, 41
Outreach genetic counseling, 101,
    102

Parent support groups/individual parent support, 89, 175, 178, 179, 189, 190, 232, 233, 249, 255, 261, 265, 266

Parental wish to see dead child, 58, 59, 272

Phenotype, 108, 157, 194

Polydactyly, 113–115, 117, 135

Postmortem examination, 55, 56, 136, 141, 167, 168, 170, 181, 204

Postnatal confirmation of prenatal diagnosis, 132, 199

Potter syndrome, 53–65

Prenatal diagnosis, 13, 22, 24–26, 34, 60, 65, 70, 71, 74, 76, 77, 89, 91, 113–129, 131, 133, 143, 145, 149–151, 153–155, 169–191, 177, 178, 180–188, 195, 197, 199, 200, 205, 209, 215, 216, 247, 248, 252, 265

Private consultation, 41, 148, 150, 155, 169, 170

Prophylactic surgery, 157, 158, 163

Psychodrama, 79, 81

Psychological defense, 99, 139

Psychotherapeutic assitance, 204, 213, 214, 216–220, 233, 235, 239, 243, 244, 276

Rapport, 46, 47, 88, 93, 100, 145, 153–156, 182, 190, 204, 244

Reciprocal translocation, 263, 265

Religious impact, 63, 148, 153–155, 200–202, 212, 219

Satellite clinic, 137

Seeking help from alternative sources, 80–83, 90, 92, 95, 201, 211–213, 220

Self-esteem, 18, 35, 247, 265

Serum aldolase, 74

Serum creatine phosphokinase, 74

Skeletal survey, 108

Social isolation, self-imposed, 20, 33

Spina bifida, 180, 183–191

Sporadic occurrence, 38, 42, 53, 142, 145, 168, 196, 250

Spouses'
protection of each other, 70, 71, 85, 93, 99
shared responsibility, 143

Staff
behavior following tragedy, 54, 58, 59, 60, 86
pressure of decision-making, 73, 79–80
support, 15, 63, 76, 77
See also Counselor

Stillbirth, 136, 138, 140–142, 169, 170

Subclinical infection, 70

Subjective reactions to a particular disorder, 39, 40, 42, 47

Suicide, 43, 224, 228

Temporary respite care, 177–179, 275

Teratogenic potential, 181

Tessier procedure, 252–254, 256

Thanatophoric dwarfism, 168, 170

Time
intervals between counseling appointments 39, 50
limitation, 104, 112, 167, 171

Truth-telling, 91, 94–97, 228, 229, 240

Tubal ligation, 62–65, 149, 212–219, 274

Turner syndrome, 157, 158, 162–164

Ultrasonography/sonography, 27, 56, 58, 60, 62, 122–124, 127, 129, 143, 167, 169, 171, 184, 187, 215, 216

Unbalanced translocation, 70, 91

Understanding versus acceptance, 35

Undiagnosable disorder, 246–267

Variable expression, 236, 241

Vasectomy, 210, 212, 213, 216, 220

Warnings against marriage where genetic defect is in question, 49, 51

Werdnig-Hoffmann disease, 204–221

Williams syndrome, 196, 249, 250, 263

X-linked dominant inheritance, 145–148

X-linked recessive inheritance, 74, 76, 121, 122, 133, 157

XO/XY mosaicism, 157–165

XXX chromosome aneuploidy, 194–202

XYY chromosome aneuploidy, 101–111